Robotic Surgery of the Bladder

Erik P. Castle • Raj S. Pruthi
Editors

Robotic Surgery of the Bladder

Springer

Editors
Erik P. Castle, M.D., F.A.C.S.
Department of Urology
Mayo Clinic
Phoenix, AZ, USA

Raj S. Pruthi, M.D., F.A.C.S.
Department of Urology
The University of North Carolina
at Chapel Hill
Chapel Hill, NC, USA

ISBN 978-1-4614-4905-8 ISBN 978-1-4614-4906-5 (eBook)
DOI 10.1007/978-1-4614-4906-5
Springer New York Heidelberg Dordrecht London

Library of Congress Control Number: 2013944895

Printed on acid-free paper

Springer is part of Springer Science+Business Media (www.springer.com)

Preface

Since the introduction of the surgical robot into the armamentarium of urological surgeons, there has been a rapid adoption of the robotic approach to urological procedures. Until recently, prostate and kidney surgery have been the primary techniques to which robotic surgery has been implemented. Over the last few years there has been an increase in robotic surgery for the management of bladder pathology, particularly bladder cancer and radical cystectomy. While the acceptance has been much slower than what was witnessed with radical prostatectomy, many surgeons are now embarking on robot-assisted radical cystectomy (RARC) and other surgical procedures of the bladder.

In *Robotic Surgery of the Bladder*, the reader can expect to benefit from the shared experience of established experts in the field of robotic surgery and bladder cancer. Topics contained within the text range from a review of the history of minimally invasive surgery of the bladder to contemporary issues such as cost. Early in the text, the principles of bladder cancer surgery are reviewed and set the bar for all surgeons planning on performing RARC. Chapters such as these reflect the comprehensive nature of the text.

With a large portion dedicated to preparation and technique, we expect that surgeons interested in moving from robot-assisted radical prostatectomy to radical cystectomy will find the detailed technical descriptions and accompanying videos to be very useful. Technical nuances including, female cystectomy, nerve sparing, and pelvic lymphadenectomy will be covered, among others. Three chapters cover urinary diversion and different approaches to one of the more complex aspects of radical cystectomy. The authors of the technical chapters are all well known within the field of robot-assisted radical cystectomy and provide the reader with a collective experience that spans more than 8 years and resulted in established reproducible steps.

Several chapters are dedicated to getting started and preparation and are of particular importance when setting oneself up for success. Two chapters covering perioperative outcomes and complications complement these sections as setup and outcomes are intimately related. Oncological outcomes, one of the most important metrics used to rate success following radical cystectomy, are extensively reviewed in Chap. 14. Surgery for benign disorders of the bladder is also covered. In order to present a balanced text covering robotic surgery of the bladder, criticisms and concerns that have been raised in the past are also thoughtfully reviewed. Finally, a discussion of future directions can be found in the end and demonstrates the limitless possibilities.

We expect that you will find this book to be both informative and instructional and look forward to your contribution to the field of robotic surgery of the bladder.

Phoenix, AZ, USA Erik P. Castle, M.D., F.A.C.S.
Chapel Hill, NC, USA Raj S. Pruthi, M.D., F.A.C.S.

Contents

Contributors

Piyush K. Agarwal Urologic Oncology Branch, National Cancer Institute, National Institute of Health, Bethesda, MD, USA

Christopher B. Anderson Department of Urologic Surgery, Vanderbilt University Medical Center, Nashville, TN, USA

Magnus Annerstedt Sophiahemmet Hospital, Urology Clinic, Stockholm, Sweden

Daniel A. Barocas Department of Urologic Surgery, Center for Surgical Quality and Outcomes Research, Vanderbilt University Medical Center, Nashville, TN, USA

Michele Billia Department of Urology, Kings College London, Kings Health Partners, Guy's Hospital, London, UK

Erik P. Castle Department of Urology, Mayo Clinic, Phoenix, AZ, USA

Kevin G. Chan Department of Surgery, Division of Urology and Urologic Oncology, City of Hope Medical Center, Duarte, CA, USA

Sam S. Chang Department of Urologic Surgery, Vanderbilt University Medical Center, Nashville, TN, USA

Jan Colli Department of Urology, Tulane University Health Sciences Center, New Orleans, LA, USA

Michael S. Cookson Department of Urologic Surgery, Vanderbilt University Medical Center, Nashville, TN, USA

Prokar Dasgupta Kings College London, Kings Health Partners, Guy's Hospital, MRC Centre for Transplantation NIHR Biomedical Research Centre, London, UK

John W. Davis Urology Director, Urosurgical Prostate Cancer Program, MD Anderson Cancer Center, Houston, TX, USA

Vincenzo Ficarra Department of Urology, University of Padova, Padova, Italy

Kris E. Gaston Department of Urologic Oncology, Carolinas Medical Center, Levine Cancer Institute, Charlotte, NC, USA

Mark L. Gonzalgo Department of Urology, Sylvester Comprehensive Cancer Center, University of Miami Miller School of Medicine, Miami, FL, USA

David A. Green Department of Urology, Weill Medical College of Cornell University, New York, NY, USA

Joshua G. Griffin University of Kansas Medical Center, Kansas City, KS, USA

Ken Haberman Department of Urology, University of Minnesota, Minneapolis, MN, USA

Ashok K. Hemal Wake Forest Baptist Health, Winston-Salem, NC, USA

Anthony N. Hoang Urologic Oncology Branch, National Cancer Institute, National Institute of Health, Bethesda, MD, USA

Jeffrey Holzbeierlein Department of Urology, University of Kansas Medical Center, Kansas City, KS, USA

Mitchell R. Humphreys Department of Urology, Mayo Clinic, Phoenix, AZ, USA

George S. Kallingal Department of Urology, Martin Army Community Hospital, Fort Benning, GA, USA

Muhammad Shamim Khan Department of Urology, Kings College London, Kings Health Partners, Guy's Hospital, London, UK

Badrinath R. Konety Department of Urology, Institute for Prostate and Urologic Cancers, University of Minnesota, Minneapolis, MN, USA

Raj Kurpad Department of Urology, The University of North Carolina at Chapel Hill, Chapel Hill, NC, USA

Alexander Mottrie Department of Urology, O.L.V. Hospital, Aalst, Belgium

Matthew E. Nielsen Department of Urology, The University of North Carolina at Chapel Hill, Chapel Hill, NC, USA

Jeffrey W. Nix Urologic Oncology Branch, National Cancer Institute, National Institutes of Health, Bethesda, MD, USA

Rafael N. Nunez Department of Urology, Mayo Clinic, Phoenix, AZ, USA

Mathew Oommen Department of Urology, Tulane University Health Sciences Center, New Orleans, LA, USA

Dipen Parekh Department of Urology, University of Texas Health Sciences Center at San Antonio, San Antonio, TX, USA

Raj S. Pruthi Department of Urology, The University of North Carolina at Chapel Hill, Chapel Hill, NC, USA

Douglas S. Scherr Department of Urology, Weill Medical College of Cornell University, New York, NY, USA

Angela Smith Department of Urology, The University of North Carolina at Chapel Hill, Chapel Hill, NC, USA

Katherine Theisen Department of Urology, University of Minnesota, Minneapolis, MN, USA

David D. Thiel Department of Urology, Mayo Clinic, Jacksonville, FL, USA

Raju Thomas Department of Urology, Tulane University Health Sciences Center, New Orleans, LA, USA

Matthew K. Tollefson Department of Urology, Mayo Clinic, Rochester, MN, USA

Stavros I. Tyritzis Department of Molecular Medicine & Surgery, Section of Urology, Karolinska University Hospital, Karolinska Institutet, Solna, Stockholm, Sweden

Eric M. Wallen Department of Urology, The University of North Carolina at Chapel Hill, Chapel Hill, NC, USA

Peter Wiklund Department of Urology, Karolinska University Hospital, Stockholm, Sweden

Timothy G. Wilson Department of Surgery, Division of Urology and Urologic Oncology, City of Hope Medical Center, Duarte, CA, USA

Christopher E. Wolter Department of Urology, Mayo Clinic, Phoenix, AZ, USA

Michael Woods Division of Urology, The University of North Carolina at Chapel Hill, Chapel Hill, NC, USA

Paul R. Young Department of Urology, Mayo Clinic, Jacksonville, FL, USA

History of Minimally Invasive Techniques for Radical Cystectomy with Urinary Diversion

1

Jan Colli, Mathew Oommen, and Raju Thomas

Introduction

Radical cystectomy with urinary diversion is the most effective treatment for non-metastatic, muscle-invasive bladder cancer [1]. Most cystectomies are performed via open surgical technique; however, laparoscopic and robotic cystectomies have recently gained popularity at various centers. Minimally invasive techniques are well established in the field of urology and are increasingly being used for a variety of indications ranging from benign to malignant urologic diseases [2].

Even in skilled and experienced hands, open radical cystectomy is associated with complication rates as high as 30–60 % [3]. Laparoscopic and robotic cystectomies have the advantage of smaller incisions, lower pain scores, and potentially shorter hospital stays, quicker recoveries, and lower overall morbidities, lower blood loss, while at the same time aiming to achieve similar oncologic outcomes as open surgical techniques [4].

Few studies have reported on the long-term efficacy of minimally invasive techniques in the treatment of muscle-invasive bladder cancer. In this chapter, we will outline the history of laparoscopic and robot-assisted radical cystectomy as having a growing role in the management of muscle-invasive bladder cancer. In addition, we will also present an overview of the literature regarding outcomes for laparoscopic and robotic cystectomies.

History of Laparoscopic Radical Cystectomy

Laparoscopic radical cystectomy preceded the robotic era and the first laparoscopic radical cystectomy (LRC) with ileal conduit was performed in 1993 in Malaga, Spain [5]. This was duplicated at other centers and in 2000, Gill et al. [6] reported on two patients who underwent LRC with intracorporeal ileal conduit. And, in 2002, Gill et al. [7] published his series on LRC with continent orthotopic ileal neobladder performed completely intracorporeally. Following that, two groups reported their series on LRC with laparoscopic continent reconstruction of rectosigmoid pouch [8, 9]. Currently, the largest series of patients ($N=171$) who underwent LRC with intracorporeal orthotopic ileal neobladder, is from China, with a median follow-up of 3 years [10]. LRC, however, did not gain traction except in select centers because of the physically demanding nature of the procedure and skills needed.

J. Colli, MD • M. Oommen, MD (✉)
R. Thomas, MD, FACS, MHA
Department of Urology, Tulane University Health Sciences Center, 1430 Tulane Avenue, SL-42, New Orleans, LA 70112, USA
e-mail: matt.oommen@gmail.com

E.P. Castle and R.S. Pruthi (eds.), *Robotic Surgery of the Bladder*, DOI 10.1007/978-1-4614-4906-5_1,

History of Robot-Assisted Radical Cystectomy

After the formal approval of the Robotic surgical device in 2001, many hospitals gained access to the Da Vinci™ Robotic System (Intuitive Surgical Inc., Sunnyvale, CA). Though approved for radical prostatectomy, robot-assisted radical cystectomies (RARC) were performed, using the Da Vinci™, with the first series of robot-assisted radical cystectomies with extracorporeal ileal conduit published in 2003 by Menon et al. [11] Centers, which were well versed in Robotic Radical prostatectomy, ventured into RARC, and soon this procedure was increasingly used and is now an acceptable treatment option. With increased experience, surgeons started performing the urinary diversion intracorporeally and thus another milestone in advancing MIS in bladder cancer was reached. The first reported case of RARC with intracorporeal neobladder was performed in Germany in 2003 [12]. Since that time, several robot-assisted radical cystectomy series have been reported, some with intracorporeal [13] and others with extracorporeal urinary diversion [14]. To date, outcomes studies comparing intracorporeal versus extracorporeal urinary diversion have been sparingly reported, and surgeon experience largely guides the decision for patient selection and which urinary diversion is performed. Thus, over the past decade, there has been a slow but steady trend towards applying RARC techniques for bladder cancer. The acceptance rate for RARC has been slower and limited, compared to robotic radical prostatectomy for prostate cancer.

Outcomes for Laparoscopic and Robot-Assisted Radical Cystectomy

Complications

Radical cystectomy is known to have a high rate of morbidity and relative mortality. Rates of complications in LRC range between 10 and 40 % in recent LRC series [15–17], which is slightly lower than the reported complication rates (30–60 %) found for open radical cystectomies (ORC) [3].

Prior studies have revealed an 8 % incidence of uretero–ileal anastomotic strictures in RARC, which is generally higher than the ureteral stricture rates seen in ORC [18]. This may be because of challenges in performing an extracorporeal urinary diversion if there are tension or exposure problems, especially at the left uretero-enteric anastomosis. In a series of robot-assisted radical cystectomies, Ng et al. [19] found decreased blood loss, lower transfusion rates, shorter hospital stays, and decreased complications compared to open radical cystectomies. However, many patients who undergo radical cystectomy were not found to be candidates for minimally invasive techniques, which may lead to selection bias in many of these comparative studies. For example, severe cardiopulmonary compromise is a relative contraindication to undergo minimal invasive radical cystectomy, because patients who undergo LRC and RARC need to be able to withstand steep Trendelenburg position with pneumoperitoneum, and some patients with cardiopulmonary disease may not be healthy enough to tolerate CO_2 pneumoperitonium [20].

Oncological Control

Extended pelvic lymphadenectomy during minimally invasive surgery is safe and equivalent to the open lymph node dissection technique in most series [21]. A nonrandomized study by Richards et al. found equivalent lymph node counts between ORC and RARC (15 versus 16) [22]. A small-randomized prospective trial found equal node counts, with a mean of 18 removed in the open group and 19 in the robotic group [23].

The rates of local tumor recurrence after open cystectomy are approximately 10 % [1]. Overall the 5-year survival for patients with organ-confined, lymph-node negative disease approaches 89 % [1]. LRC and RARC appears equivalent, however, follow-up data have been limited with the majority RARC series reporting less than 2-year follow-up of outcomes [4].

In addition, there have been slightly higher positive margin rates (4 %) found in the minimally invasive surgery (LRC and RARC) group compared to open radical cystectomy rates (1–2 %) [23]. Guru et al. has found higher positive margin rates in high stage bladder tumors treated with RARC [14]. However, the International Robotic Cystectomy Consortium Registry found the positive margin rate to be only 2 %, which is similar to open cystectomy rates [24].

Overall survival in the LRC cohorts was 90–100 % at 1–2 years and 63–79 % at 2–3 years [15–17]. RARC reported a 90–96 % survival rate at 1–2-year follow-up [25]. These figures should be compared to a larger series of ORC, showing a 62–68 % recurrence-free survival at 5 years and 50–60 % rate at 10 years [1].

The oncological outcomes data slants favorably for minimally invasive radical cystectomy, however the selection bias could be skewing the results. For example, most centers avoid bulky disease and T3-plus tumors early in their series [26].

History of Modifications in Techniques and Steps of Minimally Invasive Radical Cystectomy

The RARC surgical technique developed by Menon et al. [11] in 2003 has been widely accepted. This report describes posterior dissection, lateral dissection, followed lastly by anterior dissection with urethral isolation, and followed by the prostatectomy. Extended pelvic lymphadenectomy can be performed before the cystectomy; however, in obese patients or those with bulky tumors, the pelvic lymph node dissection is generally performed after the cystectomy [11] Modifications of the robot-assisted radical cystectomy have been described by various authors over the past 9 years [13, 14]. One such adaptation includes early robotic tagging of the bowel and ureteral segments, for ease in identification of these segments while performing the extracorporeal urinary diversion [14]. Pruthi et al. [27] has recently described alterations in performing intracorporeal urinary diversion, with his current robotic neobladder rates at 40 %, compared to his intracorporeal ileal conduit rates of 60 %. Patient selection and surgical experience usually drive urinary diversion choice.

Conclusions

Minimally invasive radical cystectomy and urinary diversion techniques (LRC, RARC) are increasingly being used to manage surgical candidates with bladder cancer. However, long-term data from large cohorts are lacking, which contributes to the controversy surrounding minimally invasive radical cystectomy. Furthermore, many LRC and RARC reports are not randomized, with patients in the MIS series generally not equivalent to open cystectomy series, therefore outcomes data may be considered biased. However, single-institution LRC and RARP series have reported favorable short-term and intermediate oncologic outcomes [17–19, 25]. Moreover, as experience and operative times continue to decrease, there appears to be a steady increase in interest in robot-assisted radical cystectomy, with a growing interest in intracorporeal urinary reconstruction. Multicentered data collection and analyses, directed by entities such as the International Robotic Cystectomy Consortium, is crucial to further advancing the role of RARC, in managing bladder cancer.

References

1. Stein JP, Lieskovsky G, Cote R, et al. Radical cystectomy in the treatment of invasive bladder cancer: long-term results in 1,054 patients. J Clin Oncol. 2001;19:666–75.
2. Berryhill R, Jhaveri J, Yadav R, et al. Robotic prostatectomy: a review of outcomes compared with laparoscopic and open approaches. Urology. 2008;72(1):15–23.
3. Herr H, Lee C, Chang S, Bladder cancer Collaborative Group. Standardization of radical cystectomy and pelvic lymph node dissection for bladder cancer. A collaborative report. J Urol. 2004;171:1823–8.
4. Haber G, Crouzet S, Gill IS. Laparoscopic and robotic assisted radical cystectomy for bladder cancer: a critical analysis. Eur Urol. 2008;54:54–62.
5. Sanchez de Badajoz E, Gellego Perales JL, Reche Rosado A, et al. Radical cystectomy and laparoscopic ileal conduit. Arch Esp Urol. 1993;46:621–4.

6. Gill IS, Fergany A, Klein EA, et al. Laparoscopic radical cystoprostaectomy with ileal conduit performed completely intracorporeally: the initial 2 cases. Urology. 2000;56:26–9.
7. Gill IS, Fergany A, Klein EA. Laproscopic radical cystectomy and continent orthotopic ileal neobladder performed intracorporeally: the initial experience. J Urol. 2002;168:13–8.
8. Turk I, Deger S, Winkelmann B, et al. Laparoscopic radical cystectomy with continent urinary diversion (rectosigmoid pouch) performed completely intracorporeally: the initial 5 cases. J Urol. 2001;165: 1863–6.
9. Deger S, Peters R, Roigers J, et al. Laparoscopic radical cystectomy with continent urinary diversion (rectosigmoid pouch) performed completely intracorporeall: an intermediate functional and oncological analysis. Urology. 2004;64:935–6.
10. Huang L, Lin T, Liu H, et al. Laparoscopic radical cystectomy with orthotopic ileal neobladdder for bladder cancer: oncologic results of 171 cases with a median 3 year follow-up. Eur Urol. 2010;58:442–9.
11. Menon M, Hemal AK, Tewari A, et al. Nerve-sparing robot assisted radical cysto-prostatectomy and urinary diversion. BJU Int. 2003;92:232–6.
12. Beeken W-D, Wolfram M, Engl T, et al. Robotic-assisted laparoscopic radical cystectomy and intra-abdominal formation of an orthotopic ileal neobladder. Eur Urol. 2003;44:337–9.
13. Murphy DG, Challacombe BJ, Elhage O, et al. Robotic- assisted laparoscopic radical cystectomy with extracorporeal urinary diversion: initial experience. Eur Urol. 2008;54:570–80.
14. Guru K, Seixas-Mikelus SA, Hussain A, et al. Robot-assisted radical cystectomy: short to medium-term oncological and functional outcomes. Int J Clin Prat. 2008;62:1709–14.
15. Haber GP, Gill ISE. Laparoscopic radical cystectomy with orthotopic ileal neobladder for bladder cancer: oncologic outcomes up to 5 years. BJU Int. 2007;100: 137–42.
16. Cathelineau X, Arroyo C, Rozet F, et al. Laparoscopic assisted radical cystectomy: the Montsouris experience after 84 cases. Eur Urol. 2005;47:780–4.
17. Hemal AK, Kolla SB, Wadhwa P, et al. Laparoscopic radical cystectomy and extracorporeal urinary diversion: a single center experience of 48 cases with three years of follow-up. Urology. 2008;71:41–6.
18. Khan MSA, Elhage O, Challacombe B, et al. Analysis of early complications of robotic-asisted radical cystectomy using standardized reporting system. Urology. 2011;77:357–62.
19. Ng CK, Kauffman EC, Lee MM, et al. A comparison of postoperative complications in open versus robotic cystectomy. Eur Urol. 2010;57:274–82.
20. Hemal AK, Abol-Enein H, Tewari A, et al. Robotic radical cystectomy and urinary diversion in the management of bladder cancer. Urol Clin North Am. 2004;31:719–29.
21. Schumacher MC, Jonsson MN, Wiklund NP. Does extended lymphadenopathy preclude laparoscopic or robotic-assisted radical cystectomy in advanced bladder cancer? Curr Opin Urol. 2009;19:527–32.
22. Richards KA, Hemal AK, Kader AK. Robot assisted laparoscopic pelvic lymphadenopathy at the time of radical cystectomy rivals that of open surgery: single institution report. Urology. 2010;76:1400–4.
23. Nix J, Smith A, Kurpad R, et al. Prospective randomized controlled trial of robotic versus open radical cystectomy for bladder cancer: perioperative and pathological results. Eur Urol. 2010;57:196–201.
24. Hyne MH, Helleenthal NJ, Hussain A, et al. Does previous robot-assisted radical prostatectomy affect outcomes of robot-assisted radical cystectomy? Results from the International Robotic Cystectomy Consortium. Eur Urol. 2010;58:197–202.
25. Wang GJ, Barocas DA, Raman JD, et al. Robotic versus open radical cystectomy: prospective comparison of perioperative outcomes and pathological measures of early oncological efficacy. BJU Int. 2008;101:89–93.
26. Ismail AF, Elhage O, Rimington P, et al. Initial experience with a randomized controlled trial of open, robotic and laparoscopic (CORAL) cystectomy. BJU Int. 2010;106:51–7.
27. Pruthi RS, Nielsen ME, Nix J, et al. Robotic radical cystectomy for bladder cancer: surgical and pathological outcomes in 100 consecutive cases. J Urol. 2010;183:510–4.

Principles of Bladder Cancer Surgery

2

Christopher B. Anderson, Michael S. Cookson, and Sam S. Chang

Introduction

Despite contemporary refinements in the diagnosis and management of invasive bladder cancer, it remains a potentially lethal disease that will account for nearly 15,000 deaths in the USA in 2012 alone [1]. Radical cystectomy is the gold-standard treatment for most patients with muscle invasive bladder cancer and is also appropriate for those with high-risk noninvasive disease that have failed conservative treatments. When it was first introduced for treatment of bladder cancer, cystectomy was associated with significant morbidity and mortality [2]. However, with advances over the past 60 years in patient selection, perioperative management and surgical technique, it currently has relatively low perioperative mortality rate and an acceptable rate of complications [3].

A successful outcome with radical cystectomy is not only related to surgical technique and safe extirpation of the bladder but also to factors such as patient selection, coordinated perioperative care, and use of adjunctive treatments. In this chapter, we will outline the essential principles of radical cystectomy for bladder cancer, which are equally as important for robot-assisted radical cystectomy (RARC) as for open radical cystectomy (ORC).

C.B. Anderson, M.D. (✉) • M.S. Cookson • S.S. Chang
Department of Urologic Surgery, Vanderbilt University Medical Center, A-1302 Medical Center North, Nashville, TN 37232-2765, USA
e-mail: c.anderson@vanderbilt.edu

Surgical Indications

Radical cystectomy for bladder cancer is indicated in any fit patient with clinically organ-confined muscle-invasive disease and no evidence of metastasis. Patients with advanced disease may also be offered radical cystectomy, however, the goal of surgery is typically local disease control and symptom palliation, as the prospect of cure is much less likely [4]. Furthermore, patients with high-risk noninvasive disease that have failed intravesical therapy or have adverse pathologic features, such as variant histology or lymphovascular invasion, may be offered radical cystectomy. In fact, up to one-third of patients with clinical stage ≤ T1 are found to have muscle-invasive tumors at cystectomy and 15 % may have nodal involvement, prompting some to argue for "timely" cystectomy in select high-risk patients [5–7].

Patient Selection

Deciding which patients are candidates for radical cystectomy is of paramount importance given the potential morbidity and mortality of surgery. The first aspect of patient selection is proper disease *staging*. This includes physical exam, a thorough transurethral resection (TUR), pathologic analysis of the tumor biopsies, and cross-sectional imaging. Despite this evaluation, there is still a significant risk of clinical under-staging. A repeat TUR is generally recommended for any high-grade

E.P. Castle and R.S. Pruthi (eds.), *Robotic Surgery of the Bladder*, DOI 10.1007/978-1-4614-4906-5_2,

T1 tumor given the substantial risk of residual disease and tumor upstaging, particularly in patients without muscle in the original TUR specimen [5, 8–10]. In men, biopsies of the prostatic urethra should be obtained, especially if there is consideration for orthotopic neobladder (ONB). Although computed tomography (CT) imaging has limited sensitivity to detect locally advanced disease, it is important to identify features of aggressive disease, such as hydronephrosis [11]. While there is some evidence that magnetic resonance imaging (MRI) is useful for clinical staging [12], we do not routinely order MRI or positron emission tomography (PET) in this setting.

Once patients are properly staged and deemed surgical candidates, they must undergo a *risk assessment* to identify and manage comorbidities and determine if the risks of surgery are less than that of untreated bladder cancer. Many patients presenting for surgery are elderly and have significant medical comorbidities, including pulmonary and cardiovascular disease, which increase their operative risk. Cardiologists consider radical cystectomy an intermediate risk procedure, as it is associated with a 1–5 % risk of perioperative cardiac events [13]. According to the current cardiac risk assessment guidelines, patients with preexisting cardiac disease, cardiac risk factors, or a poor functional capacity generally require preoperative cardiac risk evaluation in order to optimize cardiac function and assess the need for revascularization [14]. For patients with cardiac stents, the risk of intraoperative bleeding is generally considered higher than the risk of stent thrombosis, and discontinuation of antiplatelet therapy is preferred. Surgery is delayed a minimum of 30 days and 6 months for patients who have bare metal stents and drug eluding stents, respectively [15, 16]. If the risk of discontinuing antiplatelet therapy is acceptably low, aspirin and thienopyridine agents are discontinued 7 days preoperatively, although some argue for perioperative continuation of low-dose aspirin in certain high-risk patients [15]. Patients on anticoagulant therapy with a history of vascular thrombosis or atrial fibrillation also require preoperative evaluation to determine their risk of recurrent thrombosis with the discontinuation of anticoagulation. For patients in whom anticoagulation may be safely discontinued, it is usually held 5–7 days preoperatively, however, certain patients may require heparin or low-molecular weight heparin bridging [15, 17]. The final preoperative dose of intravenous heparin and subcutaneous low-molecular weight heparin is approximately 4–6 h and 24 h preoperatively, respectively.

Poor nutritional status, a prevalent condition among bladder cancer patients, is associated with increased perioperative morbidity and mortality [18, 19]. Gregg et al. determined that nutritional deficiency in cystectomy patients was strongly associated with 90-day mortality [20]. Malnutrition may be related to a variety of factors including paraneoplastic tumor effects or poor oral intake due to disease symptomatology or patient anxiety. In the perioperative setting, poor nutrition can impair immune status and decrease the capability for tissue repair. Therefore, preoperative enteral nutritional supplementation and the selective use of perioperative total parenteral nutrition are strategies to improve nutritional status in malnourished patients. However, the benefit from such measures has yet to be demonstrated [21].

Obesity is another nutritional factor that can increase perioperative complications. In addition to poor wound healing and increased risks of wound infections and hernias [22–24], obesity is known to be associated with higher intraoperative blood loss and postoperative complications after cystectomy [25, 26]. Obesity can also produce challenges for anesthesiologists, such as difficulty intubating, ventilating, and positioning. While it is often impractical to recommend preoperative weight loss, knowledge of these risks is important for patient counseling.

Patient age may also factor into the decision to undergo cystectomy, yet it is clear that advanced age alone should not be an independent exclusion criteria. Although certain characteristics of elderly patients are associated with increased 90-day mortality [27], certain elderly patients, even some with significant medical comorbidities [28–30], do benefit from radical cystectomy. Elderly patients can tolerate the procedure and have complication rates similar to younger patients [31].

Although indications for RARC are similar to ORC, the choice of approach should be based on a combination of patient characteristics, shared patient and physician preference and physician experience. A robotic approach should only be considered if it can safely provide optimal oncologic control. Our preference has been to selectively offer RARC to healthier and thinner patients that have had less pelvic and/or intra-abdominal surgery and less bulky disease, especially early in our experience. Understandably, this has also been the trend at other institutions [32–34]. However, with continued experience and increased surgeon comfort, the types of patients eligible for RARC will continue to expand.

One of the final, and arguably most important, aspects of patient selection is establishing *realistic expectations*. While the majority of patients do not have the luxury to forego cystectomy, it is important that they understand the ways in which it will alter their functionality, impact their quality of life, and the complications they are at risk for. Many patients will be significantly debilitated, weakened, and experience substantial weight loss postoperatively. An extensive body of literature exists regarding the measurement of health-related quality of life in cystectomy patients, which, in large part, measures the impact of the urinary diversion. If a patient has multiple options for urinary diversion, a conversation should occur regarding the relative benefits and drawbacks for each type of diversion. Although each diversion is associated with a unique spectrum of risks and benefits, the relative impact of diversion type on overall health-related quality of life may be modest [35]. Using disease-specific instruments, such as the FACT-VCI [36], health-related quality of life in cystectomy patients can be assessed and used during patient counseling.

Preoperative Planning

Given the aggressive nature of high-risk bladder cancer, it is important to recommend a *timely cystectomy* to all surgical candidates. A delay of greater than 90 days from diagnosis of muscle-invasive disease to cystectomy is associated with higher pathologic tumor stage and worse overall and disease-specific survival [37, 38]. Thus, all preoperative planning and coordination of care should begin promptly upon diagnosis so as not to unnecessarily delay cystectomy.

In preparation for surgery, all patients visit the enterostomal nurse for *ostomy site evaluation* [39]. The nurse examines the patient in the supine, seated and standing positions, and identifies the preferred site in the right lower quadrant for an ileal conduit. Patients who have chosen an ONB also have an ostomy site marked, given the small risk of being unable to safely form a neobladder, and a colostomy site can be marked for patients that require a total pelvic exenteration. We also recommend all smokers *cease smoking*, as this has been shown to decrease several perioperative complications including respiratory complications and wound infections [40–42].

The day prior to surgery we start patients on a clear liquid diet and administer a *mechanical bowel preparation* with an oral laxative, such as magnesium citrate or GoLYTELY™. This is intended to reduce fecal load and enhance intraoperative bowel retraction. There is no single mechanical bowel preparation that has demonstrated superiority over another, however, oral antibiotics are no longer administered. Because a bowel preparation can cause dehydration, especially in the elderly, patients must undergo aggressive perioperative hydration. While the utility of a mechanical bowel preparation has been disputed and there is insufficient evidence to support its routine use [43], it is still practiced at our institution, especially in patients with planned colon reconstructive procedures.

It is important to *communicate with the anesthesia team* preoperatively and for the anesthesiologists to assess perioperative anesthesia risk [44]. All cystectomy patients must have their blood typed and screened and the anesthesia team must be made aware of the risks of blood loss. They also must be made aware of the inability to monitor the patient's vital status using urine output for the majority of the case, as the ureters will be clipped. As such, all patients will require two large-bore intravenous lines and, in some cases, an arterial or central line depending on anesthesia preference.

Patients must be positioned with all pressure points well padded and the surgical and anesthesia teams must understand the risks of nerve and limb injury due to improper patient positioning.

To *prevent surgical site infections* all patients are shaved with electrical clippers, receive intravenous antibiotic prophylaxis, and are cleansed with a chlorhexidine-based skin preparation [45, 46]. Because many patients have risk factors for deep vein thrombosis (older age, cigarette smoking, obesity, malignancy, pelvic surgery), and thromboembolic events are a significant source of morbidity and mortality among cystectomy patients, deep vein thrombosis *(DVT) prophylaxis* is critical and may significantly reduce the likelihood of a DVT and fatal pulmonary embolus [47–49]. We use sequential compression devices on all patients, although some higher risk patients may require chemothromboprophylaxis with subcutaneous heparin or low-molecular weight heparin [49]. In fact, continuing DVT prophylaxis after hospital discharge may help protect against the substantial rate of out-of-hospital thromboembolic events [50, 51].

Oncologic Principles

The improved outcomes of radical cystectomy over the past half-decade are largely thought to be secondary to improvements in surgical and anesthetic care. Meticulous surgical technique not only limits potential morbidity but also contributes to improved oncologic outcomes. While RARC may further temper the morbidity of cystectomy, it can only be feasible if it preserves the same oncologic efficacy as ORC. In order to achieve both, surgeons must adhere to strict surgical principles.

Basic principles of intra-abdominal cancer surgery include exploration of the peritoneal cavity for unrecognized metastasis, early vasculature ligation, minimization of tumor spillage, and a complete tumor resection with en bloc specimen removal. Given the risk of peritoneal seeding of bladder cancer, *minimization of tumor spillage* is very important. Occlusion of the ureteral stump with a clip is performed, due to the small risk of vesicoureteral reflux, and careful control of the transected urethra is strongly recommended. In RARC, the specimen is contained in an Endocatch™ bag (Covidien Surgical, Mansfield, MA) to avoid intraperitoneal spillage and port site metastasis [52]. In addition, one must carefully handle any grossly enlarged lymph nodes to avoid damage and resultant spillage of metastatic tumor cells.

To achieve a *complete tumor resection* and negative surgical margins, one must pay careful attention to tissue planes and extend the dissection widely if there is any concern for extravesical extension. Intraoperative frozen section analysis of the distal urethral margin is standard practice at our institution, regardless of diversion type. In patients who desire an ONB, it is essential to rule out disease in the proximal urethra, as this is generally a contraindication to ONB. Alternatively, involvement of the urethra may prompt a concurrent urethrectomy for those receiving a non-orthotopic diversion.

More controversy exists regarding the utility of intraoperative *ureteral frozen section analysis*. Advocates argue that by obtaining a negative distal frozen section there may be decreased anastomotic and upper tract recurrences and that patients with positive margins can be followed more closely [53, 54]. Those against contend that the result does little to change the risk of local recurrence and distant disease failure [54–56]. Furthermore, a negative ureteral frozen section is not associated with a clear survival benefit, does not exclude proximal carcinoma in situ (CIS) and conversion from a positive to a negative margin can be difficult, and does not eliminate the risk of local recurrence [56–59]. Upper tract recurrence after radical cystectomy is a rare event and, excluding obvious ureteral involvement, is more common with aggressive tumors and the presence of CIS [56, 59, 60]. Patients with these findings should be counseled preoperatively that they are at higher risk for upper tract recurrence and will require close postoperative surveillance, however, we do not routinely obtain a ureteral frozen section analysis.

Pelvic Lymphadenectomy

Pelvic lymphadenectomy is a critical element of a radical cystectomy. Approximately 20–25 % of patients undergoing cystectomy are found to have lymph node invasion at the time of pathologic analysis [61]. While patients with extravesical disease have a higher likelihood of positive lymph nodes (42–75 %), a significant percentage of patients with organ-confined tumors also have node positive disease (6–22 %), suggesting lymphadenectomy is indicated regardless of clinical tumor stage [62–66]. Lymphadenectomy is important for accurate disease staging, improves local control, and identifies those patients that might benefit from adjuvant therapy. Furthermore, approximately 30 % of patients with pathologically positive lymph nodes demonstrate long-term, durable responses after cystectomy, suggesting lymphadenectomy may be therapeutic for some patients [63, 67, 68].

The boundaries of a standard pelvic lymphadenectomy are the genitofemoral nerve laterally, wall of the detrusor medially, node of Cloquet distally, bifurcation of the common iliac artery proximally, and the internal iliac vessels posteriorly (Fig. 2.1). Some surgeons prefer to extend the lymphadenectomy cranially to the aortic bifurcation or even further to the inferior mesenteric artery. Several reports have demonstrated improved survival in patients with more lymph nodes removed, and some have suggested using lymph node yield as a proxy for surgical quality [67, 69–72]. Interestingly, this association has been demonstrated in both pathologically node positive and node negative patients [67]. Removal of more lymph nodes likely eliminates any micrometastatic disease, allows for wider surgical margins, and provides more tissue for pathologic staging [73, 74].

Still, using nodal yield as a quality indicator is controversial and is an imperfect measure of dissection adequacy. Similarly experienced surgeons using identical templates can produce a highly variable number of lymph nodes, indicating nodal yield may, in part, be associated with nonsurgical factors [62]. For example, nodal yield is highly dependent on methods of pathological analysis, such as the technique of lymph node identification and whether nodal tissue is submitted en bloc or in packets [75, 76]. Furthermore, there can be

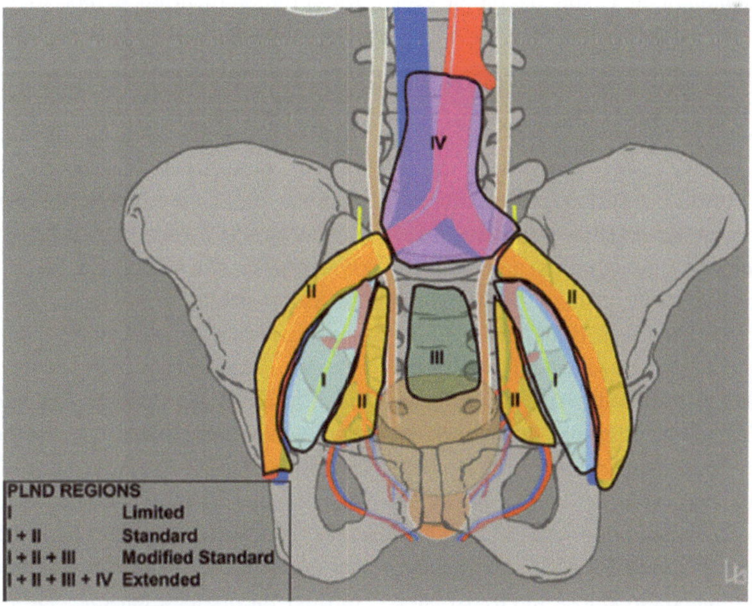

Fig. 2.1 Pelvic lymphadenectomy boundaries. Reprinted, with permission, from Elsevier Limited, Hurle, R., Naspro, R.: Pelvic lymphadenectomy during radical cystectomy: a review of the literature. Surg Oncol, 19: 208, 2010

significant intraobserver variability among pathologists in identifying what constitutes nodal tissue [77] and there is no standardized process of pathologic analysis consistently used across different institutions [78]. Finally, although recommendations have been put forth, there is no accepted minimum number of lymph nodes that defines an "adequate" lymphadenectomy [79].

Because nodal yield is an imperfect measure of surgical quality, an adequate pelvic lymphadenectomy must be defined as the removal of all nodal tissue within the bounds of the chosen template [62]. Still, the template boundaries and extent of dissection have been debated. An extended dissection has a higher nodal yield relative to a standard dissection, which may translate to improvements in recurrence and mortality with little added morbidity [80–82]. However, with the rarity of skip metastasis, a standard lymph node dissection may provide adequate staging for most patients [81, 83]. There is unlikely a survival benefit of a super extended lymphadenectomy over an extended dissection [84]. Regardless of the template chosen, a lymphadenectomy should include meticulous removal of all tissue in regions known to harbor lymph nodes that drain the bladder. Such a dissection is possible with RARC and is mandatory to ensure oncologic efficacy [85, 86].

Hemostasis

Hemostasis is essential during radical cystectomy, and there are several ways to control the vascular pedicles including clips and sutures, staplers, and bipolar electrocautery devices such as the Ligasure™ (Covidien, Boulder, CO). The use of a stapler is associated with lower blood loss than with the traditional suture and clips technique [87] and the Ligasure appears to be equally effective as a stapler, but more cost efficient [88]. One purported benefit to RARC is decreased intraoperative blood loss [33, 89], and we recently determined that RARC is associated with a lower estimated blood loss and transfusion requirement than ORC (*authors data, unpublished*). Regardless of the technique used to secure the vascular pedicles, every effort should be taken to avoid excess blood loss given the risks of a blood transfusion and its association with increased mortality after cystectomy [90].

Special Considerations in Men

Recently, new techniques have been introduced to manage the prostate and urethra during cystectomy in efforts to improve postoperative functionality and quality of life in men. Historically, *urethrectomy* was universally recommended at the time of cystectomy, however, given the low risk of urethral recurrence, the popularization of the ONB, and the possible protective effect of ONB on urethral recurrence, patients are now risk stratified to determine if urethrectomy is required [91, 92]. The primary risk factor for anterior urethral recurrence is cancer involvement of the prostate, a finding in upwards of 40 % of cystectomy specimens [91, 93]. Furthermore, CIS, multifocal tumors, and tumors involving the trigone or bladder neck are known to increase the risk of prostatic involvement [93, 94]. Thus, we generally do not perform a urethrectomy in men in the absence of risk factors for urethral recurrence. For those patients not receiving an orthotopic diversion that have a high risk of urethral recurrence, we recommend a urethrectomy at the time of cystectomy.

More recently, a *nerve sparing* approach to radical cystectomy has been proposed in an attempt to preserve potency and possibly continence with a neobladder. Initially described by Walsh [95], the technique for a nerve sparing radical cystectomy is similar to that of a nerve sparing radical prostatectomy. Some believe that sparing either one or both sets of nerves should be offered to all patients that do not have an oncologic contraindication, whether or not they receive an ONB [96]. Advocates of this approach believe that sparing the neurovascular bundle does not sacrifice the oncologic efficacy of radical cystectomy, as bladder cancer rarely extends through the prostatic capsule [97–99]. Schoenberg et al. presented 10-year data on 101 men who underwent this procedure and demonstrated no positive margins at the site of nerve sparing, survival outcomes similar to that of historic cohorts, and a significant proportion of patients who were able to engage in sexual activity postoperatively [98]. Other series have similarly shown that approximately 80 % of men who were potent prior to cystectomy had good postoperative sexual function with a nerve-sparing procedure [99, 100]. Kessler et al. demonstrated that attempted nerve sparing was associated with improved postoperative erectile function as well as continence with an ONB [101]. Thus, for properly selected sexually active men, nerve-sparing radical cystectomy appears to provide good oncologic control while increasing the likelihood of preserving erectile function and continence. There are no randomized studies of nerve sparing versus non-nerve-sparing cystectomy, thus no firm conclusions regarding these purported functional benefits can be made.

By maximally protecting the neurovascular bundle and rhabdosphincter, a *prostate capsule-sparing* radical cystectomy is an even more aggressive measure to preserve functionality in patients with an ONB. During this operation, the prostatic urethra, prostatic adenoma, and bladder are removed, a distal urethral frozen section margin is sent, and the prostatic capsule is left in place. Indications for capsule-sparing cystectomy include good preoperative sexual function with tumors that appear to be resectable without requiring a wide periprostatic margin. Contraindications include extravesical tumor extension, bladder cancer involvement of the prostate or bladder neck, CIS, hydronephrosis and biopsy-proven prostate cancer [102, 103]. Clinical staging with transrectal and transurethral evaluation of the prostate and bladder will identify most men that have contraindications to the procedure [104–106].

Although most studies are relatively small and nonrandomized, the functional outcomes with capsule-sparing cystectomy and ONB appear encouraging. Vallancien et al. reported that of 100 capsule-sparing cystectomy patients, over 80 % of previously sexually active men were able to have intercourse postoperatively [105]. In another series, Nieuwenhuijzen et al. reported 78 % of their 44 patients had satisfactory postoperative sexual function [107]. Postoperative daytime and nighttime continence in patients with ONBs also appear to be quite high with this procedure [102]. Still, capsule-sparing cystectomy is controversial given the oncologic concerns of leaving prostatic tissue behind and any conclusions regarding functional and oncological outcomes relative to traditional radical cystectomy are inferences, as no comparative studies exist.

Although urethral and prostatic fossa recurrences in capsule-sparing cystectomy series are low, the risk is cause for concern [105]. Urothelial carcinoma involvement of the prostate may be as high as 40 %, with an increased likelihood in patients with CIS or trigonal tumors [93, 94, 103, 108]. While most of these tumors can be identified preoperatively [106], urothelial carcinoma involving the prostatic capsule and periprostatic tissue (areas not well sampled during clinical staging) has been identified in cystectomy specimens [109]. Thus, advocats of this technique advise urethral and prostatic surveillance as would normally be done with an ONB, and to treat any such recurrences either endoscopically or with undiversion, if necessary [110].

Incidental prostatic adenocarcinoma can be identified in approximately 30 % of cystectomy specimens, up to one quarter of which are clinically significant, and some are located in areas that would be left behind with a capsule-sparing procedure [109, 111–115]. While there is a report of prostate cancer metastasis after radical cystectomy [116], the risk of prostate cancer-specific mortality and biochemical recurrence is low [117–120]. There are no reports of prostate cancer deaths in capsule-sparing cystectomy patients found to harbor occult prostate cancer, and most could be effectively treated, if required [121, 122].

Most importantly, oncologic outcomes with capsule-sparing cystectomy appear comparable to that of traditional radical cystectomy. In one of the largest series of capsule-sparing cystectomy patients, Rozet et al. reported a 4.7 % and 34 % rate of local and distant recurrence, respectively [122]. Despite these encouraging results, some argue that leaving the prostatic capsule is inappropriate, distant failure with capsule-sparing cystectomy is higher than would be expected, and the supporting data are limited by selection bias [123, 124]. Therefore, for properly motivated patients, capsule-sparing cystectomy with ONB may help preserve continence and sexual function, but the risk of residual or recurrent cancer must be understood and, until large randomized studies with extended follow-up exist, it cannot be considered oncologically equal to traditional radical cystectomy [124].

Special Considerations in Women

With the increasing use of ONBs in women [125], the preferred *management of the urethra* at the time of cystectomy has been called into question. While there is a relatively low risk of female urethral involvement (<10 %) by bladder cancer, patients with bladder neck and trigonal tumors are at higher risk [126–128]. In women at low risk for urethral involvement that have a negative intraoperative urethral frozen section analysis, the risk of urethral recurrence can be considered minimal and an ONB may be safely fashioned [129]. Otherwise, urethrectomy is generally performed along with radical cystectomy.

In an effort to improve functionality after cystectomy, some have recommended sparing the *gynecologic organs*. As vaginal shortening can lead to significant sexual dysfunction, young, sexually active women who desire ONBs and have minimal risk for vaginal wall involvement may be candidates of vaginal wall-sparing cystectomy [130]. Sparing the anterior vaginal wall and maximally preserving paravaginal and periurethral supporting tissues may decrease the risk of pelvic organ prolapse, maintain vaginal length, and reduce the risk of neobladder–vaginal fistula. Chang et al. demonstrated that preservation of the anterior vaginal wall in women with ONBs was associated with a low rate of complications and resulted in satisfactory functional voiding outcomes [131]. Furthermore, sparing the uterus is associated with improved incontinence in women with ONBs, further supporting the utility of preserving uninvolved gynecologic organs [132]. Importantly, sparing these organs does not appear to sacrifice the oncologic efficacy of radical cystectomy. Pathologic analysis of gynecologic organs taken during radical cystectomy demonstrated that, in the absence of gross tumor extension, they are unlikely to be involved by bladder cancer [133]. Ali-El-Dein et al. noted a 2.6 % prevalence of gynecologic organ involvement in cystectomy specimens, with a higher risk in women that had aggressive tumor characteristics [134]. Thus, it does not appear necessary to routinely remove all female gynecologic organs during radical cystectomy.

The *neurovascular bundles* that provide autonomic innervation to the vagina, clitoris, and proximal urethra run lateral to the vaginal walls and damage can result in sexual and urinary dysfunction [96, 135–137]. With an interest in improving postoperative quality of life in women, some have suggested preservation of these bundles [138, 139]. Several small case–series suggest that, in properly selected patients, sparing one or both of these nerve bundles may help preserve postoperative sexual function and urinary continence in women with ONBs [125, 140, 141]. Vaginal wall and gynecologic organ-sparing procedures may help avoid damage to these nerves.

Postoperative Care

Postoperative care is an essential element to any operation, no more so than with radical cystectomy. At our institution, we pioneered a *collaborative care pathway* for cystectomy patients, which incorporates evidence-based guidelines and standardizes patients' hospital course (Appendix). As a result, the cost and length of hospital stay after cystectomy decreased significantly with no impairment in quality of care [142, 143]. Part of this pathway was exclusion of routine postoperative surgical intensive care unit placement. While it is important to have the resources available to admit a cystectomy patient to an intensive care unit, it is not routine practice. In fact, with the use of a collaborative care pathway, only 6.5 % of radical cystectomy patients required postoperative intensive care unit admission [144].

Another component to postoperative patient care is *patient disposition* at the time of hospital discharge. With shorter lengths of inpatient stay, there is an increasing use of postoperative home healthcare services and rehabilitation facilities [145]. Aghazadeh et al. recently reported that approximately a third of cystectomy patients are discharged home with services and 9 % to an inpatient facility [146]. In fact, older age, lower preoperative albumin, being unmarried, and a higher Charlson comorbidity index (CCI) were independently associated with discharge to home with services, while older age, poor preoperative exercise tolerance, and a longer hospital stay were associated with discharge to a rehabilitation facility. It is important to educate patients preoperatively that only half are discharged home without services and patients at higher risk of requiring postdischarge care should be appropriately counseled.

Complications

Due to the substantial perioperative morbidity of radical cystectomy (Table 2.1), surgeons must be familiar with all possible complications and be prepared to recognize and manage them expediently. Importantly, patients should be counseled about the prevalence and spectrum of these risks preoperatively.

Historically, perioperative complications were reported within 30 days of cystectomy. One large series reported 30-day morbidity, readmission, and mortality rates of 45 %, 18 %, and 1.7 %, respectively [3]. However, given the considerable risk of additional complications in the months following surgery, there has been a trend to report up to 90 days postoperatively. Stimson et al. identified increases in readmission and mortality rates to 27 % and 7 %, respectfully, when following patients to 90 days [147]. Given the nonstandardized methods for reporting complications, it is difficult to compare different series and accurately define the morbidity of radical cystectomy [148]. Thus, using stringent criteria [149] to report 90-day complications, there was a 64 % prevalence of any complication, 26 % risk of readmission, and 2.7 % mortality rate (Table 2.2) [150]. Gastrointestinal, infectious, and wound complications were the most common diagnoses and 11 % required an interventional radiology procedure.

While studies reporting perioperative morbidity after RARC are limited by patient numbers and procedural selection bias, there appears to be

Table 2.1 Perioperative morbidity and mortality in contemporary radical cystectomy series

Series	Procedure	Time of assessment (days)	Number of patients	Mortality	Morbidity
Lee [1]	ORC	30	498	1.6	45
Hollenbeck [2]	ORC	30	2,538	–	30.5
Novotny [3]	ORC	30	516	0.8	27.3
Lowrance [4]	ORC	30	553	1.7	41
Stimson [5]	ORC	90	753	6.9	–
Stein [6]	ORC	90	1,054	2.5	28
Novarra [7]	ORC	90	358	3	49
Hautmann [8]	ORC	90	923	2.3	58
Svatek [9]	ORC	90	283	0	54
Shabsigh [10]	ORC	90	1,142	2	64
Smith [11]	RARC	30	227	0	30
Jonsson [12]	RARC	30	45	0	40
Ng [13]	RARC	90	79	0	49
Khan [14]	RARC	90	50	0	34
Hayn [15]	RARC	90	156	5.8	52

Table 2.2 Perioperative complications after open and robot-assisted radical cystectomy

Category	ORC [10]	RARC [15]
Number of patients	1,142	156
Number of complications	1,637	186
Number of patients with a complication	735	102
Gastrointestinal	29 %	31 %
Infectious	25 %	25 %
Wound/skin	15 %	7 %
Genitourinary	11 %	13 %
Cardiac	11 %	3 %
Pulmonary	9 %	4 %
Bleeding	9 %	
Hematologic/vascular		5 %
Thromboembolic	8 %	
Metabolic		3 %
Nervous	5 %	0.5 %
General		7 %
Miscellaneous	3 %	
Surgical	1 %	
Head and neck		1 %
Endocrine		0.5 %

a similar rate of complications. Hayn et al. reported perioperative complications on 156 RARC patients and found that 52 % of patients experienced at least one complication within 90 days of surgery [151]. Gastrointestinal, infectious, and genitourinary were the most common types of complications and 21 %, 8.3 %, and 5.8 % of patients were readmitted, required an interventional radiology procedure, and died, respectively. Thus, despite the purported benefits of RARC, it is clearly associated with a similar frequency and spectrum of complications as ORC (Table 2.2).

Quality Indicators for Radical Cystectomy

Although there have been vast improvements in the management of patients with bladder cancer, differences still exist in the quality of surgery delivered. Quality surgical care can be analyzed within the Donabedian framework of structure, process, and outcome [152]. While the components of this framework are interrelated, structural aspects (physical facilities, hospital/surgeon volume) help drive clinical processes (adequacy of lymphadenectomy, use of ONB), which, in turn, are related to outcomes (perioperative morbidity and mortality) [153]. Though certain outcomes may be impacted by patient factors, such as comorbidity and disease severity, some potentially modifiable surgical factors may also impact outcomes. Currently, there are no accepted quality of care indicators for radical cystectomy, thus proxies must be used to estimate surgical quality.

Surgeon and Hospital Volume

Hospital and/or surgeon case volume appear to be associated with several surgical outcomes and have been proposed as indicators for surgical quality [154–156]. In a seminal article by Birkmeyer, higher hospital volume was associated with lower perioperative mortality for several operations, including a greater than 50 % decrease in mortality for radical cystectomy [157]. In a subsequent study specifically examining the relationship between hospital volume and radical cystectomy outcomes, Hollenbeck et al. determined that patients treated at low volume hospitals were 46 % more likely to suffer a perioperative death than patients treated at high volume hospitals [158]. Potential explanations for improved outcomes at higher volume hospitals include employment of more specialized surgeons, more consistent postoperative processes of care, better intensive care unit staffing, greater resources for managing complications, and the practice of a more complete Donabedian framework [159, 160].

Higher surgeon volume may also be related to cystectomy outcomes, although this association does not appear to be as consistent. In another Birkmeyer article, higher surgeon volume was associated with lower perioperative mortality for several operations, including radical cystectomy, even when controlling for hospital volume [161]. However, a recent analysis of post-cystectomy survival suggested that the impact of surgeon volume is attenuated when accounting for hospital

Table 2.3 Standards for radical cystectomy and PLND stratified by patient age and stage [16]

			Margins		Lymph nodes		
Age at presentation	pT stage	Number of patients	Positive *N* (%)	Negative	Mean	SD	Median
<65							
No	<T2	203	3 (1.5)	200	15.3	10.5	14
	≥T3	143	23 (16)	120	13.9	9.6	12
Yes	<T2	30	0 (0)	30	10.7	9.9	8
	≥T3	20	5 (25)	15	5.8	6.7	4
65–75							
No	<T2	202	4 (2)	198	13.5	10.8	12
	≥T3	161	17 (11)	144	14.7	9.4	13
Yes	<T2	32	1 (2)	31	7.6	6.3	9.5
	≥T3	22	4 (18)	18	6.4	6.2	6
>75							
No	<T2	105	2 (1)	103	10.5	7.8	9
	≥T3	108	10 (9)	98	10.2	7.9	10
Yes	<T2	25	0 (0)	25	7.6	6.4	7
	≥T3	40	2 (5)	38	5.3	5.6	4
Totals	All	1,091	71 (6.5)		12.5	9.7	11
	≥T3	494	61 (12)				

Reproduced, with permission, from Elsevier Limited, Herr, H. W., Faulkner, J. R., Grossman, H. B. et al.: Surgical factors influence bladder cancer outcomes: a cooperative group report. J Clin Oncol, 22: 2781, 2004

volume [155]. Still, there does appear to be a learning curve with RARC such that more surgeon experience is associated with improved outcomes [33, 162]. Together, these data imply differences in surgical quality based on hospital and/or surgeon volume, although the root causes remain to be explained and no definition of what "high" volume should be currently exists. Therefore, while it may be related to cystectomy outcomes in some way, the use of volume as a proxy for surgical quality is imperfect and remains a topic of debate.

Surgical Factors

In an effort to establish surgical parameters to define quality for radical cystectomy, Herr et al. led a collaborative effort to benchmark "reasonable standards" of care [163]. They proposed that a 75–80 % utilization of pelvic lymphadenectomy, 10–14 lymph nodes removed, a positive margin rate ≤10 % (preferably <5 %) and a minimum annual surgeon volume of ten cases could be considered as standards of care (Table 2.3). In a subsequent study, Herr et al. attempted to determine which surgical factors were most important for survival and local recurrence after cystectomy [67]. Negative surgical margins and ≥10 lymph nodes removed were independently associated with survival, while positive margins and <10 lymph nodes removed were independently associated with local recurrence. Interestingly, the type of surgeon (urologic oncologist) and type of institution (academic) were each inversely associated with positive margin status and removal of <10 lymph nodes. In all, surgical quality appeared to be related to survival and recurrence, and nontechnical factors, namely surgeon training and hospital setting, influenced surgical quality.

Adjunctive Therapies

Urothelial carcinoma is a chemosensitive malignancy and data over the past decade has solidified the use of chemotherapy in its management. Given the high rate of distant recurrences, there is no question that systemic therapy plays a role in the management of bladder cancer [164]. Chemotherapy can either be administered preoperatively or postoperatively, and there are advocates for each approach [165]. While neoadjuvant chemotherapy can allow for tumor downstaging, provide early treatment for systemic micrometastasis, is delivered to the tumor with an intact vasculature and may be tolerated better, it also may lead to overtreatment and unintentionally delay cystectomy. Adjuvant chemotherapy can be used selectively for high-risk patients and allows for immediate cystectomy but may be poorly tolerated and delays administration of systemic therapy to patients who may fail surgery due to distant recurrences [166].

Current level 1 data clearly demonstrates a survival benefit of neoadjuvant chemotherapy [167]. Based on a meta-analysis of over 3,000 patients from 11 randomized control trials, the use of multiagent cisplatin neoadjuvant therapy resulted in a 14 % relative risk reduction in mortality and a 22 % reduction in disease specific mortality at 5 years [168]. Patients with a good performance status and clinical factors concerning for high-risk and locally advanced disease are the best candidates for neoadjuvant chemotherapy [169]. However, despite supporting data, neoadjuvant chemotherapy remains relatively underutilized, providing a target for improvement in the quality of care delivered to cystectomy patients [170, 171]. While adjuvant chemotherapy may be beneficial, its use is not strongly supported based on a recent meta-analysis [172, 173]. Because there are no trials directly comparing adjuvant and neoadjuvant chemotherapy, the relative benefit of one over another is speculative.

Survivorship

The last element to a successful cystectomy is survivorship care. One such element of survivorship is cancer surveillance. At 5 years approximately 30–40 % of patients experience a recurrence, but most occur within 2 years of surgery [68, 174, 175]. Depending on pathologic risk factors, there is a small risk of urethral recurrence [91, 176] and an even smaller risk of upper tract recurrence [177]. Boorjian et al. demonstrated that post-cystectomy patients experienced improved survival if their recurrence was detected asymptomatically through routine surveillance imaging, and patients who presented symptomatically fared poorer, supporting the value in routine postoperative surveillance imaging [178]. Unfortunately, there are no set guidelines about the recommended frequency and method for postoperative surveillance and there remains tremendous variation in how patients are monitored [179]. At our institution we image the abdomen and pelvis, typically using CT with intravenous contrast, every 6 months for the first 2 years and then annually thereafter. We do not routinely screen for urethral recurrences in patients with incontinent diversions and retained urethras [180, 181].

Other elements of survivorship include management of late treatment effects, quality of life issues, and physical and psychosocial rehabilitation [169]. As these issues are unquestionably important to cystectomy patients and their families, instituting multidisciplinary survivorship programs continues to be a growing effort among urologists.

Conclusion

Radical cystectomy is the gold-standard treatment for high-risk bladder cancer and a successful result is dependent on multiple patient, surgeon, and institutional factors. The outcome of radical cystectomy can be optimized through proper patient selection, adherence to surgical principles, the use of adjunctive treatments, and regular postoperative follow-up. Regardless of the surgical approach chosen, these principles must be followed as they undoubtedly translate to improved surgical quality.

Editors' Commentary

Erik P. Castle and Raj S. Pruthi

Most who care for patients with bladder cancer understand that the ultimate goal of radical cystectomy is oncologic success and patient safety—irrespective of operative technique. As the authors state, a successful outcome with radical cystectomy is not only related to surgical technique and safe extirpation of the bladder but also to factors such as patient selection, coordinated perioperative care, and use of adjunctive treatments. Such principles are nicely outlined in this chapter by experts in the field of bladder cancer. Such principles are simply mandatory for all who perform this operation and care for the patient with bladder cancer.

Robotic techniques in bladder cancer surgery must continue to duplicate the surgical principles of open radical cystectomy with regard to the extirpative portion of the procedure and to the ability to perform adequate lymphadenectomy. Fortunately, the robotic approach to cystectomy appears to provide acceptable operative, pathological, and short-term clinical outcomes—seemingly duplicating the principles and practices of the time-tested open surgical technique.

Appendix

A. Radical cystectomy with ileal conduit pathway orders
  a. Admission
    i. Diagnosis: malignant neoplasm of bladder (188); s/p radical cystectomy with ileal conduit
    ii. Diagnosis: possible, probable, or r/o cancer/malignancy
    iii. Admit to: urology
    iv. Condition:
    v. Allergies:
  b. Nursing
    i. Vital signs q4h × 2 days
      1. Convert to vital signs q8h on POD 2
    ii. Strict I&O q4h
    iii. Drain: Jackson-Pratt to self-suction. Empty and record q4h. Change dressing around drain PRN daily starting POD 1
      1. Discontinue JP drain 4 h after stent removal prior to discharge
    iv. Ureteral stents to gravity drainage
    v. Volurex incentive spirometer q1h while awake
    vi. Sequential compression devices bilaterally
    vii. Notify house officer for Temp >101, SBP > 160, DBP > 100, HR > 120, UOP < 60 mL/2 h
    viii. Activity: out of bed to chair day of surgery with assistance
      1. Ambulate in halls TID POD 1 and POD 2
      2. Ambulate q2h while awake starting POD 3
  c. Diet
    i. NPO POD 0 × 24 h
    ii. POD 1: may chew gum while awake PRN, otherwise NPO
    iii. Begin restricted clear liquid diet POD 2: 8 oz q8h
    iv. Clear liquid diet POD 3
  d. Ostomy orders
    i. Wound ostomy nurse consult
  e. Medications
    i. D5LR at 150 mL/h × 1 bag
      1. Then, D5 1/2NS + 20 mEq/L KCl at 150 mL/h
    ii. Cefoxitin 2,000 mg IV q8h × 3 doses
      1. If allergic to PCN or cephalosporins and serum Cr < 1.3
        a. Gentamicin 3 mg/kg IV
        b. Clindamycin 900 mg IV
      2. If allergic to PCN or cephalosporins and serum Cr > 1.3
        a. Aztreonam 2,000 mg IV
        b. Clindamycin 900 mg IV
    iii. Bisacodyl 10 mg PR BID, start POD 3
    iv. Milk of Magnesia 30 mL PO BID, start POD 4
    v. Levofloxacin 500 mg PO ×1 with stent removal
    vi. *Pain medications*
      1. Ketorolac 30 mg IV in recovery room
        a. Then, 15 mg IV q6h × 24 h
      2. Hydromorphone 1 mg/mL PCA: 0.1 mg q8h × 3 days
      3. Oxycodone 5 mg/acetaminophen 325 mg POD q4h PRN × 3 days PRN pain score 2–5

4. Oxycodone 10 mg/acetaminophen 325 mg POD q4h PRN×3 days PRN pain score 6–10

vii. *Prophylaxis*

1. Enoxaparin 40 mg subcut qday10
   a. Or for renal insufficiency: heparin 5,000 U subcut q8h
2. Famotidine 20 mg IV q12h×5 days
3. Esomeprazole 20 mg PO daily when famotidine is discontinued

viii. *As needed medications*

1. Ondensetron 4 mg IV q6h PRN nausea
2. Acetaminophen 650 mg PO/PR q4h PRN temp > 101
3. Chloroseptic spray at bedside for PRN use

f. Labs

i. Hematocrit POD 1, 2, 4

ii. Basic metabolic panel POD 1, 4

g. Patient/family education

i. Instruction on changing pouch and wafer

B. Radical cystectomy with continent diversion pathway orders

a. Admission

i. Diagnosis: malignant neoplasm of bladder (188); s/p radical cystectomy with continent diversion

ii. Diagnosis: possible, probable, or r/o cancer/malignancy

iii. Admit to: urology

iv. Condition:

v. Allergies:

b. Nursing

i. Vital signs q4h×2 days

1. Convert to vital signs q8h on POD 2

ii. Strict I&O q4h

iii. Drain: Jackson-Pratt to self-suction. Empty and record q4h. Change dressing around drain PRN daily starting POD 1.

iv. Ureteral stents to gravity drainage

v. Foley catheter to bedside bag drainage

1. Irrigate Foley catheter with 60 mL normal saline TID starting POD 1

vi. Volurex incentive spirometer q1h while awake

vii. Sequential compression devices bilaterally

viii. Notify house officer for Temp > 101, SBP > 160, DBP > 100, HR > 120, UOP < 60 mL/2 h

ix. Activity: out of bed to chair day of surgery if possible, with assistance

1. Ambulate in halls TID POD 1 and POD 2
2. Ambulated q2h while awake starting POD 3

c. Diet

i. Strict NPO until POD 5, no ice chips

d. Medications

i. D5LR at150 mL/h×1 bag

1. Then, D5 1/2NS + 20 mEq/L KCl at150 mL/h

ii. Cefoxitin 2,000 mg IV q8h×3 doses

1. If allergic to PCN or cephalosporins and serum Cr < 1.3
   a. Gentamicin 3 mg/kg IV
   b. Clindamycin 900 mg IV
2. If allergic to PCN or cephalosporins and serum Cr > 1.3
   a. Aztreonam 2,000 mg IV
   b. Clindamycin 900 mg IV

iii. Bisacodyl 10 mg PR BID, start POD 4

iv. Milk of Magnesia 30 mL PO BID, start POD 5

v. Levofloxacin 500 mg PO ×1 with stent removal

vi. *Pain medications*

1. Ketorolac 30 mg IV in recovery room
   a. Then, 15 mg IV q6h×24 h
2. Hydromorphone 1 mg/mL PCA: 0.1 mg q8h×3 days
3. Oxycodone 5 mg/acetaminophen 325 mg POD q4h PRN×3 days PRN pain score 2–5
4. Oxycodone 10 mg/acetaminophen 325 mg POD q4h PRN×3 days PRN pain score 6–10

vii. *Prophylaxis*

1. Enoxaparin 40 mg subcut qday10

a. Or for renal insufficiency: heparin 5,000 U subcut q8h
2. Famotidine 20 mg IV q12h×5 days
3. Esomeprazole 20 mg PO daily when famotidine is discontinued

viii. *As needed medications*
1. Ondensetron 4 mg IV q6h PRN nausea
2. Acetaminophen 650 mg PO/PR q4h PRN temp > 101
3. Chloroseptic spray at bedside for PRN use

ix. *When taking PO, start one of the following*
1. Nitrofurantoin monohydrate 100 mg PO q12h × 14 days
2. Trimethoprim–sulfamethoxazole DS PO qHS × 14 days

e. Labs
i. Hematocrit POD 1, 2, 4
ii. Potassium POD 1
iii. Basic metabolic panel POD 4

f. Patient/family education
i. Begin teaching patient/family catheter care and instructions for irrigations of catheter with normal saline starting POD 1.

References

1. Siegel R, Naishadham D, Jemal A. Cancer statistics, 2012. CA Cancer J Clin. 2012;62:10.
2. Marshall VF, Whitmore Jr WF. The present position of radical cystectomy in the surgical management of carcinoma of the urinary bladder. J Urol. 1956;76:387.
3. Lowrance WT, Rumohr JA, Chang SS, et al. Contemporary open radical cystectomy: analysis of perioperative outcomes. J Urol. 2008;179:1313.
4. Quek ML, Stein JP, Clark PE, et al. Natural history of surgically treated bladder carcinoma with extravesical tumor extension. Cancer. 2003;98:955.
5. Dutta SC, Smith Jr JA, Shappell SB, et al. Clinical under staging of high risk nonmuscle invasive urothelial carcinoma treated with radical cystectomy. J Urol. 2001;166:490.
6. Fritsche HM, Burger M, Svatek RS, et al. Characteristics and outcomes of patients with clinical T1 grade 3 urothelial carcinoma treated with radical cystectomy: results from an international cohort. Eur Urol. 2010;57:300.
7. Stein JP, Penson DF. Invasive T1 bladder cancer: indications and rationale for radical cystectomy. BJU Int. 2008;102:270.
8. Herr HW. The value of a second transurethral resection in evaluating patients with bladder tumors. J Urol. 1999;162:74.
9. Hall MC, Chang SS, Dalbagni G, et al. Guideline for the management of nonmuscle invasive bladder cancer: (Stages Ta, T1, and Tis): 2007 update. J Urol. 2007;178:2314–30.
10. Kulkarni GS, Hakenberg OW, Gschwend JE, et al. An updated critical analysis of the treatment strategy for newly diagnosed high-grade T1 (previously T1G3) bladder cancer. Eur Urol. 2010;57:60.
11. Stimson CJ, Cookson MS, Barocas DA, et al. Preoperative hydronephrosis predicts extravesical and node positive disease in patients undergoing cystectomy for bladder cancer. J Urol. 2010;183:1732.
12. Giannarini G, Petralia G, Thoeny HC. Potential and limitations of diffusion-weighted magnetic resonance imaging in kidney, prostate, and bladder cancer including pelvic lymph node staging: a critical analysis of the literature. Eur Urol. 2012;61:326.
13. Fleisher LA. Cardiac risk stratification for noncardiac surgery: update from the American College of Cardiology/American Heart Association 2007 guidelines. Cleve Clin J Med. 2009;76 Suppl 4:S9.
14. Freeman WK, Gibbons RJ. Perioperative cardiovascular assessment of patients undergoing noncardiac surgery. Mayo Clin Proc. 2009;84:79.
15. Douketis JD, Spyropoulos AC, Spencer FA, et al. Perioperative management of antithrombotic therapy: antithrombotic therapy and prevention of thrombosis, 9th ed: American College of chest physicians evidence-based clinical practice guidelines. Chest. 2012;141:e326S.
16. Eberli D, Chassot PG, Sulser T, et al. Urological surgery and antiplatelet drugs after cardiac and cerebrovascular accidents. J Urol. 2010;183:2128.
17. Jaffer AK. Perioperative management of warfarin and antiplatelet therapy. Cleve Clin J Med. 2009;76 Suppl 4:S37.
18. Karl A, Rittler P, Buchner A, et al. Prospective assessment of malnutrition in urologic patients. Urology. 2009;73:1072.
19. Terry WJ, Bueschen AJ. Complications of radical cystectomy and correlation with nutritional assessment. Urology. 1986;27:229.
20. Gregg JR, Cookson MS, Phillips S, et al. Effect of preoperative nutritional deficiency on mortality after radical cystectomy for bladder cancer. J Urol. 2011;185:90.
21. Baldwin C, Spiro A, Ahern R, et al. Oral nutritional interventions in malnourished patients with cancer: a systematic review and meta-analysis. J Natl Cancer Inst. 2012;104:371.
22. Kouba E, Sands M, Lentz A, et al. Incidence and risk factors of stomal complications in patients undergoing cystectomy with ileal conduit urinary diversion for bladder cancer. J Urol. 2007;178:950.

23. Lee JS, Terjimanian MN, Tishberg LM, et al. Surgical site infection and analytic morphometric assessment of body composition in patients undergoing midline laparotomy. J Am Coll Surg. 2011;213:236.
24. Sugerman HJ, Kellum Jr JM, Reines HD, et al. Greater risk of incisional hernia with morbidly obese than steroid-dependent patients and low recurrence with prefascial polypropylene mesh. Am J Surg. 1996;171:80.
25. Chang SS, Jacobs B, Wells N, et al. Increased body mass index predicts increased blood loss during radical cystectomy. J Urol. 2004;171:1077.
26. Lee CT, Dunn RL, Chen BT, et al. Impact of body mass index on radical cystectomy. J Urol. 2004; 172:1281.
27. Morgan TM, Keegan KA, Barocas DA, et al. Predicting the probability of 90-day survival of elderly patients with bladder cancer treated with radical cystectomy. J Urol. 2011;186:829.
28. Chang SS, Alberts G, Cookson MS, et al. Radical cystectomy is safe in elderly patients at high risk. J Urol. 2001;166:938.
29. Farnham SB, Cookson MS, Alberts G, et al. Benefit of radical cystectomy in the elderly patient with significant co-morbidities. Urol Oncol. 2004;22:178.
30. Stroumbakis N, Herr HW, Cookson MS, et al. Radical cystectomy in the octogenarian. J Urol. 1997;158:2113.
31. Clark PE, Stein JP, Groshen SG, et al. Radical cystectomy in the elderly: comparison of clincal outcomes between younger and older patients. Cancer. 2005;104:36.
32. Pruthi RS, Nielsen ME, Nix J, et al. Robotic radical cystectomy for bladder cancer: surgical and pathological outcomes in 100 consecutive cases. J Urol. 2010;183:510.
33. Wang GJ, Barocas DA, Raman JD, et al. Robotic vs open radical cystectomy: prospective comparison of perioperative outcomes and pathological measures of early oncological efficacy. BJU Int. 2008;101:89.
34. Richards KA, Hemal AK. Current status and outcomes of robot-assisted laparoscopic radical cystectomy and urinary diversion. Curr Urol Rep. 2011;12:107.
35. Porter MP, Penson DF. Health related quality of life after radical cystectomy and urinary diversion for bladder cancer: a systematic review and critical analysis of the literature. J Urol. 2005;173:1318.
36. Cookson MS, Dutta SC, Chang SS, et al. Health related quality of life in patients treated with radical cystectomy and urinary diversion for urothelial carcinoma of the bladder: development and validation of a new disease specific questionnaire. J Urol. 2003;170:1926.
37. Chang SS, Hassan JM, Cookson MS, et al. Delaying radical cystectomy for muscle invasive bladder cancer results in worse pathological stage. J Urol. 2003;170:1085.
38. Gore JL, Lai J, Setodji CM, et al. Mortality increases when radical cystectomy is delayed more than 12 weeks: results from a surveillance, epidemiology, and end results-medicare analysis. Cancer. 2009;115:988.
39. AUA and wocn joint position statement on the value of preoperative stoma marking for patients undergoing urinary ostomy surgery. http://www.auanet.org/content/media/uostomystoma.pdf (2008).
40. Gourgiotis S, Aloizos S, Aravosita P, et al. The effects of tobacco smoking on the incidence and risk of intraoperative and postoperative complications in adults. Surgeon. 2011;9:225.
41. Myles PS, Iacono GA, Hunt JO, et al. Risk of respiratory complications and wound infection in patients undergoing ambulatory surgery: smokers versus nonsmokers. Anesthesiology. 2002;97:842.
42. Nakagawa M, Tanaka H, Tsukuma H, et al. Relationship between the duration of the preoperative smoke-free period and the incidence of postoperative pulmonary complications after pulmonary surgery. Chest. 2001;120:705.
43. Tabibi A, Simforoosh N, Basiri A, et al. Bowel preparation versus no preparation before ileal urinary diversion. Urology. 2007;70:654.
44. Correll DJ, Bader AM, Hull MW, et al. Value of preoperative clinic visits in identifying issues with potential impact on operating room efficiency. Anesthesiology. 2006;105:1254.
45. Wolf JS, Bennett CJ, Dmochowski RR, et al. AUA best practice policy statement on: urologic surgery antimicrobial prophylaxis. http://www.auanet.org/content/media/antimicroprop08.pdf (2012).
46. Darouiche RO, Wall Jr MJ, Itani KM, et al. Chlorhexidine-alcohol versus povidone-iodine for surgical-site antisepsis. N Engl J Med. 2010;362:18.
47. Goldhaber SZ. Risk factors for venous thromboembolism. J Am Coll Cardiol. 2010;56:1.
48. Kibel AS, Loughlin KR. Pathogenesis and prophylaxis of postoperative thromboembolic disease in urological pelvic surgery. J Urol. 1995;153:1763.
49. Forrest J, Clemens J, Finamore P, et al. AUA best practice statement for the: prevention of deep vein thrombosis in patients undergoing urologic surgery. http://www.auanet.org/content/media/antimicroprop08.pdf (2008).
50. Rasmussen MS, Jorgensen LN, Wille-Jorgensen P. Prolonged thromboprophylaxis with low molecular weight heparin for abdominal or pelvic surgery. Cochrane Database Syst Rev. 2009:CD004318.
51. Spencer FA, Lessard D, Emery C, et al. Venous thromboembolism in the outpatient setting. Arch Intern Med. 2007;167:1471.
52. El-Tabey NA, Shoma AM. Port site metastases after robot-assisted laparoscopic radical cystectomy. Urology. 2005;66:1110.
53. Stein JP. Should frozen section examination of the ureteral margins be routinely performed during cystectomy? Nat Clin Pract Urol. 2007;4:536.

54. Donat SM. Argument against frozen section analysis of distal ureters in transitional cell bladder cancer. Nat Clin Pract Urol. 2008;5:538.
55. Schumacher MC, Studer UE. Ureteric frozen sections during radical cystectomy for transitional cell carcinoma of the bladder – to do or not to do? BJU Int. 2009;103:1149.
56. Raj GV, Tal R, Vickers A, et al. Significance of intraoperative ureteral evaluation at radical cystectomy for urothelial cancer. Cancer. 2006;107:2167.
57. Tollefson MK, Blute ML, Farmer SA, et al. Significance of distal ureteral margin at radical cystectomy for urothelial carcinoma. J Urol. 2010;183:81.
58. Gakis G, Schilling D, Perner S, et al. Sequential resection of malignant ureteral margins at radical cystectomy: a critical assessment of the value of frozen section analysis. World J Urol. 2011;29:451.
59. Herr HW, Whitmore Jr WF. Ureteral carcinoma in situ after successful intravesical therapy for superficial bladder tumors: incidence, possible pathogenesis and management. J Urol. 1987;138:292.
60. Solsona E, Iborra I, Ricos JV, et al. Upper urinary tract involvement in patients with bladder carcinoma in situ (Tis): its impact on management. Urology. 1997;49:347.
61. Hurle R, Naspro R. Pelvic lymphadenectomy during radical cystectomy: a review of the literature. Surg Oncol. 2010;19:208.
62. Dorin RP, Daneshmand S, Eisenberg MS, et al. Lymph node dissection technique is more important than lymph node count in identifying nodal metastases in radical cystectomy patients: a comparative mapping study. Eur Urol. 2011;60:946.
63. Ghoneim MA, Abdel-Latif M, el-Mekresh M, et al. Radical cystectomy for carcinoma of the bladder: 2,720 consecutive cases 5 years later. J Urol. 2008; 180:121.
64. Leissner J, Ghoneim MA, Abol-Enein H, et al. Extended radical lymphadenectomy in patients with urothelial bladder cancer: results of a prospective multicenter study. J Urol. 2004;171:139.
65. Mills RD, Turner WH, Fleischmann A, et al. Pelvic lymph node metastases from bladder cancer: outcome in 83 patients after radical cystectomy and pelvic lymphadenectomy. J Urol. 2001;166:19.
66. Stein JP, Skinner DG. Results with radical cystectomy for treating bladder cancer: a 'reference standard' for high-grade, invasive bladder cancer. BJU Int. 2003;92:12.
67. Herr HW, Faulkner JR, Grossman HB, et al. Surgical factors influence bladder cancer outcomes: a cooperative group report. J Clin Oncol. 2004;22:2781.
68. Stein JP, Lieskovsky G, Cote R, et al. Radical cystectomy in the treatment of invasive bladder cancer: long-term results in 1,054 patients. J Clin Oncol. 2001;19:666.
69. Konety BR, Joslyn SA, O'Donnell MA. Extent of pelvic lymphadenectomy and its impact on outcome in patients diagnosed with bladder cancer: analysis of data from the surveillance, epidemiology and end results program data base. J Urol. 2003;169:946.
70. Leissner J, Hohenfellner R, Thuroff JW, et al. Lymphadenectomy in patients with transitional cell carcinoma of the urinary bladder; significance for staging and prognosis. BJU Int. 2000;85:817.
71. May M, Herrmann E, Bolenz C, et al. Association between the number of dissected lymph nodes during pelvic lymphadenectomy and cancer-specific survival in patients with lymph node-negative urothelial carcinoma of the bladder undergoing radical cystectomy. Ann Surg Oncol. 2011;18:2018.
72. Wright JL, Lin DW, Porter MP. The association between extent of lymphadenectomy and survival among patients with lymph node metastases undergoing radical cystectomy. Cancer. 2008;112:2401.
73. Marin-Aguilera M, Mengual L, Burset M, et al. Molecular lymph node staging in bladder urothelial carcinoma: impact on survival. Eur Urol. 2008; 54:1363.
74. Kurahashi T, Hara I, Oka N, et al. Detection of micrometastases in pelvic lymph nodes in patients undergoing radical cystectomy for locally invasive bladder cancer by real-time reverse transcriptase-PCR for cytokeratin 19 and uroplakin II. Clin Cancer Res. 2005;11:3773.
75. Bochner BH, Herr HW, Reuter VE. Impact of separate versus en bloc pelvic lymph node dissection on the number of lymph nodes retrieved in cystectomy specimens. J Urol. 2001;166:2295.
76. Stein JP, Penson DF, Cai J, et al. Radical cystectomy with extended lymphadenectomy: evaluating separate package versus en bloc submission for node positive bladder cancer. J Urol. 2007;177:876.
77. Parkash V, Bifulco C, Feinn R, et al. To count and how to count, that is the question: interobserver and intraobserver variability among pathologists in lymph node counting. Am J Clin Pathol. 2010;134:42.
78. Meijer RP, Nunnink CJ, Wassenaar AE, et al. Standard lymph node dissection for bladder cancer: significant variability in the number of reported lymph nodes. J Urol. 2012;187:446.
79. Koppie TM, Vickers AJ, Vora K, et al. Standardization of pelvic lymphadenectomy performed at radical cystectomy: can we establish a minimum number of lymph nodes that should be removed? Cancer. 2006;107:2368.
80. Bochner BH, Cho D, Herr HW, et al. Prospectively packaged lymph node dissections with radical cystectomy: evaluation of node count variability and node mapping. J Urol. 2004;172:1286.
81. Abol-Enein H, Tilki D, Mosbah A, et al. Does the extent of lymphadenectomy in radical cystectomy for bladder cancer influence disease-free survival? A prospective single-center study. Eur Urol. 2011; 60:572.
82. Dhar NB, Klein EA, Reuther AM, et al. Outcome after radical cystectomy with limited or extended pelvic lymph node dissection. J Urol. 2008;179:873.

83. Jensen JB, Ulhoi BP, Jensen KM. Lymph node mapping in patients with bladder cancer undergoing radical cystectomy and lymph node dissection to the level of the inferior mesenteric artery. BJU Int. 2010;106:199.
84. Zehnder P, Studer UE, Skinner EC, et al. Super extended versus extended pelvic lymph node dissection in patients undergoing radical cystectomy for bladder cancer: a comparative study. J Urol. 2011; 186:1261.
85. Abaza R, Dangle PP, Gong MC, et al. Quality of lymphadenectomy is equivalent with robotic and open cystectomy using an extended template. J Urol. 2012;187:1200.
86. Hellenthal NJ, Hussain A, Andrews PE, et al. Lymphadenectomy at the time of robot-assisted radical cystectomy: results from the International Robotic Cystectomy Consortium. BJU Int. 2011; 107:642.
87. Chang SS, Smith Jr JA, Cookson MS. Decreasing blood loss in patients treated with radical cystectomy: a prospective randomizes trial using a new stapling device. J Urol. 2003;169:951.
88. Thompson IMI, Barocas DA, Bischoff CJ, et al. Blood loss associated with radical cystectomy: a prospective randomized study comparing impact ligasure versus stapling device. Society of Urologic Oncology Annual Meeting, Podium #1; 2011.
89. Nix J, Smith A, Kurpad R, et al. Prospective randomized controlled trial of robotic versus open radical cystectomy for bladder cancer: perioperative and pathologic results. Eur Urol. 2010;57:196.
90. Morgan TM, Barocas DA, Chang SS, et al. The relationship between perioperative blood transfusion and overall mortality in patients undergoing radical cystectomy for bladder cancer. Urol Oncol. 2013;31(6):871–7.
91. Stein JP, Clark P, Miranda G, et al. Urethral tumor recurrence following cystectomy and urinary diversion: clinical and pathological characteristics in 768 male patients. J Urol. 2005;173:1163.
92. Hassan JM, Cookson MS, Smith Jr JA, et al. Urethral recurrence in patients following orthotopic urinary diversion. J Urol. 2004;172:1338.
93. Patel SG, Cookson MS, Barocas DA, et al. Risk factors for urothelial carcinoma of the prostate in patients undergoing radical cystoprostatectomy for bladder cancer. BJU Int. 2009;104:934.
94. Nixon RG, Chang SS, Lafleur BJ, et al. Carcinoma in situ and tumor multifocality predict the risk of prostatic urethral involvement at radical cystectomy in men with transitional cell carcinoma of the bladder. J Urol. 2002;167:502.
95. Walsh PC, Mostwin JL. Radical prostatectomy and cystoprostatectomy with preservation of potency. Results using a new nerve-sparing technique. Br J Urol. 1984;56:694.
96. Kessler TM, Burkhard FC, Studer UE. Clinical indications and outcomes with nerve-sparing cystectomy in patients with bladder cancer. Urol Clin North Am. 2005;32:165.
97. Colombo R, Bertini R, Salonia A, et al. Nerve and seminal sparing radical cystectomy with orthotopic urinary diversion for select patients with superficial bladder cancer: an innovative surgical approach. J Urol. 2001;165:51.
98. Schoenberg MP, Walsh PC, Breazeale DR, et al. Local recurrence and survival following nerve sparing radical cystoprostatectomy for bladder cancer: 10-year followup. J Urol. 1996;155:490.
99. Zippe CD, Raina R, Massanyi EZ, et al. Sexual function after male radical cystectomy in a sexually active population. Urology. 2004;64:682.
100. Hekal IA, El-Bahnasawy MS, Mosbah A, et al. Recoverability of erectile function in post-radical cystectomy patients: subjective and objective evaluations. Eur Urol. 2009;55:275.
101. Kessler TM, Burkhard FC, Perimenis P, et al. Attempted nerve sparing surgery and age have a significant effect on urinary continence and erectile function after radical cystoprostatectomy and ileal orthotopic bladder substitution. J Urol. 2004; 172:1323.
102. Lake A, Weizer AZ. Prostate sparing approaches for radical cystectomy: functional and oncological outcomes. AUA Update Ser. 2009;28:186.
103. Weizer AZ, Schuster T. Prostate capsule sparing cystectomy. In: Lee CT, Wood DP, editors. Current clinical urology: bladder cancer. Humana Press; 2010. p. 147–58.
104. Donat SM, Wei DC, McGuire MS, et al. The efficacy of transurethral biopsy for predicting the long-term clinical impact of prostatic invasive bladder cancer. J Urol. 2001;165:1580.
105. Vallancien G, Abou El Fettouh H, Cathelineau X, et al. Cystectomy with prostate sparing for bladder cancer in 100 patients: 10-year experience. J Urol. 2002;168:2413.
106. Wood Jr DP, Montie JE, Pontes JE, et al. Identification of transitional cell carcinoma of the prostate in bladder cancer patients: a prospective study. J Urol. 1989;142:83.
107. Nieuwenhuijzen JA, Meinhardt W, Horenblas S. Clinical outcomes after sexuality preserving cystectomy and neobladder (prostate sparing cystectomy) in 44 patients. J Urol. 2005;173:1314.
108. Barocas DA, Patel SG, Chang SS, et al. Outcomes of patients undergoing radical cystoprostatectomy for bladder cancer with prostatic involvement on final pathology. BJU Int. 2009;104:1091.
109. Weizer AZ, Shah RB, Lee CT, et al. Evaluation of the prostate peripheral zone/capsule in patients undergoing radical cystoprostatectomy: defining risk with prostate capsule sparing cystectomy. Urol Oncol. 2007;25:460.
110. Pinthus JH, Nam RK, Klotz LH. Prostate sparing radical cystectomy – not for all, but an option for some. Can J Urol. 2006;13 Suppl 1:81.
111. Singh A, Kinoshita Y, Rovito Jr PM, et al. Higher than expected association of clinical prostate and bladder cancers. J Urol. 2005;173:1526.

112. Chun TY. Coincidence of bladder and prostate cancer. J Urol. 1997;157:65.
113. Kurokawa K, Ito K, Yamamoto T, et al. Comparative study on the prevalence of clinically detectable prostate cancer in patients with and without bladder cancer. Urology. 2004;63:268.
114. Autorino R, Di Lorenzo G, Damiano R, et al. Pathology of the prostate in radical cystectomy specimens: a critical review. Surg Oncol. 2009;18:73.
115. Revelo MP, Cookson MS, Chang SS, et al. Incidence and location of prostate and urothelial carcinoma in prostates from cystoprostatectomies: implications for possible apical sparing surgery. J Urol. 2008;179:S27.
116. Winkler MH, Livni N, Mannion EM, et al. Characteristics of incidental prostatic adenocarcinoma in contemporary radical cystoprostatectomy specimens. BJU Int. 2007;99:554.
117. Abbas F, Hochberg D, Civantos F, et al. Incidental prostatic adenocarcinoma in patients undergoing radical cystoprostatectomy for bladder cancer. Eur Urol. 1996;30:322.
118. Delongchamps NB, Mao K, Theng H, et al. Outcome of patients with fortuitous prostate cancer after radical cystoprostatectomy for bladder cancer. Eur Urol. 2005;48:946.
119. Moutzouris G, Barbatis C, Plastiras D, et al. Incidence and histological findings of unsuspected prostatic adenocarcinoma in radical cystoprostatectomy for transitional cell carcinoma of the bladder. Scand J Urol Nephrol. 1999;33:27.
120. Kouriefs C, Fazili T, Masood S, et al. Incidentally detected prostate cancer in cystoprostatectomy specimens. Urol Int. 2005;75:213.
121. Muto G, Bardari F, D'Urso L, et al. Seminal sparing cystectomy and ileocapsuloplasty: long-term followup results. J Urol. 2004;172:76.
122. Rozet F, Lesur G, Cathelineau X, et al. Oncological evaluation of prostate sparing cystectomy: the Montsouris long-term results. J Urol. 2008;179:2170.
123. Ghoneim MA. Radical cystectomy in men. In: Graham SDJ, Keane TE, editors. Glenn's urologic surgery. Philadelphia, PA: Lippincott Williams & Wilkins; 2010. p. 97–104.
124. Hautmann RE, Stein JP. Neobladder with prostatic capsule and seminal-sparing cystectomy for bladder cancer: a step in the wrong direction. Urol Clin North Am. 2005;32:177.
125. Stenzl A, Jarolim L, Coloby P, et al. Urethra-sparing cystectomy and orthotopic urinary diversion in women with malignant pelvic tumors. Cancer. 2001;92:1864.
126. Coloby PJ, Kakizoe T, Tobisu K, et al. Urethral involvement in female bladder cancer patients: mapping of 47 consecutive cysto-urethrectomy specimens. J Urol. 1994;152:1438.
127. Stein JP, Cote RJ, Freeman JA, et al. Indications for lower urinary tract reconstruction in women after cystectomy for bladder cancer: a pathological review of female cystectomy specimens. J Urol. 1995; 154:1329.
128. Stenzl A, Draxl H, Posch B, et al. The risk of urethral tumors in female bladder cancer: can the urethra be used for orthotopic reconstruction of the lower urinary tract? J Urol. 1995;153:950.
129. Stein JP, Penson DF, Lee C, et al. Long-term oncological outcomes in women undergoing radical cystectomy and orthotopic diversion for bladder cancer. J Urol. 2009;181:2052.
130. Schover LR, von Eschenbach AC. Sexual function and female radical cystectomy: a case series. J Urol. 1985;134:465.
131. Chang SS, Cole E, Cookson MS, et al. Preservation of the anterior vaginal wall during female radical cystectomy with orthotopic urinary diversion: technique and results. J Urol. 2002;168:1442.
132. Anderson CB, Cookson MC, Chang SS, et al. Voiding function in women with orthotopic neobladder urinary diversion. J Urol. 2012;188:200.
133. Chang SS, Cole E, Smith Jr JA, et al. Pathological findings of gynecologic organs obtained at female radical cystectomy. J Urol. 2002;168:147.
134. Ali-El-Dein B, Abdel-Latif M, Mosbah A, et al. Secondary malignant involvement of gynecologic organs in radical cystectomy specimens in women: is it mandatory to remove these organs routinely? J Urol. 2004;172:885.
135. Moszkowicz D, Alsaid B, Bessede T, et al. Neural supply to the clitoris: immunohistochemical study with three-dimensional reconstruction of cavernous nerve, spongious nerve, and dorsal clitoris nerve in human fetus. J Sex Med. 2011;8:1112.
136. Volkmer BG, Gschwend JE, Herkommer K, et al. Cystectomy and orthotopic ileal neobladder: the impact on female sexuality. J Urol. 2004; 172:2353.
137. Zippe CD, Raina R, Shah AD, et al. Female sexual dysfunction after radical cystectomy: a new outcome measure. Urology. 2004;63:1153.
138. Bhatta Dhar N, Kessler TM, Mills RD, et al. Nerve-sparing radical cystectomy and orthotopic bladder replacement in female patients. Eur Urol. 2007; 52:1006.
139. Stenzl A, Colleselli K, Poisel S, et al. Rationale and technique of nerve sparing radical cystectomy before an orthotopic neobladder procedure in women. J Urol. 1995;154:2044.
140. Bhatt A, Nandipati K, Dhar N, et al. Neurovascular preservation in orthotopic cystectomy: impact on female sexual function. Urology. 2006;67:742.
141. Nandipati KC, Bhat A, Zippe CD. Neurovascular preservation in female orthotopic radical cystectomy significantly improves sexual function. Urology. 2006;67:185.
142. Chang SS, Cookson MS, Baumgartner RG, et al. Analysis of early complications after radical cystectomy: results of a collaborative care pathway. J Urol. 2002;167:2012.
143. Koch MO, Seckin B, Smith Jr JA. Impact of a collaborative care approach to radical cystectomy and urinary reconstruction. J Urol. 1995;154:996.

144. Chang SS, Cookson MS, Hassan JM, et al. Routine postoperative intensive care monitoring is not necessary after radical cystectomy. J Urol. 2002;167:1321.
145. Taub DA, Dunn RL, Miller DC, et al. Discharge practice patterns following cystectomy for bladder cancer: evidence for the shifting of the burden of care. J Urol. 2006;176:2612.
146. Aghazadeh MA, Barocas DA, Salem S, et al. Determining factors for hospital discharge status after radical cystectomy in a large contemporary cohort. J Urol. 2011;185:85.
147. Stimson CJ, Chang SS, Barocas DA, et al. Early and late perioperative outcomes following radical cystectomy: 90-day readmissions, morbidity and mortality in a contemporary series. J Urol. 2010; 184:1296.
148. Donat SM. Standards for surgical complication reporting in urologic oncology: time for a change. Urology. 2007;69:221.
149. Martin 2nd RC, Brennan MF, Jaques DP. Quality of complication reporting in the surgical literature. Ann Surg. 2002;235:803.
150. Shabsigh A, Korets R, Vora KC, et al. Defining early morbidity of radical cystectomy for patients with bladder cancer using a standardized reporting methodology. Eur Urol. 2009;55:164.
151. Hayn MH, Hellenthal NJ, Hussain A, et al. Defining morbidity of robot-assisted radical cystectomy using a standardized reporting methodology. Eur Urol. 2011;59:213.
152. Donabedian A. Evaluating the quality of medical care. Milbank Mem Fund Q. 1966;44(Suppl):166.
153. Cooperberg MR, Konety BR. Quality of care indicators for radical cystectomy. In: Lee CT, Wood DP, editors. Current clinical urology: bladder cancer. Humana Press; 2010. p. 177–86.
154. Goossens-Laan CA, Gooiker GA, van Gijn W, et al. A systematic review and meta-analysis of the relationship between hospital/surgeon volume and outcome for radical cystectomy: an update for the ongoing debate. Eur Urol. 2011;59:775.
155. Morgan TM, Barocas DA, Keegan KA, et al. Volume-Outcome in cystectomy: is it the surgeon or the setting? American Urological Association Annual Meeting, Abstract #127, 2012.
156. Elting LS, Pettaway C, Bekele BN, et al. Correlation between annual volume of cystectomy, professional staffing, and outcomes: a statewide, population-based study. Cancer. 2005;104:975.
157. Birkmeyer JD, Siewers AE, Finlayson EV, et al. Hospital volume and surgical mortality in the United States. N Engl J Med. 2002;346:1128.
158. Hollenbeck BK, Wei Y, Birkmeyer JD. Volume, process of care, and operative mortality for cystectomy for bladder cancer. Urology. 2007;69:871.
159. Hollenbeck BK, Daignault S, Dunn RL, et al. Getting under the hood of the volume-outcome relationship for radical cystectomy. J Urol. 2007; 177:2095.
160. Trinh QD, Sun M, Sammon J, et al. Leapfrog volume thresholds and perioperative complications after radical prostatectomy. Cancer. 2012;118:4991–8.
161. Birkmeyer JD, Stukel TA, Siewers AE, et al. Surgeon volume and operative mortality in the United States. N Engl J Med. 2003;349:2117.
162. Hayn MH, Hussain A, Mansour AM, et al. The learning curve of robot-assisted radical cystectomy: results from the International Robotic Cystectomy Consortium. Eur Urol. 2010;58:197.
163. Herr H, Lee C, Chang S, et al. Standardization of radical cystectomy and pelvic lymph node dissection for bladder cancer: a collaborative group report. J Urol. 2004;171:1823.
164. Hassan JM, Cookson MS, Smith Jr JA, et al. Patterns of initial transitional cell recurrence in patients after cystectomy. J Urol. 2006;175:2054.
165. Clark PE. Neoadjuvant versus adjuvant chemotherapy for muscle-invasive bladder cancer. Expert Rev Anticancer Ther. 2009;9:821.
166. Donat SM, Shabsigh A, Savage C, et al. Potential impact of postoperative early complications on the timing of adjuvant chemotherapy in patients undergoing radical cystectomy: a high-volume tertiary cancer center experience. Eur Urol. 2009;55:177.
167. Grossman HB, Natale RB, Tangen CM, et al. Neoadjuvant chemotherapy plus cystectomy compared with cystectomy alone for locally advanced bladder cancer. N Engl J Med. 2003;349:859.
168. Advanced Bladder Cancer (ABC) Meta-analysis Collaboration. Neoadjuvant chemotherapy in invasive bladder cancer: update of a systematic review and meta-analysis of individual patient data advanced bladder cancer (ABC) meta-analysis collaboration. Eur Urol. 2005;48:202.
169. Wheat JC, Lee CT. Contemporary management of muscle invasive bladder cancer. AUA Update Series. 2010;29:338.
170. Miles BJ, Fairey AS, Eliasziw M, et al. Referral and treatment rates of neoadjuvant chemotherapy in muscle-invasive bladder cancer before and after publication of a clinical practice guideline. Can Urol Assoc J. 2010;4:263.
171. Raj GV, Karavadia S, Schlomer B, et al. Contemporary use of perioperative cisplatin-based chemotherapy in patients with muscle-invasive bladder cancer. Cancer. 2011;117:276.
172. Advanced Bladder Cancer (ABC) Meta-analysis Collaboration. Adjuvant chemotherapy in invasive bladder cancer: a systematic review and meta-analysis of individual patient data Advanced Bladder Cancer (ABC) Meta-analysis Collaboration. Eur Urol. 2005;48:189.
173. Smith S, Gilligan T. Adjuvant chemotherapy in bladder cancer: a good concept but where's the proof? In: Lee CT, Wood DP, editors. Current clinical urology: bladder cancer. Humana Press; 2010. p. 239–45.
174. Shariat SF, Karakiewicz PI, Palapattu GS, et al. Outcomes of radical cystectomy for transitional cell

carcinoma of the bladder: a contemporary series from the Bladder Cancer Research Consortium. J Urol. 2006;176:2414.
175. Hautmann RE, Gschwend JE, de Petriconi RC, et al. Cystectomy for transitional cell carcinoma of the bladder: results of a surgery only series in the neobladder era. J Urol. 2006;176:486.
176. Boorjian SA, Kim SP, Weight CJ, et al. Risk factors and outcomes of urethral recurrence following radical cystectomy. Eur Urol. 2011;60:1266.
177. Sanderson KM, Cai J, Miranda G, et al. Upper tract urothelial recurrence following radical cystectomy for transitional cell carcinoma of the bladder: an analysis of 1,069 patients with 10-year followup. J Urol. 2007;177:2088.
178. Boorjian SA, Tollefson MK, Cheville JC, et al. Detection of asymptomatic recurrence during routine oncological followup after radical cystectomy is associated with improved patient survival. J Urol. 2011;186:1796.
179. Dalbagni G, Bochner BH, Cronin A, et al. A plea for a uniform surveillance schedule after radical cystectomy. J Urol. 2011;185:2091.
180. Clark PE, Stein JP, Groshen SG, et al. The management of urethral transitional cell carcinoma after radical cystectomy for invasive bladder cancer. J Urol. 2004;172:1342.
181. Lin DW, Herr HW, Dalbagni G. Value of urethral wash cytology in the retained male urethra after radical cystoprostatectomy. J Urol. 2003;169:961.

Robot-Assisted Cystectomy: Getting Started: Prior Experience, Learning Curve, and Initial Patient Selection

3

Matthew K. Tollefson and Mitchell R. Humphreys

None of our men are 'experts.' We have most unfortunately found it necessary to get rid of a man as soon as he thinks himself an expert because no one ever considers himself expert if he really knows his job. A man who knows a job sees so much more to be done than he has done that he is always pressing forward and never gives up an instant of thought to how good and how efficient he is. Thinking always ahead thinking always of trying to do more brings a state of mind in which nothing is impossible. The moment one gets into the 'expert' state of mind a great number of things become impossible.

—Henry Ford

Introduction

The task of learning and incorporating robot-assisted cystectomy into a busy surgical practice is a daunting proposition, particularly for surgeons well versed in open surgical techniques. The promise of a minimally invasive alternative to open surgery, especially for bladder cancer, is significant due to the purported benefits of fewer complications, decreased blood losses, and a shorter hospital stay. The development of robot-assisted cystectomy represents the first widespread challenge to open cystectomy. Yet, the procedure remains technically challenging even for surgeons experienced in robot-assisted pelvic surgery. Indeed, how does a surgeon transition from a practice dominated by open surgery to one that offers the benefits of minimally invasive surgery?

Abandoning one technique with which a surgeon is comfortable, and transitioning to another in which that surgeon is a novice, creates potential concerns regarding ethical responsibility, patient safety, oncologic efficacy, and surgical training. This task seems particularly intimidating in the group of patients undergoing surgery for invasive urothelial carcinoma, where few salvage therapies exist for those with inadequate initial surgical extirpation. Furthermore, the patients themselves frequently possess significant medical comorbidities making lengthy and complicated procedures undesirable.

With these concerns in mind, it is important for the entire surgical team to prepare for the challenges of robot-assisted bladder surgery prior to the first case. Critical members of this surgical team include all of the personnel that bring this procedure to clinical fruition in the preoperative, intraoperative, and postoperative setting. In this chapter, we review our experience in converting a high volume practice with robotic prostatectomy and open radical cystectomy to one that offers robot-assisted cystectomy. In addition, we describe some technical modifications to both robot-assisted radical prostatectomy and open radical cystectomy that made our transition to

M.K. Tollefson, M.D. (✉)
Department of Urology, Mayo Clinic, Rochester, MN 55905, USA

Department of Urology, Mayo Clinic, Gonda 7 South, 200 First Street Southwest, Rochester, MN 55905, USA
e-mail: tollefson.matthew@mayo.edu

M.R. Humphreys, M.D.
Department of Urology, Mayo Clinic, Phoenix, AZ 85054, USA

E.P. Castle and R.S. Pruthi (eds.), *Robotic Surgery of the Bladder*, DOI 10.1007/978-1-4614-4906-5_3,

robot-assisted cystectomy easier. Finally, we review the existing literature regarding the evidence for a learning curve in robot-assisted cystectomy and provide tips for surgeons embarking upon their initial experience in robot-assisted bladder surgery.

Initial Patient Selection: The Ideal Patient

We remain convinced that the ideal patient exists who does not have medical comorbidities, is at their ideal body weight and poses no unsurprising demographic, anatomic, or pathologic characteristics. However, we are equally convinced that the ideal patient does not need to have their bladder removed or have bladder cancer. While that ideal patient may not be available there are certain factors within your control to maximize outcomes with robot-assisted cystectomy. Optimal patient selection can reduce operative time and complication rates for a surgeon's initial experience. Yet, this desire lies in direct contradiction to the reality that most patients that require a cystectomy have invasive bladder cancer and most patients present with significant comorbidities. There is an important balance between identifying perfect candidates for the early robot-assisted cystectomy experience and maintaining adequate case volume to prevent catastrophic complications as well as to develop and maintain surgical expertise that must be considered.

We recommend beginning with patients who are not obese and may require a simple cystectomy for chronic cystitis or a nonfunctional bladder. Additionally, while the female pelvis is generally more accessible and less confining than the male pelvis, many urologists are more comfortable beginning the operation in men due to extensive experience in robotic-assisted radical prostatectomy. Based on the rarity of simple cystectomy, the next patients that should be considered ideally have non-bulky urothelial disease with organ confined, low tumor burden, with no identifiable lymphadenopathy on preoperative imaging, and who do not have significant cardiopulmonary disease. Patients should have no evidence of extravesical disease, history of prior pelvic surgery or radiation, as these complex cases are better treated after the robotic team has gained significant experience. Neoadjuvant chemotherapy is becoming more commonplace and can decrease the tumor burden to aid in patient selection, but it is important to wait a sufficient time (4 to 6 weeks) to allow adequate patient recovery prior to surgical intervention. Infact it has been shown in a retrospective series that waiting up to 10 weeks after neoadjuvant chemotherapy did not adversely affect oncological outcomes at time of cystectomy [1].

Patient height, weight, and body habitus are important considerations in early patient selection. For patients with a body mass index exceeding 35 kg/m^2, it can be more difficult to identify landmarks, expose the necessary structures, pass instruments, and it may be more problematic to maintain Trendelenberg positioning for the duration of the case. Central obesity can pose significant challenges of instrument reach and trocar placement, even with extralong trocars available. The normal robotic trocars are 100 mm in length, while the extralong trocars are 150 mm in length. Additionally, for larger patients undergoing intracorporeal urinary diversion, the thick broad mesentery may present a unique challenge as staple loads may not adequately provide hemostasis.

Finally, consideration of prior abdominal surgery and radiation are important. While experienced surgeons may be able to complete these procedures safely, patients with multiple prior abdominal operations are at an increased risk of intraoperative complications. This tends to occur most commonly with accessing the abdominal cavity in the face of multiple prior midline surgeries where adhesions are present or after ventral hernia mesh repair. If these cases are selected for the robot-assisted approach, it is advisable to first gain some experience and comfort with the technology and the steps of the procedure before embarking on these demanding circumstances. The preferred method of access is with direct visualization utilizing the Hassan technique [2] or in other circumstances putting a 5 mm trocar and laparoscope in a naïve part of the abdomen to access the feasibility of proceeding with normal trocar placement. Similarly, just as in open surgery, patients with a history of prior pelvic radiation are at increased risk of perioperative complications and should be informed of the small but real risk of bowel injury requiring a fecal diversion. Indeed, patients with a history of prostate cancer are more likely to require bladder cancer surgery. While we have completed these procedures in patients with prior prostate irradiation and prior radical prostatectomy, these operations are significantly more complicated and necessitate the maintenance of good oncological principals to prevent tumor spillage. When embarking on a new program in robot-assisted bladder cancer surgery, it is best to initially avoid patients with extensive prior abdominal surgery and patients with a history of pelvic irradiation.

The Decision to Offer Robotic Bladder Cancer Surgery

The decision to offer robot-assisted bladder cancer surgery is a difficult one; particularly while randomized trial data demonstrating significant benefits are immature. Robot-assisted radical cystectomy (RARC) is significantly different than other robot-assisted procedures. For example, even the highest volume radical cystectomy centers usually perform fewer than 200 radical cystectomies annually (an annual incidence in the USA of less than 10,000) [3]. This contrasts with over 100,000 radical prostatectomies and greater than 600,000 hysterectomies performed annually in the USA [3, 4]. Therefore, the decision to pursue robot-assisted bladder cancer surgery must be considered in the context of medical centers that offer robotic surgery for other disease states. It is unlikely that robotic bladder cancer surgery alone will be sufficient to justify the substantial initial capital investment required for robotic surgery [5, 6]. Furthermore, adequate surgical volume is necessary to improve upon the learning curve [7, 8]. Frequent robotic procedures allow the entire robotic team (including nurses, assistants, technologists, anesthesia providers, and surgeons) to exercise ease and expertise with the fundamentals of the robotic set up, anesthetic concerns, positioning, and technique. Most urologists have the capability and comfort of performing robot-assisted radical prostatectomy, and such an experience is critical in starting to offer robot-assisted bladder surgery. The number one priority of any operation, especially for one as deadly as bladder should be the quality of the operation rather than the approach, and it is a display of good judgment by the surgeon if they recognize the failure to progress and convert the operation to an open approach before risking unnecessary complications or outcomes.

The Robotic Team

Surgeons who perform open or robotic bladder cancer surgery are dependent upon a number of other providers, each of whom has an important role to optimize patient care. We organized our robotic bladder cancer team around the individuals that assist in robot-assisted radical prostatectomy (Table 3.1). This team includes nurses, a Certified Surgical Technologist, a Certified Surgical Assistant, specific anesthesiologists, urology residents or fellows, and a fellowship-trained surgeon. We found it extremely helpful to travel with critical members of this team to other hospitals completing these procedures to observe and ask task specific questions to lessen anxiety before beginning the procedures ourselves. Each member of the robotic team was able to focus upon their role in making the procedure work and

Table 3.1 Characteristics of a successful robot-assisted radical cystectomy team

Comfort with steps of robotic prostatectomy
Experience with open radical cystectomy and urinary diversion
Laparoscopic experience
Understanding of patient positioning
Review of other surgeon experience
Anesthesiology support
Ease in troubleshooting robotic issues
Monitoring of surgical results

transfer that experience to our institution. Additionally we found it helpful to perform mock procedures in our operating room setting to rehearse member specific roles and responsibilities to ensure a smooth transition to our first patient. Finally, during the initial 20–30 cases, our team modified the procedures based on experience and observation of what worked at our institution to develop a consistent technique.

While the surgeon receives most of the accolades and burdens for the outcomes of these procedures, the bedside assistant is a particularly important member of the surgical team. We have used both urology residents and fellows, but also found that having a dedicated surgical assistant is helpful. These assistants provide some stability to the surgical team. Whoever fills the role of bedside assistant; it is important that they are comfortable with basic laparoscopic techniques, safe torcar placement, suctioning, tissue handling, retraction, placement of clips, passing suture material, and providing essential exposure. These are not easy tasks and are not quickly mastered by assistants that are infrequently exposed to robotic or laparoscopic procedures. Therefore, consistency and repetition in this role is particularly important.

Similarly, anesthesia providers play a critical role in the successful completion of these procedures. Registry data has shown that about 60 % of all new cancer patients older than 65 years suffer form at least one other serious disease [9]. Bladder cancer patients frequently have comorbid health conditions that directly impact parts of the procedure. For example, the prevalence of chronic obstructive pulmonary disease (COPD) is common in both men (19 %) and women (8.9 %) with bladder cancer [10], likely secondary to the increased risk of disease associated with smoking. This has significant implications upon pneumoperitoneum and carbon dioxide retention. Similarly, obesity in combination with steep Trendelenberg positioning can create increased pulmonary pressures. Furthermore, patients must be draped and padded in such a fashion that they will not suffer complications from the extended duration of these procedures. Techniques to manage these potential issues are critical to the successful completion of the procedure and to prevent unnecessary complications.

Finally, circulating and scrub nurses are critical to the efficient completion of these cases. They are responsible for the efficient sterile draping of the robotic arms and preparing the patient and robot for the procedure. They are also needed to quickly and accurately identify and provide equipment and supplies that are commonly required for the completion of these procedures. Quick and efficient nursing practice can alter a procedure from lasting many hours to one that provides efficient and improved patient care.

The ability of the team to effectively communicate and prepare for these procedures will play a major role in patient safety and the quality of the surgical intervention. The integrated approach and education of all the team members is essential to the successful adoption of robot-assisted bladder surgery.

Lessons to Take from Prior Surgical Experience

As discussed previously, comfort in robot-assisted pelvic surgery, specifically robot-assisted radical prostatectomy, is a prerequisite for a urologist looking to add robot-assisted bladder cancer surgery to their armamentarium. While significant and important differences between the procedures exist, experience gained from robot-assisted radical prostatectomy translates to robot-assisted bladder cancer surgery particularly with respect to pelvic lymphadenectomy, neurovascular bundle preservation (if performed), and apical prostate dissection. Furthermore, ease and understanding of basic robotic maneuvers (such as suturing, knot tying, and cautery) and visualization (with different angle lenses) within the confines of the pelvis facilitates quicker adaptation for the surgeon and the surgical team alike. Finally, the anatomic approach and landmarks in the pelvis are exactly the same. For these reasons, we feel that comfort with robotic radical prostatectomy is critical prior to adopting robotic bladder cancer surgery.

Similarly, familiarity and comfort in performing open radical cystectomy with urinary diversion are a prerequisite in adapting the robot assisted approach. Such familiarity is obviously critical should a conversion to open radical cystectomy be necessary. Beyond that, however, the basic surgical and oncological principles and anatomy are similar between the open and the robotic approaches. Finally, the majority of surgeons starting an experience with robot-assisted radical cystectomy perform the urinary diversion in an open fashion. Therefore, expertise with open urinary diversion is imperative as it may be performed through a smaller incision, an incision positioned higher in the abdomen, and/or from a different angle.

While many of these concepts are discussed in detail elsewhere in this text, it is important to highlight portions of both open cystectomy and robotic prostatectomy that impact upon a surgeon transitioning to a practice offering RARC. The specific technical aspects of the procedure are discussed in detail throughout this textbook and are beyond the scope of this chapter. However, there are several important points that relate to prior experience and starting a robot-assisted cystectomy program that warrant discussion. Therefore, here we outline several portions of both RARP and open cystectomy and discuss how they impact the adoption of RARC.

Surgical Concepts to Bridge RARP to RARC

Lymphadenectomy

Lymphadenectomy is likely the most difficult portion of RARC for most practitioners to master. While the importance of an extended pelvic lymphadenectomy is debatable for patients with prostate cancer, its importance for patients with invasive urothelial carcinoma is well established. Numerous studies have now demonstrated improved survival with extended lymphadenectomy and adequate nodal dissection templates are vital. Indeed, lymph node yield is perhaps the most commonly utilized marker of surgical quality. Therefore, it is critical for surgeons embarking upon RARC to perform an adequate lymphadenectomy and also demonstrate comfort with the extent and degree of lymphadenectomy necessary for patients with invasive bladder cancer.

As high-volume RARP providers, we found it helpful to extend the boundaries of lymphadenectomy during RARP for patients with intermediate- and high-risk prostate cancer. This allowed more familiarity with handling the pelvic vessels and allowed us to develop safe and efficient techniques for dealing with bleeding situations. Over time, we expanded our RARP practice to routinely include lymph node packets in the obturator, internal iliac, and external iliac regions. We found it useful to begin this dissection posteriorly to the iliac vessels between the lymph node packet and the pelvic side wall. This experience was important in developing and maintaining a program in RARC due to the huge volume discrepancies that exist between RARP and RARC.

Posterior Dissection

Dissection of the seminal vesicles and developing a plane between the prostate and the rectum are essential components of RARP as well as RARC. While we have typically performed the seminal vesicle dissection during RARP from an anterior approach, familiarity with the transperitoneal posterior-based approach to RARP would facilitate the conversion to RARC. Posterior-based approaches to RARP enable surgeons to more accurately identify the vascular pedicles at the time of RARC as well as to perform selective neurovascular bundle preservation during RARC when clinically appropriate. We found it helpful after performing the ureteral dissection and lymphadenectomy with the 30° lens that switching to the 0° lens enabled more caudal dissection between the prostate and the rectum during RARC where it was almost possible to reach the apex of the prostate. This caudal dissection is important during RARC as it decreases the risk of rectal injury and enables easier dissection for the remainder of the procedure. Furthermore, the sheer bulk of a cystoprostatectomy specimen is much more challenging to manage after the bladder has been dropped off the anterior abdomenal wall (we would recommend this as one of the last steps in RARC) than the smaller specimen obtained at the time of prostatectomy. This bulk makes the cystoprostatectomy specimen more difficult to maneuver particularly for residual posterior and rectal attachments.

Anterior and Apical Dissection

Developing the space of Retzius and dissection of the apex of the prostate are routine procedures during both RARC and RARP. Surgeons comfortable with RARP should be able to transition these skills easily to RARC. Differences do exist, in part due to location of the tumor and the possibility of extravesical disease that make comfort with this portion of the procedure important. Specifically, surgeons must be comfortable with subtle modifications of the anterior dissection to ensure a negative surgical margin, even in patients with anterior-based T3 tumors. Furthermore, apical dissection remains important (particularly in the setting of orthotopic urinary diversion), though surgeons comfortable with control of the dorsal venous complex and apical prostate dissection should be able to transfer this to their expertise expeditiously. Unlike in prostatectomy it is important to prevent urine spillage. For this we recommend that after the prostate apex has been carefully dissected that the urethra be identified so that a large Hemo-o-lok® polymer clip (Teleflex, Limerick, PA) or stapler can be used to ensure a hermetic seal and prevent possible tumor or urine leakage after removal of the Foley catheter.

Surgical Concepts Bridging Open Cystectomy to RARC

Lymphadenectomy

Just as comfort with lymphadenectomy from a robotic approach is important when starting RARC, familiarity open pelvic lymphadenectomy is important. This experience is critical to define and replicate the landmarks and limits of dissection. Cystectomy surgeons have for years defined the role of extended lymphadenectomy and it is critical not to lose any progress that may influence the outcome from the disease and intervention. Accordingly, lymphadenectomy at a minimum should include the obturator, internal iliac, external iliac, and distal 1/3 of the common iliac. We recommend that extended pelvic lymphadenectomy be performed as the new standard to include all lymphatic tissue including the common iliacs, proximally to the aortic bifurcation and pre-sacral tissue as well [11]. An important landmark that we use to limit the cranial aspect of the dissection is the take off of the inferior mesenteric artery (IMA).

Control of Vascular Pedicles

One of the primary advantages of robot assistance during cystectomy or prostatectomy is decreased venous bleeding, largely attributed to the pneumoperitoneum used during the procedure. However, even patients undergoing RARC may experience significant bleeding. Nearly 20 % of patients in the International Robotic Cystectomy Consortium report receiving a blood transfusion. Therefore adequate control of the vascular pedicle to the bladder and prostate is critical.

We have found that Hemo-o-lok® polymer clips (Teleflex, Limerick, PA) are useful in this setting as they provide a secure mechanism to control the vascular pedicles. Laparoscopic staple devices are also useful in this setting. The development of a robot-assisted stapler device is underway, but we have not used this device to date. Alternative energy sources are also useful adjunctive measures to provide hemostatic control. Indeed, one of the first modifications we made to our robot-assisted cystectomy procedure was the addition of a LigaSure™ device (Covidien, Boulder, CO) for the vascular pedicle and the bowel mesentery. The combined force and energy application with the tissue sensing impedance allows for excellent hemostasis, minimal char, and efficient progress of the procedure. Other advanced energy platforms compatible with the robot-assisted approach include: monopolar and bipolar cautery, mechanical (harmonic), and lasers.

Urinary Diversion

Most surgeons early in their adoption of robot-assisted radical cystectomy perform the necessary urinary diversion through an open approach.

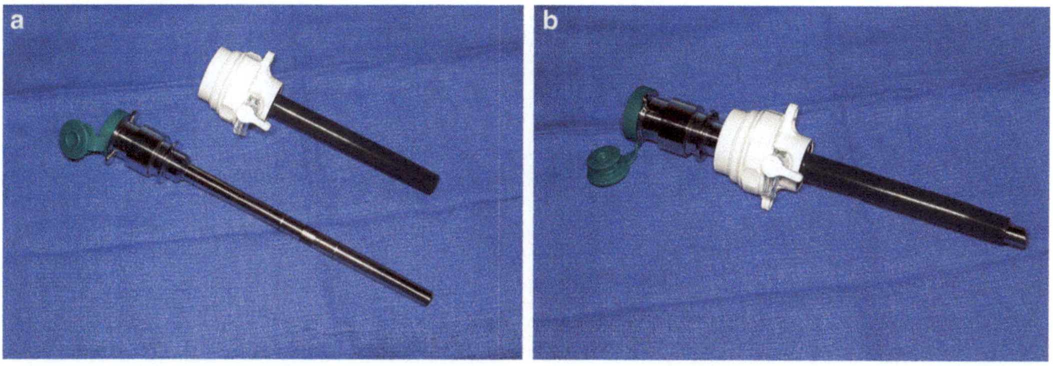

Fig. 3.1 Configuration of lateral port for intracorporeal diversion. (**a**) Standard 10–12 mm laparoscopic port with extralong robotic trocar. (**b**) Robotic trocar going through 10–12 mm port

Indeed for the first 20–30 of these cases, we felt most secure performing the urinary diversion through an open approach. This allowed us to focus our initial robotic experience exclusively upon the cystectomy and pelvic lymphadenectomy. It is useful to first start RARC by identifying the ureters and doing the proximal and distal dissections first. This will help to identify relevant vascular structures and provide important landmarks for the rest of the procedure. We would recommend that the proximal dissection of the left ureter be taken more proximally than you would normally perform, being sure to take a wide margin of tissue around the ureter in order to provide as much vascular supply as possible. If you do your diversion extracorporally the extra length of the left ureter will prevent traction injury and potential vascular compromise as it transverses below the mesentery to limit the potential for the subsequent development of an anastamotic stricture. It is also helpful to pre-tag the Hemo-o-lok® polymer clips (Teleflex, Limerick, PA) with different colored suture so that they can be readily identified later in the case. Proximal and distal uses of these clips on the ureter prevent urine or tumor spillage and allow immediate frozen section pathological analysis of the ureteral margin.

When transitioning to an intracorporeal urinary diversion, we found it helpful to have the assistant on the left side of the patient. The angle from the left side of the patient makes division of the ileal bowel segment and its associated vascular supply much easier. However, this is in contradiction of our normal practice of having the surgical assistant on the right side of the patient for RARP. Therefore, we place a 10–12 mm laparoscopic port in the left lateral-most port site and kept the surgical assistant on the right. It is then quite easy to deploy the normal or even extralong robotic port through this laparoscopic port, making sure to align with the rotational point (Fig. 3.1a, b), without compromise of the pneumoperitoneum. Then, a second surgical assistant may scrub in for the urinary diversion, or the surgical assistant on the right may transition over to the left to complete any necessary staple work on the bowel or associated mesentery. We have found this approach to be beneficial in allowing us to maintain our expertise in RARP while incorporating the techniques and experience into the practice of RARC. It is also helpful to first identify the relevant segments of the bowel (depending on the planned type of diversion) and tagging them with different colored sutures at the beginning of the case prior to any dissection to prevent later confusion. The Hemo-o-lok® polymer clips (Teleflex, Limerick, PA) are useful to bundle the sutures together for later manipulation and prevent distraction during the rest of the procedure. Our initial intracorporeal diversions were primarily aimed at female patients as it avoided an otherwise necessary abdominal incision for specimen extraction (generally extracted through the vagina). However, independent of the type of diversion we would recommend making the incision, if needed, that best provides the surgical team with the best exposure need to quickly complete the operation, which in most cases does not coincide with existing trocar placement.

The Learning Curve: Are We There Yet?

The concept of a learning curve is based upon the premise that practice makes perfect. In urology, a number of studies have evaluated the learning curve regarding robot-assisted radical prostatectomy [12–14]. In general, these studies demonstrate improvements in the margin negative rate, blood loss, and operative time in the first 40–50 cases with a more gradual improvement after that time. It is important to accurately reflect on patient outcomes and experiences to improve surgical training, enhance hospital credentialing, and reassure patients.

However, identification of a learning curve associated with robot-assisted radical cystectomy has been elusive due to the many factors that individually can influence this parameter. Indeed, some authors have questioned whether such a learning curve exists given that surgeons performing bladder cancer surgery are generally well-trained surgeons prior to embarking on the procedure for bladder cancer. Thus far, studies have focused efforts to characterize the learning curve based upon several early postoperative parameters including blood loss, lymph node yield, operative time, surgical margin status, and early complications [7, 15–17]. While most of these studies have demonstrated an improvement with time, it is clear that if a learning curve exists, it is different for each surgeon (Table 3.2). Furthermore, techniques for these procedures are constantly evolving and even providers considered to be experts in robot-assisted bladder surgery are continually searching for mechanisms and methods to simplify and improve the procedure. We have found that the learning curve can be dramatically shortened building on personal experience not only with robot-assisted and prior pelvic surgery, but with video review as well. Not everyone has the luxury of an in-house mentor who is already expert at these procedures. We have discovered that reviewing the successful procedures of others and learning from them is critical to adoption. Additionally we routinely record all our procedures then review them to see what we liked and did not like about the procedure and what we would change. We found that this exercise in reflection with the advantage of the pathology report has helped us to improve our technique and disease outcomes. If there are several surgeons, both open and robot assisted, available, the exchange of ideas and criticism can further push everyone to maximize their surgical outcomes.

Table 3.2 Factors impacting length of learning curve

Prior robotic surgical experience
Mentoring of initial robotic cystectomy cases
Patient factors (tumor extent, BMI, prior surgeries, pelvic irradiation, etc.)
Robotic set-up time
Type of urinary diversion
Experience of robotic team
Self evaluation

Outcome Measurement: How Are We Doing?

A commitment to robot-assisted bladder cancer surgery must be continually critical of perioperative and postoperative outcomes. While we continue to await data from randomized trials, robot-assisted radical cystectomy will continue to be scrutinized. Therefore, it is essential for surgeons to be aware of how they are doing relative to their own experience and the only way to do so is to continually monitor outcomes. The development of a prospectively maintained database should be created prior to the completion of the first procedure and is an important aspect of beginning the practice. Preoperative, intraoperative, and postoperative data are collected from all patients undergoing robot-assisted bladder surgery at our institution. Fundamental components of this data collection include patient demographics, clinical tumor characteristics, comorbidities, neoadjuvant chemotherapy, operative time, blood loss, pathologic characteristics (including positive margins), and hospital stay (Table 3.3). Although such collection can be time consuming, it is important to continually reflect upon one's outcome in order to improve with time. It is impossible to experience

Table 3.3 Necessary elements for database collection

Preoperative components
Age
Sex
Clinical stage
BMI
Neoadjuvant therapies
Surgical components
Estimated blood loss
Operative time (separate for node dissection, cystectomy, and urinary diversion)
Type of urinary diversion
Intraoperative complications
Pathologic stage
Surgical margin status
Nodal yield
Postoperative components
Length of hospital stay
Postoperative complications (including Clavien classification)
Disease recurrence and location

a "learning curve" if one is not aware of their outcomes.

Final Thoughts

Getting started is frequently the most difficult portion of adopting any new procedure or technology. Establishment of a robust robot-assisted surgical program requires commitment from hospital administration (for console time), surgeons, anesthesiology, and the development of a robotic team. Adequate preparation, patient selection, equipment availability, and dedication of the whole team, however, can make the difference between a successful experience and one that flounders. As surgeons, we owe it to our patients to make the procedure as safe and efficacious as possible.

References

1. Alva AS, Tallman CT, He C, et al. Efficient delivery of radical cystectomy after neoadjuvant chemotherapy for muscle-invasive bladder cancer: a multidisciplinary approach. Cancer. 2012;118:44.
2. Gould JC, Philip A. Principles and techniques of abdominal access and physiology of pneumoperitoneum. Chapter 22. In: Souba WW, Fink MP, Jurkovich GJ, Kaiser KR, Pearce WH, Pemberton JH, Soper NJ, editors. ACS surgery, principals and practice. Danbury, Connecticut: WebMD professional Publishing; 2007.
3. Siegel R, Desantis C, Virgo K, et al. Cancer treatment and survivorship statistics, 2012. CA Cancer J Clin. 2012;62:220–41.
4. Siegel R, Naishadham D, Jemal A. Cancer statistics, 2012. CA Cancer J Clin. 2012;62:10.
5. Martin AD, Nunez RN, Castle EP. Robot-assisted radical cystectomy versus open radical cystectomy: a complete cost analysis. Urology. 2011;77:621.
6. Kahn Z, Nadelson E, Mieza M, et al. Causes of post-prostatectomy retention. Urology. 1991;37:263.
7. Richards KA, Kader K, Pettus JA, et al. Does initial learning curve compromise outcomes for robot-assisted radical cystectomy? A critical evaluation of the first 60 cases while establishing a robotics program. J Endourol. 2011;25:1553.
8. Hellenthal NJ, Hussain A, Andrews PE, et al. Lymphadenectomy at the time of robot-assisted radical cystectomy: results from the International Robotic Cystectomy Consortium. BJU Int. 2011;107:642.
9. Janssen-Heihnen ML, Houterman S, Lemmens VE, et al. Prognostic import of increasing age and co-morbidity in caner patients: a population-based approach. Crit Rev Oncol Hematol. 2005;55:231.
10. van de Schans SA, Janssen-Heijnen ML, Biesma B, et al. COPD in cancer patients: higher prevalence in the elderly, a different treatment strategy in case of primary tumours above the diaphragm, and a worse overall survival in the elderly patient. Eur J Cancer. 2007;43:2194.
11. Dorin RP, Skinner EC. Extended lymphadenectomy in bladder cancer. Curr Opin Urol. 2010;20:414.
12. Lebeau T, Rouprêt M, Ferhi K, et al. The role of a well-trained team on the early learning curve of robot-assisted laparoscopic procedures: the example of radical prostatectomy. Int J Med Robot. 2012; 8:67–72.
13. Trinh QD, Sammon J, Sun M, et al. Perioperative outcomes of robot-assisted radical prostatectomy compared with open radical prostatectomy: results from the nationwide inpatient sample. Eur Urol. 2012;61:679.
14. Atug F, Castle EP, Srivastav SK, et al. Positive surgical margins in robotic-assisted radical prostatectomy: impact of learning curve on oncologic outcomes. Eur Urol. 2006;49:866.
15. Hayn MH, Hellenthal NJ, Seixas-Mikelus SA, et al. Is patient outcome compromised during the initial experience with robot-assisted radical cystectomy? Results of 164 consecutive cases. BJU Int. 2011;108:882.
16. Pruthi RS, Smith A, Wallen EM. Evaluating the learning curve for robot-assisted laparoscopic radical cystectomy. J Endourol. 2008;22:2469.
17. Guru KA, Kim HL, Piacente PM, et al. Robot-assisted radical cystectomy and pelvic lymph node dissection: initial experience at Roswell Park Cancer Institute. Urology. 2007;69:469.

Robot-Assisted Radical Cystectomy: Room Setup, Patient Positioning, Instrumentation, and Anesthetic Considerations

4

David D. Thiel and Paul R. Young

Room Setup

Robot-assisted radical cystectomy (RARC) can be performed in the same operating theater as robot-assisted prostatectomy. The limiting factor in all robotic surgery with regard to operating room setup is space. Care must be taken to secure as much space in the room as needed for robot cart docking/undocking, surgeon console, and sterile tables sufficient for robotic instruments as well as those necessary for open cystectomy/urinary diversion. Sufficient anesthesia working space is also required. There should also be sufficient space to allow for the flow of anesthesia personnel, blood products, and other items to the patient's bedside. Our current robotic suite is 750 sq. ft (25 ft × 35 ft), and we find it offers sufficient space to safely perform the operation.

It is important that all assistants be able to clearly see the operative monitors. Since our surgical assistant is on the patient's right-hand side, it is imperative that a monitor be placed directly across from the assisting surgeon/technician (Fig. 4.1a). It is easiest if the assistant does not have to torque his or her neck or trunk to get a clean view of the monitor. Some OR suites have a large monitor mounted on the wall across from the assistant position. Others have mobile ceiling-mounted booms available to move the assistant's monitor directly into view. It is also important that nonassisting technicians and nurses also have a view of the operative field either through large mounted monitors or boom-mounted mobile monitors (Fig. 4.1b). Some of our assistants find it more comfortable to sit on a high stool while assisting during the operation.

Patient Positioning

Proper patient positioning is a big key to safe and effective performance of robot-assisted radical cystectomy. Proper positioning is necessary to allow for full range of motion of the robotic arms as well as to prevent harm to the patient in the form of neuropraxias and compartment syndromes. Proper positioning must also be used to secure safe, effective access to the abdomen for the bedside assistant. Given the implications for positioning in RARC, the surgeon should be actively involved in patient positioning for the procedure. All patients should have appropriate intravenous access and possibly even central line access before positioning is completed. We adduct the patient's arms in a tuck position in all our cystectomy patients using foam pads and the patient's draw sheet (Fig. 4.2a–c). Leaving the arms out in a "crucifix" position carries the risk of brachial plexus injury in prolonged robotic cases [1]. Care is taken to cushion all pressure points with padding. The arms should be low

D.D. Thiel, M.D. (✉) • P.R. Young, M.D.
Department of Urology, Mayo Clinic,
3 East Urology, 4500 San Pablo Road South,
Jacksonville, FL 32224, USA
e-mail: Thiel.David@mayo.edu

E.P. Castle and R.S. Pruthi (eds.), *Robotic Surgery of the Bladder*, DOI 10.1007/978-1-4614-4906-5_4,

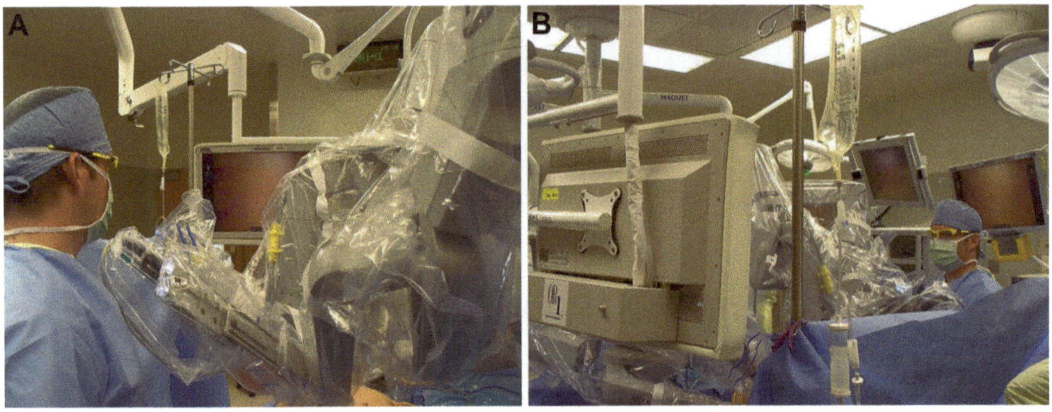

Fig. 4.1 Room monitors. (**a**) Demonstrated the assistant on the patient's right-hand side with a monitor directly across from their position to prevent neck and trunk torque during the case. These monitors are on mobile booms anchored from the ceiling. Certainly, large monitors can be anchored to the wall. (**b**) Demonstrates that other monitors are available on both sides of the bed to allow surgical techs and assistants to view the intra-abdominal events

enough on the patient's sides to not interfere with the robotic working arms and to allow the surgical field to be prepared lateral to the patient's anterior-superior iliac spine (ASIS).

Patients can be positioned in one of four ways for RARC. The four variations in positioning depend on necessity of surgeon access to the perineum, patient anatomic limitations, and robot docking preference. All robot-assisted radical cystectomy operations require the patient to be in the steep Trendelenburg position and care must be taken to secure the patient to the bed to prevent patient movement towards the head of the bed during surgery. We tape the patient's chest over foam padding to prevent slippage in the steep Trendelenburg position (Fig. 4.3). Once the patient is secured to the bed, the position is tested by placing the patient in Trendelenburg to see if movement ensues before the patient is sterilely prepared and draped for the operation. If the patient's chest is secured to the bed with tape, it must not be so tight as to prevent chest wall movement during ventilation. Some have proposed using a desufflated "bean bag" (Olympic Vac Pac, Olympic Medical, Seattle, WA) under the patient to prevent slippage during steep Trendelenburg position as opposed to taping the patient's chest to the bed [1]. The patient should be sterile draped and prepared from the sub-xiphoid region down to the mid-thigh region including the perineum (Fig. 4.4). The genitals should be prepared in the field to allow for intraoperative manipulation and catheter placement. The sterile urethral catheter is placed once the patient is prepared and draped. Some surgeons require a Mayo stand over the patient's face to place instruments during the procedure and to protect the patient's face. We do not place a Mayo stand over the patient's face during the operation.

The standard robotic prostatectomy/robot-assisted radical cystectomy position is to have the patient in the low dorsal lithotomy position with the legs in Allen stirrups (Allen Medical Systems, Acton, MA). Once the patient is placed in steep Trendelenburg position, the robot is docked between the split legs. Success of this position requires that the patient's buttocks be directly at the break in the table. Prolonged dorsal lithotomy positioning is known to carry an increased risk of lower extremity neuropathies [2]. In fact, Warner et al. [2] noted that for each hour in lithotomy position, the risk of motor neuropathy increased 100-fold. Prolonged hip flexion, abduction, and external rotation, as well as pressure point injuries, are all thought to contribute to the morbidity of the dorsal lithotomy position. Care should be taken to secure all pressure points and to insure the legs stay bent at a 45° angle. Leg straightening during the procedure can lead to debilitating neuropathies. It is important to evaluate all pressure points

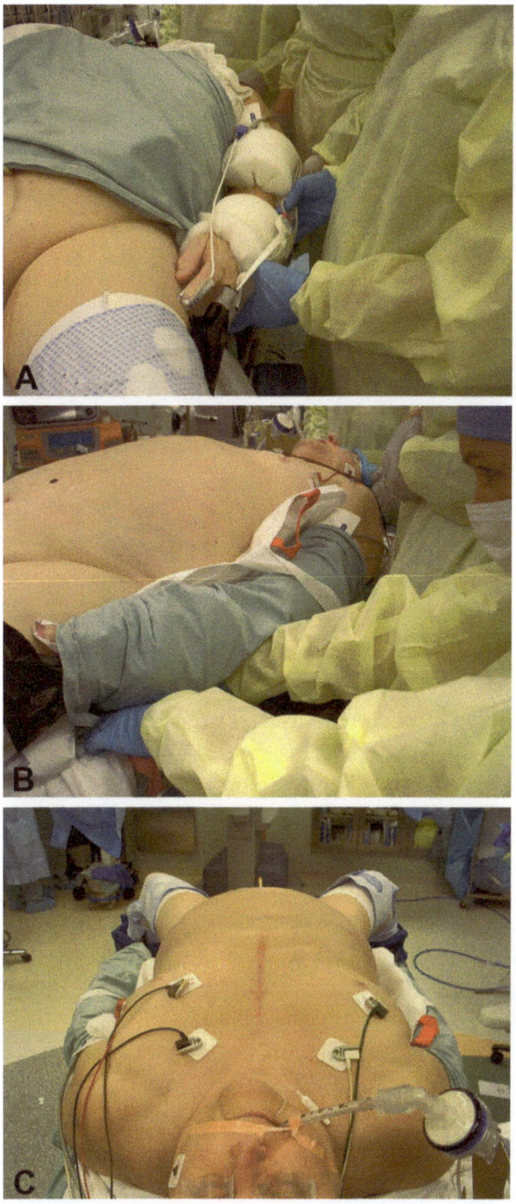

Fig. 4.2 Arm tucking. (**a–c**) Demonstrate how the patient's arms are tucked to their side with cushioning around the arms. The arms are tucked with the aid of the patient's draw sheet under their trunk

and leg positioning before the patient is draped because operative drapes will hide the patient's true position once the case begins (Fig. 4.5a, b). Regardless of approach used, pneumatic compression boots should be placed. The popliteal region should be inspected following positioning to

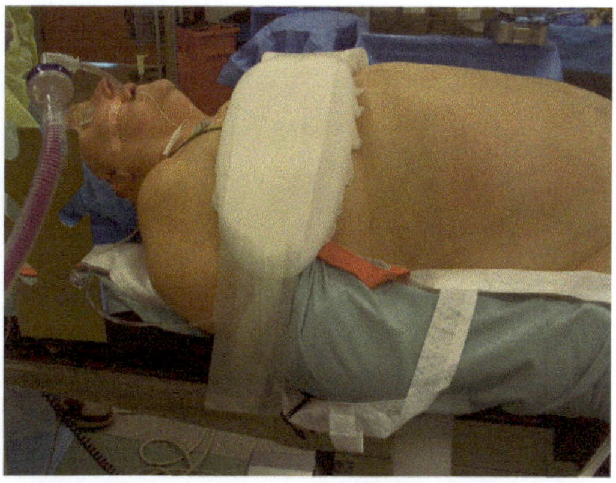

Fig. 4.3 Chest tape to prevent patient slippage. Demonstrates the patient's chest taped to the table over foam padding to prevent slippage during steep Trendelenburg positioning. Care must be taken not to make the tape so tight as to prevent chest wall motion for ventilation

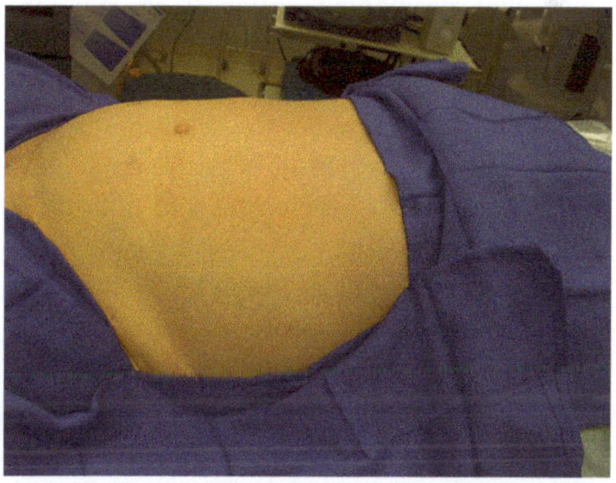

Fig. 4.4 Patient draping. The operative field should be the xiphoid process down to the mid-thigh region with the genitals prepared into the field. The field should be wide enough to include the patient ASIS to allow for lateral port placement

insure that there is no pressure in this region from stirrups. Rosevear et al. wisely noted that a potential pressure point exists between the robotic fourth arm and the patient's left leg [3]. They reported a case of lower extremity compartment syndrome secondary to the pressure exerted by the robotic fourth arm on a patient's left leg. The authors concluded that surgeons should maintain a high level of suspicion for compartment syndrome or potential neuropathies in all patients exposed to

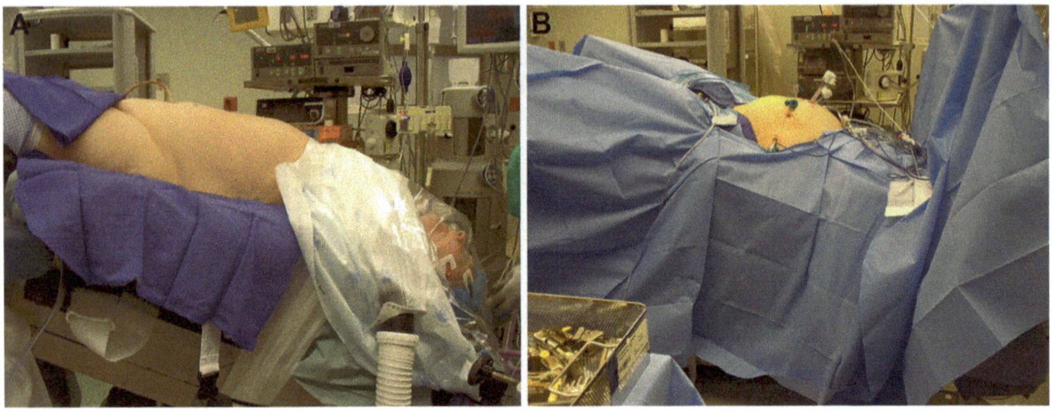

Fig. 4.5 Importance of position check before patient draping. (**a**, **b**) Are pictures of the same patient in Trendelenburg position and it demonstrates how drapes can hide abnormalities in positioning

Trendelenburg positioning for long periods of time, especially if the operating room time is prolonged.

Another positioning option is to have the patient on a split leg table. This allows the legs to stay straight without lithotomy positioning. The robot is docked in between the split straight legs. If this option is elected, it is preferred to have straps at the level of the calves and mid thighs with padding between them and the patient [3]. The theoretical advantage of this positioning is to allow the patient to lie in a more anatomical position with the absence of popliteal pressure exerted by stirrups as seen in low lithotomy positioning. However, the lack of lithotomy positioning does not guarantee absence of lower extremity neuropathies. Koc et al. [4] reviewed 377 consecutive robot prostatectomies completed with the split leg table and found five (1.3 %) lower extremity neuropathies. Three of the five had neuropathies relating to the femoral nerve distribution. After adjusting for all variables, prolonged operative time was found to be the only risk factor for the lower extremity neuropathies. Interestingly, elevated BMI was not associated with lower extremity neuropathies in the split leg table studies, despite increased BMI being associated with lower extremity neuropathies in dorsal lithotomy patients [3, 5, 6]. This may suggest an advantage for the split leg table in those with elevated BMI who are facing prolonged operative times associated with RARC. Warner et al. [2] reviewed close to 200,000 lithotomy patients, noting the most common nerve distributions injured with dorsal lithotomy position were the peroneal, sciatic, and femoral nerves. The split leg table injuries tend to involve the femoral nerve most commonly. It is proposed that the hip hyperextension necessary to allow the robot to be docked with the split-leg table may lead to femoral nerve compression as it courses beneath the inguinal ligament [4, 7].

Another option for patient positioning is to have the patient in lithotomy positioning in preparation for docking the robot from the side of the patient. The robot is docked beside the patient as opposed to in between the patient's legs. This allows unfettered access to the patient's perineum without undocking the robot, which may be important in females requiring simultaneous transvaginal access for urethral dissection. Transvaginal access may also allow for any uterine mobilization or vaginal cuff mobilization that may become necessary during surgery. Side docking removes the perceived symmetry created by docking the robot from between the legs in the patient's midline. Port placement remains the same as the standard procedure. The robot is docked at a 45° angle to the lower torso and aligned with the outer border of the left leg stirrup [8]. Colon surgeons and gynecologists have utilized this technique for pelvic surgery with a learning curve of three to five cases and no increase in instrument clashing [8, 9]. All authors have noted that this can only be completed with the second and third generation robotic systems (S and Si units). The first generation systems do not have enough arm mobility for this type of maneuver.

A final option for patient positioning involves side docking the robot with the patient's legs flat (no lithotomy positioning or split leg). Uffort and Jensen noted this technique to be advantageous in patients with limited hip abduction, such as patients with bilateral hip implants [10]. The authors extended this technique to all robotic prostatectomies at their institution and compared the traditional robotic prostatectomy setup times to those of the above technique. They found that the side docking technique resulted in a 4.5 min improvement in setup time compared to the standard low lithotomy position. This technique did not result in increased robot arm clashing or increased operating room time. This position would not be optimal for any patient that needed perineal/vaginal access during RARC.

Instruments

Intuitive Surgical Corporation (Sunnyvale, CA, USA) offers numerous surgical instruments for their three generations of robotic systems. Most of the instruments are equipped with Intuitive Corporation's patented Endowrist® technology. Endowrist technology allows for 7 degrees of freedom, 90° of articulation, motion scaling, and tremor reduction [11]. The company divides their operative instrument selection into five categories—energy, forceps, needle drivers, retractors, and specialized instruments.

Energy instruments include monopolar and bipolar cautery instruments (electrical energy), Harmonic ACE™ (mechanical energy), PK™ dissecting forceps (advanced bipolar), and laser [12].

Standard needle drivers are available as well as devices that have internal suture cutting blades. Forceps include devices for grabbing tissue in an atraumatic fashion. Retractors are devices used to retract tissue. These instruments are usually used in the third robotic arm. Specialized instruments would include hemostatic clip appliers.

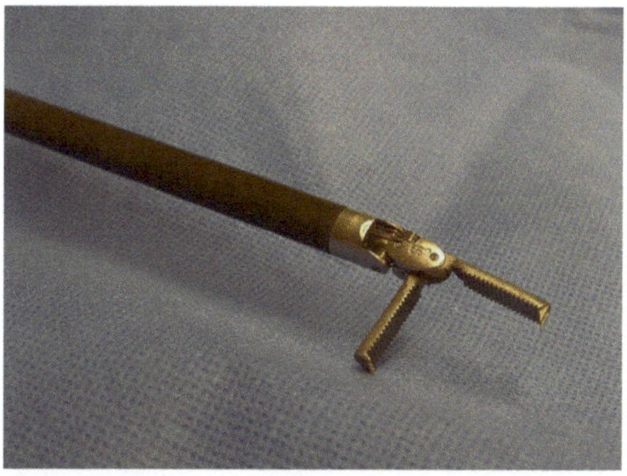

Fig. 4.6 Cobra grasper demonstrates the Cobra grasper used to manipulate the bladder to one side or another once it is mobile. This grasper is used almost exclusively in the third robotic arm. The tips can be very traumatic and we only use this on tissue that will be removed. This instrument should not be used to retract bowel

Despite the plethora of robotic instruments available, our selection is relatively simple for RARC. The cystectomy portion is almost entirely performed with monopolar scissors in the right hand and bipolar dissecting forceps in the left hand. The third robotic assistant arm usually has large Prograsp® forceps present. These instruments are seldom exchanged during cystectomy. The Cobra® grasper may be helpful when used in the third robotic arm to retract the bladder as it becomes more mobile during the operation (Fig. 4.6) The Cobra teeth are very strong and can be traumatic. We only use this device on tissue that will be removed. This device should never be used to retract bowel. The dorsal vein is sutured with standard needle drivers, although the drivers with internal suture cutting would suffice.

The bladder/prostate pedicle can cause troublesome bleeding during cystectomy, and the robotic approach is no different. When the pedicle can be thinned out nicely, Endo-GIA staplers with vascular loads do a nice job of securing the vascular pedicle. In experienced hands, Endo-GIA stapling devices can make cystectomy faster and demonstrate decreased blood loss compared to standard suturing techniques [13]. The one drawback to using Endo-GIA staplers in robot-assisted radical cystectomy is the requirement of the assistant to have sufficient experience with the device for safe application. The use of the

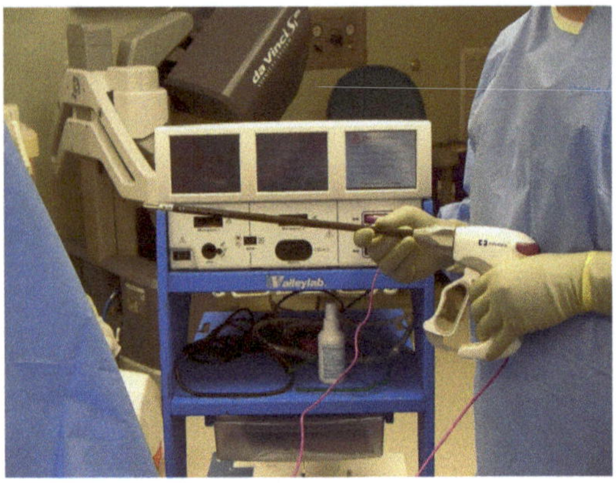

Fig. 4.7 Impact device. The Ligasure impact vessel sealing system is used to seal the bladder/prostate pedicles. It must be activated by the beside assistant

Harmonic scalpel has also been reported for control of the pedicle during cystectomy [14]. The Harmonic scalpel energy can now be utilized by the bedside assistant or via the operating surgeon with the Harmonic ACE instrument. It should be noted that the robot-mounted Harmonic ACE does not currently articulate like other Intuitive Corporation instruments. Certainly, the pedicle can be managed with clips and possibly even with bipolar cautery/monopolar cutting. Free bleeding vessels can be oversewn with suture following bladder removal.

We currently utilize the Ligasure Impact™ vessel sealing system to secure the pedicle during RARC (Fig. 4.7). The Ligasure™ vessel sealing system achieves hemostasis by reforming the collagen and elastin in vessel walls to form an autologous seal. Vessels up to and including 7 mm in diameter may be sacrificed with this technology [15]. The device is not available to the operating robotic surgeon and must be activated and the energy delivered by the bedside assistant. The Ligasure device has been shown to seal vessels with burst pressures over 400 mmHg in porcine models [16]. No matter what energy is used during the procedure, care must be taken to avoid contact with surrounding structures such as bowel. Kim et al. [17] noted that the Harmonic ACE, Ligasure device, and the Plasma Trisector all have significant residual thermal energy directly following application that could cause injury to peripheral structures if contact was made. On a similar note, a Canadian study evaluated robotic instruments and discovered that they all demonstrated stray electrical current along their shaft during use [18]. The stray electrical current was sufficient to cause unwanted bowel injury if contact occurred. The authors recommended cautious use of robotic instruments around surrounding bowel and agreed with Intuitive Surgical Corporation's recommended instrument replacement after eight to ten uses.

Anesthetic Considerations

As with all robotic surgeries, it is important that the anesthesiologist recognize the importance of complete relaxation and paralysis throughout robot-assisted radical cystectomy. Many anesthesiologists involved in robotic surgery recommend atracurium and cisatracurium for muscle relaxation given their predictable chemical breakdown and short half-lives [19]. Care should be taken to limit the use of nitrous oxide, as it may cause distension of the bowel, making visualization of the operative field difficult. As laparoscopic surgery enters its third decade, the effects of pneumoperitoneum on pulmonary physiology, cardiac output, and potential air emboli complications are well understood [19–21]. The prolonged operative time of radical cystectomy compared to robotic prostatectomy underscores the need for careful hemodynamic monitoring during surgery.

Radical cystectomy presents anesthetic challenges due to the risk of excessive blood loss, fluid shifts acquired with prolonged operative time, cardiopulmonary morbidity, and thromboembolic events. The addition of robotics to the cystectomy armamentarium adds to the morbidity associated with prolonged steep Trendelenburg positioning with lower extremities in lithotomy position and pneumoperitoneum. Comparison of anesthetic experiences acquired from robotic prostatectomy literature is difficult due to the typically younger, more physically fit population that receives robotic prostatectomy and shorter operative time associated with robotic prostatectomy compared to RARC.

Thromboembolic deterrent (TED) stockings are placed preoperatively on all patients. Pneumatic compression stockings are placed for the duration of the operation. We do not administer preprocedure fractionated heparin or subcutaneous heparin, although some have advocated this decreases intraoperative and postoperative thromboembolic risk. An arterial line is placed for hemodynamic monitoring. Large bore intravenous lines should be placed in preparation of possible blood loss anemia. A central venous catheter may be elected in cases with anticipated excessive blood loss or for advanced access in less healthy patients. All patients are covered with a forced air warming device over the upper body. All patients undergo general anesthesia with an endotracheal tube.

Trendelenburg positioning during RARC is necessary to pull the abdominal viscera away from the operative field. However, this position is nonphysiologic and may have significant physiologic effects if maintained for a long period of time. Trendelenburg positioning can cause significant changes in cardiovascular, respiratory, metabolic, and cerebral physiology [22]. The increase in intracranial pressure seen with steep Trendelenburg positioning combined with pneumoperitoneum is also seen with either event alone [23]. The $PaCo_2$ should be maintained in the normal range during RARC [22]. Mean arterial blood pressure (MAP) as well as central venous pressures (CVP) increase markedly during pneumoperitoneum with Trendelenburg position in both health patients and those with baseline cardiopulmonary disease [24]. A study of robotic prostatectomy patients of ASA physical status I–II noted two to threefold increases of right as well as left-sided filling pressures [24]. Systemic blood pressure changed during the surgery, but there was no change in cardiac output. Other studies have confirmed the absence of cardiac output change associated with robotic prostatectomy [25]. Lestar et al. propose that this maintenance of cardiac output during pneumoperitoneum with steep Trendelenburg position is maintained in healthy men due to their abundance of cardiac reserve [24]. Therefore, a patient with compromised preoperative cardiac function could experience heart failure due to excessive preload. It is not known if returning these cardiac compromised patients to horizontal position will improve the patients' normal heart function [24].

Urine production can be expected to be sluggish during robotic surgery as in other laparoscopic/robotic surgeries. The pneumoperitoneum associated with laparoscopy can be associated with a 50 % decrease in renal plasma flow and glomerular filtration leading to decreased urine output [26]. This should be considered when administering crystalloid fluid replacement. The sluggish urine output associated with this effect often responds to aggressive fluid loading, but care must be taken to avoid potentially dangerous fluid overload [27].

Serious ocular consequences, such as retinal detachment and blindness, have been associated with Trendelenburg positioning as early as 1952 [28, 29]. Visual loss secondary to posterior ischemic optic neuropathy has been reported following robotic prostatectomy [28, 30]. Impaired ocular perfusion pressure is thought to be the major contributor to visual loss following prolonged spinal surgery [31]. It is not know the impact that the addition of prolonged pneumoperitoneum has on intraocular pressures (IOP). Awad et al. [28] examined the IOP of 33 consecutive patients undergoing robotic prostatectomy. IOP was 13.3 mmHg higher after Trendelenburg positioning when compared to the supine position. Duration of surgery and tidal CO_2 were the only significant predictors of IOP increases during robotic prostatectomy. Robot-assisted radical cystectomy operative times are naturally longer than those for prostatectomy. To date there has not been reported cases of visual field loss following RARC. However, ocular consideration must be given if the case is prolonged. Due to the IOP changes associated with Trendelenburg positioning and the prolonged operative time of robotic cystectomy, glaucoma can be seen as a relative contraindication to robotic cystectomy. All patients with elevated IOP at baseline before surgery may benefit from consultation with an ophthalmologist.

Editors' Commentary

Erik P. Castle and Raj S. Pruthi

The authors have described the considerations and steps of one of the most important aspects of any robotic procedure: setup. The key to the success of any procedure is preparation. This concept is particularly true for robot-assisted radical cystectomy. The procedure has many more steps and considerations than its robotic counterpart, robot-assisted radical prostatectomy (RARP). Hence preparation is paramount to success. Room setup such as monitor placement and location of the assistant can impact the ease with which the team can support the surgeon. In cases where the surgical and anesthetic team are experience with robot assisted radical prostatectomy, setup and positioning should be relatively straightforward. However, the issue of longer operative times must be kept in mind. Even the most experienced robot-assisted radical cystectomy surgeons have operative times that range between 4 and 8 h. As was the case early on during the learning curve for RARP, long cases can translate into complications, particularly those associated with prolonged extreme positioning. Therefore, it is important that any steps to enhance efficiency and success are undertaken as are outlined within this chapter.

References

1. Carey RI, Leveillee RJ. Patient positioning for robotic urologic procedures. In: Patel V, editor. Robotic urologic surgery. London: Springer; 2007. p. 61–6.
2. Warner MA, Warner DO, Harper CM, et al. Lower extremity neuropathies associated with lithotomy positions. Anesthesiology. 2000;93:938–42.
3. Rosevear HM, Lightfoot AJ, Zahs M, Waxman SW, Winfield HN. Lessons learned from a case of calf compartment syndrome after robot-assisted laparoscopic prostatectomy. J Endourol. 2010;24(10):1597–601.
4. Koc G, Tazeh NN, Joudi FN, Winfield HN, Tracy CR, Brown JA. Lower extremity neuropathies after robot-assisted laparoscopic prostatectomy on a split-leg table. J Endourol. 2012;26:1026–9.
5. Anema JG, Morey AF, McAninch JW, et al. Complications related to the high lithotomy position during urethral reconstruction. J Urol. 2000;164:360–3.
6. Manny TB, Gorbachinsky I, Hemal AK. Lower extremity neuropathy after robot assisted laparoscopic radical prostatectomy and radical cystectomy. Can J Urol. 2010;17:5390–3.
7. Pardanani S, Barbieri RL. Neurovascular complications of the lithotomy position: the four-hour rule. J Gynecol Tech. 1998;4:143–7.
8. Einarsson JI, Hibner M, Advincula AP. Side docking: an alternative docking method for gynecological robotic surgery. Rev Obstet Gynecol. 2011;4(3/4):123–5.
9. Hellan M, Stein H, Pigazzi A. Toatally robotic low anterior resection with total mesorectal excision and splenic flexure mobilization. Surg Endosc. 2009;23:447–51.
10. Uffort EE, Jensen JC. Side docking the robot for robotic laparoscopic radical prostatectomy. JSLS. 2011;15(2):200–2.
11. Thiel DD, Winfield HN. Robotics in urology: past, present, and future. J Endourol. 2008;22(4):825–30.
12. http://www.intuitivesurgical.com/products/instruments/ – corporate website outlining all instruments.
13. Tzortzis V, Gravas S, Mitsogiannis IC, Moutzouris G, Karatzas A, Leventis A, et al. Impact of stapling devices on radical cystectomy: comparative study between low- and high-volume surgeons. Urology. 2008;71(2):337–40.
14. Simonato A, Gregori A, Lissiani A, Bozzola A, Galli S, Gaboardi F. Laparoscopic radical cystoprostatectomy: a technique illustrated step by step. Eur Urol. 2003;44(1):132–8.
15. Daskalopoulos G, Karyotis I, Heretis I, Delakas D. Electrothermal bipolar coagulation for radical prostatectomies and cystectomies: a preliminary case-controlled study. Int Urol Nephrol. 2004;36(2):181–5.
16. Hruby GW, Marruffo FC, Durak E, Collins SM, Pierorazio P, Humphrey PA, et al. Evaluation of surgical energy devices for vessel sealing and peripheral energy spread in a porcine model. J Urol. 2007;178(6):2689–93.
17. Kim FJ, Chammas Jr MF, Gewehr E, Morihisa M, Caldas F, Hayacibara E, et al. Temperature safety profile of laparoscopic devices: harmonic ACE (ACE), Ligasure V (LV), and plasma trisector (PT). Surg Endosc. 2008;22(6):1464–9.
18. Mendez-Probst CE, Vilos G, Fuller A, Fernandez A, Borg P, Galloway D, et al. Stray electrical currents in laparoscopic instruments used in da Vinci® robot-assisted surgery: an in vitro study. J Endourol. 2011;25(9):1513–7.
19. Yerington CL, Nuechterlein B. Anesthetic considerations and management. In: Patel V, editor. Robotic urologic surgery. London: Springer; 2007. p. 54–9.
20. Joris JL. Anesthesia for laparoscopic surgery. In: Miller RD, editor. Anesthesia. Philadelphia, PA: Elsevier; 2005. p. 2286.
21. Johannsen G, Andersen M, Juhl B. The effects of general anaesthesia on the haemodynamic events during laparoscopy with CO_2 insufflation. Acta Anaesthesiol Scand. 1989;33:132.

22. Park EY, Koo BN, Min KT, Nam SH. The effect of pneumoperitoneum in the steep Trendelenburg position on cerebral oxygenation. Acta Anaesthesiol Scand. 2009;53:895–9.
23. Halverson A, Buchanan R, Jacobs L, Shayani V, Hunt T, Riedel C, et al. Evaluation of mechanism of increased intracranial pressure with insufflation. Surg Endosc. 1998;12:266–9.
24. Lestar M, Gunnarsson L, Lagerstrand L, Wiklund P, Odeberg-Wernerman S. Hemodynamic perturbations during robot-assisted laparoscopic radical prostatectomy in 45° trendelenburg position. Anesth Analg. 2011;113:1069–75.
25. Falabella A, Moore-Jeffries E, Sullivan MJ, Nelson R, Lew M. Cardiac function during steep Trendelenburg position and CO_2 pneumoperitoneum for robotic-assisted prostatectomy: a trans-esophageal Doppler probe study. Int J Med Robot. 2007;3:312–5.
26. Chiu AW, Azadzoi KM, Hatztichristou DG, et al. Effects of intra-abdominal pressure on renal tissue perfusion during laparoscopy. J Endoruol. 1994;8: 99–103.
27. Costello TG, Webb P. Anaesthesia for robot-assisted anatomic prostatectomy. Experience at a single institution. Anaesth Intensive Care. 2006;34:787–92.
28. Awad H, Santilli S, Ohr M, Roth A, Yan W, Fernandez S, et al. The effects of steep Trendelenburg positioning on intraocular pressure during robotic radical prostatectomy. Anesth Analg. 2009;109: 473–8.
29. Hewer CL. The physiology and complications of the Trendelenbrug position. Can Med Assoc J. 1956;74: 285–8.
30. Weber ED, Colyer MH, Lesser RL, Subramanian PS. Posterior ischemic optic neuropathy after minimally invasive prostatectomy. J Neuroophthalmol. 2007;27: 285–7.
31. Lauer K. Visual loss after spine surgery. J Neurosurg Anesthesiol. 2004;16:77–9.

Preoperative Preparation and Care

5

Jeffrey Holzbeierlein and Joshua G. Griffin

Introduction

Bladder cancer is the sixth most common malignancy in the USA, with an estimated 73,000 new cases diagnosed in 2012 [1]. Among these, approximately 25 % will initially present with muscle invasive disease. Radical cystectomy remains the gold standard in the management of non-metastatic muscle-invasive bladder cancer and provides the best chance for cure of this disease. Nonetheless, radical cystectomy is associated with significant perioperative morbidity and mortality rate of approximately 28 % and 2 %, respectively [2]. Invasive bladder cancer typically presents in the eighth decade, in a population of patients whom may have significant comorbidities, further compromising recovery from this procedure. Robot-assisted radical cystectomy has been shown to be a technically feasible procedure that may offer some advantages over the traditional open approach. This chapter focuses on the preoperative evaluation, preparation and perioperative care of patients undergoing robot-assisted radical cystectomy (RARC), with the goal of optimizing patient outcomes and minimizing complications. While written in the context of robotic surgery, this information can easily be applied to the open approach as well.

J. Holzbeierlein, M.D. (✉)
Department of Urology, University of Kansas Medical Center, 3901 Rainbow Boulevard, Mail Stop 3016, Kansas City, KS 66160, USA
e-mail: jholzbeierlein@kumc.edu

J.G. Griffin
University of Kansas Medical Center, Kansas City, KS, USA

Evaluation

Initial evaluation for all patients includes a detailed history and physical examination followed by laboratory studies and radiographic imaging. Clinical staging with computed tomography is important to evaluate for locally advanced or metastatic disease, as this could affect decision-making regarding surgical treatment. For patients found to have locally or regionally advanced disease a bone scan may also be warranted. Although some reports also suggest utility of positron emission scans (PET scans) in diagnosing occult metastatic disease, our experience is that these have been of limited utility over traditional imaging and furthermore are not typically covered by insurance [3]. Although beyond the scope of this review, neoadjuvant chemotherapy has been demonstrated to provide a survival advantage to patients with muscle invasive disease, and thus, most of our patients will receive neoadjuvant chemotherapy prior to radical cystectomy [4]. Typically, for patients who receive chemotherapy, we advise waiting 2–4 weeks after the completion of chemotherapy to allow blood counts and platelet counts to recover.

E.P. Castle and R.S. Pruthi (eds.), *Robotic Surgery of the Bladder*, DOI 10.1007/978-1-4614-4906-5_5,

Given that the population of muscle-invasive bladder cancer patients is older and often has a long history of smoking, it is imperative that the urologist identify any factors that may suggest underlying pulmonary or cardiovascular disease, both of which may need further evaluation. Those with a history of chronic obstructive pulmonary disease (COPD) or other chronic lung disease processes should undergo at minimum pulmonary function testing and arterial blood gas analysis. Carbon dioxide insufflation leads to significant pulmonary alterations including reduced lung volumes, hypercarbia, hypercapnia, and reduced venous return. While these physiologic changes are usually of no consequence in the healthy patient, they can be poorly tolerated if there is underlying pulmonary disease and hypoxemia can develop both during and after the operation [5]. Cardiac disease, including congestive heart failure and arrhythmias should be noted as both may require more invasive monitoring during surgery due to the effect of decreased cardiac preload and resulting acidosis from CO_2 resorption, respectively. Other important factors include neurologic or musculoskeletal disease, which may affect patient positioning at the time of surgery. A history of renal insufficiency is also important and may affect the choice of continent vs. incontinent urinary reconstruction [6].

The only absolute contraindications to RARC would include an uncorrected bleeding disorder, bowel obstruction, or presence of peritonitis or intra-abdominal abscess. However, as previously mentioned, individuals with severe pulmonary disease may not tolerate laparoscopic surgery and in some cases should forego this approach. While there are no absolute contraindications to RARC in terms of previous surgeries, prior abdominal operations may pose a particular challenge to gaining intra-abdominal access. A good knowledge of the surgical history as well as all incisions will help dictate where the Veress needle should be placed. In some situations, the Hasson technique may be more appropriate.

Nutritional Status Evaluation

Nutritional deficiency is not an uncommon finding in cancer patients and may have a significant impact on surgical outcomes. Gregg et al. retrospectively reviewed a cohort of over 500 patients who underwent radical cystectomy at a single institution. Patients with preoperative nutritional deficiency, defined as albumin <3.5 g/dl, body mass index <18.5, or preoperative weight loss over 5 %, had higher 90-day mortality rates (16.5 % vs. 5.1 %) and lower overall survival at 3 years (44.5 % vs. 67.6 %) compared to non-nutrient-deficient patients. After controlling for other variables, preoperative nutritional deficiency was associated with higher all cause mortality [7]. While the role of perioperative total parenteral nutrition or enteral feedings has not been completely defined, patients should be screened for these nutritional risk factors and perhaps evaluated by a dietician before surgery.

Patient Preparation

Patient preparation begins with a thorough discussion of the surgery and expectations both during the perioperative and postoperative period. Patients should be extensively counseled regarding the options for urinary reconstruction. For those patients who select an ileal conduit, it is helpful to provide them with an appliance to wear before surgery in order to become familiar with the appliance. Consultation with an enterostomal therapist is strongly advised in efforts to determine the optimal stoma site. In instances in which a stomal therapist is not available, it is imperative for the surgeon to mark the stoma on both the left and right sides in both the sitting and recumbent positions. Additional preoperative recommendations include smoking cessation which should always be encouraged as this has been shown to reduce the risk of postoperative complications [8]. Antiplatelet medications or nonsteroidal anti-inflammatory inhibitors should be held 7–10 days prior to surgery. Urinary tract infections should be treated with a test of cure prior to surgery.

Bowel Preparation

For many years a mechanical bowel preparation (MBP) with or without the use of oral antibiotics has been used in patients undergoing radical cystectomy and urinary reconstruction. However, the role of routine MBP has been challenged by many as causing more adverse effects than benefits [9]. Bowel preparation leads to dehydration and may cause electrolyte abnormalities and in several randomized controlled trials has shown a higher incidence of complications such as anastomotic leak, wound infection, and intra-abdominal abscess for those undergoing colorectal surgery [10]. While there have been no randomized controlled trials addressing MBP for radical cystectomy and urinary diversion, several retrospective studies have demonstrated no advantage of MBP [9, 11]. Given these findings we no longer routinely use a mechanical bowel preparation, and patients are only required to be nothing per os (NPO) after midnight the evening prior to surgery. Alternatively one may wish to administer a light bowel prep consisting of magnesium citrate the day prior to surgery, or a sodium phosphate enema the morning of surgery.

Intraoperative and Postoperative Care

Prior to induction of anesthesia, pneumatic compression devices should be placed. At our institution we also administer 5,000 units of heparin subcutaneously. Deep venous thrombosis (DVT) prophylaxis with heparin is continued throughout the hospital stay and has reduced our rates of thrombotic complications to 6.7 %. A second or third general cephalosporin is given intravenously within 1 h of incision and continued for 24 h based on the American Urological Association's best practice statement [12]. Alternatives include an aminoglycoside + metronidazole/clindamycin or fluoroquinolone. Orogastric or nasogastric tubes should always be placed for stomach decompression before obtaining abdominal insufflation. Patients are placed in the dorsal lithotomy position and great attention should be placed to all bony prominences and adequately padded prior to draping the patient. Skin hair should be removed with clippers in the operating room or in the holding area.

The routine use of postoperative nasogastric tube suction (NTS) is no longer implemented. A meta-analysis evaluating 33 randomized controlled trials involving over 5,000 patients undergoing abdominal surgery demonstrated an increased rate of both pulmonary complications and delayed return to bowel functions [13]. For radical cystectomy, NTS has shown to prolong hospital stay and delay time to return of bowel function [14, 15]. At present, NTS should only be used in selective cases, such as in the setting of bowel injury or those with a history of neurogenic bowel.

The use of a perioperative care pathways has been shown to reduce time to oral diet and discharge in patients undergoing radical cystectomy and have been highlighted in several high volume centers [15–17]. Key features include early NGT removal, use of chewing gum and pro-motility agent metoclopramide, pain control using non-opioid agents, and early implementation of a regular diet. Using these "fast-track" protocols, Pruthi et al. was able to demonstrate a reduced time to discharge with a mean of 5 days. At our institution, patients are started on a clear liquid diet on postoperative day 2 and then advanced to a regular diet after return of flatus. We emphasize early ambulation as well as minimizing opioid use for pain control. A bowel regimen, consisting of dulcolax and a stool softener is also started on hospital day 2.

Prior to discharge patients should receive appropriate education regarding care of orthotopic neobladder or ileal conduit. For those with orthotopic neobladder, patients should demonstrate proficiency in bladder irrigation and catheter care. Those whom have ileal conduit diversion should be comfortable with stoma care and appliance changes.

Conclusion

Robot-assisted radical cystectomy is a minimally invasive treatment for invasive or recurrent high-grade bladder cancer and may reduce postoperative pain and convalescence after surgery, both of which may reduce hospital stay. A thorough evaluation prior to surgery, including cardiac and pulmonary tests where appropriate is imperative to reduce significant complications. Mechanical bowel prep and routine nasogastric suction are not necessary and may prolong time to bowel function return. The implementation of routine clinical pathways has the potential advantage of further reducing hospital stay and recovery time.

Editors' Commentary

Erik P. Castle and Raj S. Pruthi

In recent decades the risks and complications of cystectomy and urinary diversion have been greatly reduced. Such improvements have come due to a variety of factors including improved operative techniques, superior anesthetic management, and evolved perioperative medical care.

One such measure to help improve outcomes and minimize morbidity of this procedure is the optimization of perioperative care—i.e., the use of clinical care pathways. The authors provide a "modern" and thoughtful approach to the perioperative management of patients undergoing radical cystectomy—whether open or robotic. Such evidence-based approaches to perioperative care have allowed the successful implementation of fast-track programs in a variety of operative procedures including colorectal surgery, hepatobiliary procedures, and cardiothoracic surgery. Indeed, cystectomy and urinary diversion may be particularly suitable to a structured care pathway given its potential for high morbidity (including postoperative ileus), potential for increased post-operative stay, and overall relatively high perioperative cost. Such clinical care pathways have the potential to utilize evidence-based modifications to reduce morbidity and improve recovery with regard to early institution of oral diet and early hospital discharge. Ongoing modification and analysis of this program remain an important aspect of clinical care pathways which provide a ready mechanism by which scientific evidence translates into clinical practice.

References

1. National Cancer Institute. SEER stat fact sheets: bladder. http://www.seer.cancer.gov/csr/1975_2009_pops09. Accessed May 2012.
2. Kim SP, Boorjian SA, Shah ND, Karnes RJ, Weight CJ, Moriarty JP, et al. Contemporary trends of in-hospital complications and mortality for radical cystectomy. BJU Int. 2012;110:1163–8. doi:10.1111/j.1464-410X. 2012.10990.x.
3. Kibel AS, Dehdashti F, Katz MD, Klim AP, Grubb RL, Humphrey PA, et al. Prospective study of [18F] fluorodeoxyglucose positron emission tomography/computed tomography for staging of muscle-invasive bladder carcinoma. J Clin Oncol. 2009;27(26):4314–20.
4. Grossman HB, Natale RB, Tangen CM, Speights VO, Vogelzang NJ, Trump DL, et al. Neoadjuvant chemotherapy plus cystectomy compared with cystectomy alone for locally advanced bladder cancer. N Engl J Med. 2003;349(9):859–66.
5. Gutt CN, Oniu T, Mehrabi A, Schemmer P, Kashfi A, Kraus T, et al. Circulatory and respiratory complications of carbon dioxide insufflation. Dig Surg. 2004;21(2):95–105.
6. World Health Organization Consensus Conference on Bladder Cancer, Hautmann RE, Abol-Enein H, Hafez K, Haro I, Mansson W, et al. Urinary diversion. Urology. 2007;69(1):17–49.
7. Gregg JR, Cookson MS, Phillips S, Salem S, Chang SS, Clark PE, et al. Effect of preoperative nutritional deficiency on mortality after radical cystectomy for bladder cancer. J Urol. 2011;185(1):90–6.
8. Theadom A, Cropley M. Effects of preoperative smoking cessation on the incidence and risk of intraoperative and postoperative complications in adult smokers: a systematic review. Tob Control. 2006;15(5):352–8.
9. Shafii M, Murphy DM, Donovan MG, Hickey DP. Is mechanical bowel preparation necessary in patients undergoing cystectomy and urinary diversion? BJU Int. 2002;89(9):879–81.
10. Bucher P, Mermillod B, Gerva P, Morel P. Mechanical bowel preparation for elective colorectal surgery: a meta-analysis. Arch Surg. 2004;139:1359–64.
11. Raynor MC, Lavien G, Nielsen M, Wallen EM, Pruthi RS. Elimination of preoperative mechanical bowel

preparation in patients undergoing cystectomy and urinary diversion. Urol Oncol. 2013;31:32–5.
12. Wolf JS, Bennett, CJ, Dmochowski RR, Hollenbeck BK, Pearle MS, et al. Best practice policy statement on urologic surgery antimicrobial prophylaxis. American Urologic Association. 2008. http://www.auanet.org/content/clinical-practice-guidelines/clinical-guidelines.cfm#2. Accessed May 2012.
13. Nelson R, Edwards S, Tse B. Prophylactic nasogastric decompression after abdominal surgery. Cochrane Database Syst Rev 2007;(3):CD004929.
14. Inman BA, Harel F, Tiguert R, Lacombe L. Routine nasogastric tubes are not required following cystectomy with urinary diversion: a comparative analysis of 430 patients. J Urol. 2003;170(5):1888–91.
15. Pruthi RS, Chun J, Richman M. Reducing time to oral diet and hospital discharge in patients undergoing radical cystectomy using a perioperative care plan. Urology. 2003;62(4):661–5.
16. Maffezzini M, Campodonico F, Canepa G, Gerbi G, Parodi D. Current perioperative management of radical cystectomy with intestinal urinary reconstruction for muscle-invasive bladder cancer and reduction of the incidence of postoperative ileus. Surg Oncol. 2008;17(1):41–8.
17. Pruthi RS, Nielsen M, Smith A, Nix J, Schultz H, Wallen EM. Fast track program in patients undergoing radical cystectomy: results in 362 consecutive patients. J Am Coll Surg. 2010;210(1):93–9.

Robot-Assisted Radical Cystectomy: Male

6

Erik P. Castle and Raj S. Pruthi

Introduction

The standard treatment of muscle-invasive bladder cancer is open radical cystectomy (ORC) and urinary diversion. Radical cystectomy can be a challenging operation with significant patient morbidity and mortality. The first laparoscopic simple cystectomy was reported in 1992 by Parra et al. [1]. Since that publication there have been several reports of laparoscopic radical cystectomy for malignant disease with various methods of urinary diversion. With the introduction of the daVinci™ surgical system (Intuitive Surgical, Sunnyvale, CA) the prevalence of robot-assisted radical prostatectomies has increased dramatically. It was a natural progression to apply robotic technology to laparoscopic cystectomies. In 2003, Menon et al. published the first series of robot assisted radical cystectomy (RARC) and urinary diversion [2]. The goal of this chapter is to provide a detailed description of RARC in male patients as well as discuss pertinent literature on outcomes of this procedure.

Indications

The indications for radical cystectomy includes tumor invasion of muscularis propria, carcinoma in situ refractory to intravesical therapy, recurrent multifocal superficial disease refractory to repeat transurethral resection with or without intravesical therapy, and may be considered for initial therapy in high grade T1 disease, particularly in the setting of concurrent CIS. There are no absolute preoperative contraindications specific to patients being considered for RARC. There are two intraoperative situations that are absolute contraindications to proceeding with RARC. The first situation is hypotension or compromised ventilation with positioning and abdominal insufflation, which is of particular concern in obese patients. The second is CO_2 retention with insufflation resulting in unmanageable acidosis. This highlights the need for a careful preoperative cardiopulmonary evaluation in this patient population. Relative contraindications include abnormal anatomy (i.e., ectopic kidney, vascular aneurysm), morbid obesity, prior radiation, and prior abdominal or pelvic surgery. As with all laparoscopic oncology surgery, the principles of open surgery must be followed with RARC. If there is concern these oncologic principles will be compromised, a robot-assisted approach should not be used.

The online version of this chapter (doi:10.1007/978-1-4614-4906-5_6) contains supplementary material, which is available to authorized users.

E.P. Castle, M.D., F.A.C.S. (✉)
Department of Urology, Mayo Clinic, 5779 East Mayo Blvd, Phoenix, AZ 85054, USA
e-mail: castle.erik@mayo.edu

R.S. Pruthi, M.D., F.A.C.S.
Department of Urology, The University of North Carolina at Chapel Hill, Chapel Hill, NC, USA

E.P. Castle and R.S. Pruthi (eds.), *Robotic Surgery of the Bladder*, DOI 10.1007/978-1-4614-4906-5_6,

Technique

Port Placement

Six ports are utilized

- Four robotic ports
  - One 12 mm camera port
  - Three 8 mm robotic arm ports
- Two assistant ports
  - 15 mm and 5 mm assistant ports

The ports are arranged in an "inverted-V" fashion (Fig. 6.1). Access and establishment of the pneumoperitoneum can be performed with a Veress needle or Hassan technique. The camera port is placed in the midline cephalad to the umbilicus. If an extended lymphadenectomy is planned then placement of the camera port at least 4 cm cephalad to the umbilicus is key in order to be able to perform and adequate proximal dissection on the great vessels. The two 8 mm robotic ports (right and left arms) are placed 8–10 cm lateral to midline at or above the level of the umbilicus. Two assistant ports on the right (or left) are placed lateral to the right robotic port and the third working arm (also known as the "fourth arm") port is placed superior-lateral to the ipsilateral robotic port and on the opposite side of the assistant ports. If an intracorporeal diversion is planned, the assistant should be placed on the left side with the third robotic arm on the right side of the patient. We recommend using a 15-mm assistant port for one of the ports to make extraction of lymph nodes easier as well as the fact it allows easy passage of a 15-mm specimen retrieval bag to be used for the bladder and prostate. A list of common robotic and laparoscopic instruments used during RARC can be found in Table 6.1.

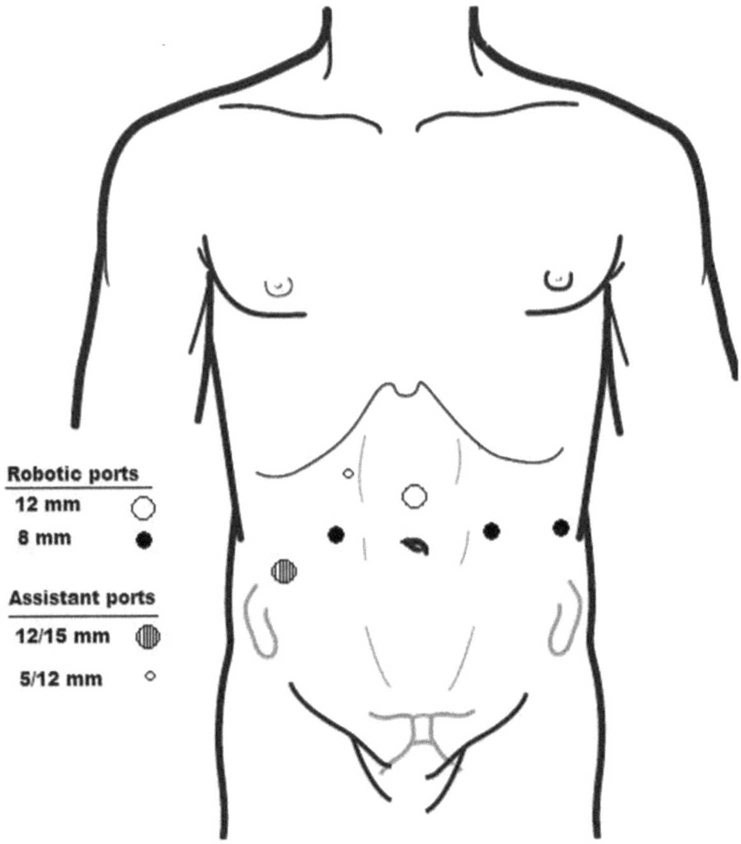

Fig. 6.1 Port placement for RARC

Table 6.1 List of commonly used instruments for RARC

Robotic instruments
Monopolar scissors
Maryland bipolar
Prograsp™ forceps
Large needle drivers × 2
Robotic locking clip applier (*optional*)
Fenestrated bipolar (*optional*)
Cadiere forceps (*optional*)
Laparoscopic instruments
Suction/aspirator
Needle driver
Locking grasper
Atraumatic grasper
Locking clip applier (*small, medium and large*)
Suture
3-0 polyglactin cut to 20 cm for ureteral and bowel tags (*pre-tie the suture to the locking clips to be used on the ureters*)
0 polyglactin cut to 15 cm for ligation of the DVC
2-0 and 3-0 polyglactin cut to 20 cm for over sewing edges of the DVC and any bleeding sites from the neurovascular bundles and pedicles

Mobilization of the Sigmoid and Left Colon

A 30° down lens can be used at the outset of the procedure. This allows for better visualization of the pelvis and retroperitoneum during the lymphadenectomy. This will be changed to a 0° lens for the posterior dissection. The procedure is begun by incising the peritoneum lateral to the left colon. The left colon and sigmoid colon should be released from the left sidewall to allow access to the left iliac vessels and left ureter.

Development of the Left Paravesical Space and Division of the Left Ureter

With the left medial umbilical ligament identified, the peritoneum lateral to the ligament and medial to the left iliac vessels should be incised. Blunt dissection is employed to expose the endopelvic fascia. In male patients, dividing the vas deferens allows the bladder to be retracted medially and facilitates exposure of the pelvic vasculature.

The left ureter is identified crossing over the iliac vessels. The ureter should be dissected free of its underlying structures while preserving as much periureteral tissue as possible. The distal end can be dissected down to its insertion into the bladder. The left umbilical artery and/or left superior vesical artery should be seen just lateral to the insertion of the ureter into the bladder and clipped/ligated to allow for more length on the ureter. The ureter can be clipped distally with a locking clip. The proximal clip on the ureter should have a suture pre-tied to the clip (10–12 in.) so no additional "tagging" or marking of the ureter is required later in the procedure. The ureter should be dissected free of its attachments cephalad. Attempt should be made to preserve any vital blood supply to the ureter from the left common iliac artery. This should be done *before* dividing the ureter as proximal dissection can be difficult once the ureter is divided. The ureter can then be divided sharply. A margin can be sent for frozen section at this point if desired. It should be noted that too much or too aggressive dissection proximal on the ureter can result in devitalization of the ureter and may contribute to anastomotic stricture in the postoperative setting. In many cases, individual vessels from the common iliac or distal aorta can be seen and preserved to maintain ureteral blood flow.

The Left Pelvic Lymphadenectomy

At this point the left pelvic lymphadenectomy can be performed. It is the preference of the authors of this chapter to perform the lymphadenectomy at this time. Please refer to Chap. 9 for details. In some cases, the lymphadenectomy can be deferred until after the cystectomy is performed. Early in a surgeon's experience, one may elect to complete the cystectomy first.

Development of the Right Paravesical Space, Right Ureter, and Right Lymphadenectomy

The right paravesical space is developed similar to the left. Dissection is similar as done on the left, but it should be noted that the incision in the retroperitoneum on this side should be extended onto the right side of the sigmoid mesentery to develop the preaortic space and allow for passage of the left ureter. It is important to develop a relatively large space in this region. Often there is fear to do aggressive blunt dissection due to concern for the mesenteric vessels; however, if the surgeon stays close to the great vessels, the space is very safe to develop.

Identification, Ligation, and Division of the Superior Vesical Arteries

The umbilical and superior vesical arteries are clearly seen at the completion of the lymphadenectomy and are clipped—locking clips are preferred. Clipping is recommended and may allow for more distal dissection of the ureters. If the ureters have not already been tagged with a pre-tied clip, then one should switch instruments to needle drivers and tag the distal ends of both ureters.

Transferring the Left Ureter Through the Sigmoid Mesentery

The left ureter can be transposed behind the sigmoid mesentery with the help of the right side assistant. The right side assistant should gently advance a blunt-tipped instrument below the mesentery along the anterior surface of the aorta. If the robotic "third arm" has been placed on the right side then it can be passed through very easily as well. The tag on the left ureter can be grasped and the ureter should easily pass through the mesenteric window.

Tagging the Distal Ileum with 8–10 in. 2-0 Vicryl Suture

The ileum should be tagged with a 2-0 Vicryl suture. This too should be left at least 10–12 in. in length. We recommend mobilizing the lateral attachments of the cecum so as to facilitate delivery of the ileum into the abdominal incision and make identification of the distal portion of the ileum easier.

Development of the Prerectal and Posterior Vesical Space

The camera lens can be changed to a 0° (degree) lens for optimal visualization. The peritoneum extending from the posterior bladder to the anterior sigmoid should be incised. Using blunt and careful cautery dissection, the prerectal space is developed. One must employ the assistant(s) to retract the bladder and its posterior structures anteriorly. In male patients, Denonvillier's fascia needs to be incised to carry the dissection as far caudad as possible. The dissection should be carried down to the rectourethralis muscle. If a nerve sparing is desired then one should dissect anterior to Denonvillier's fascia and leave it on the anterior rectal surface staying close to the prostate.

Division of the Remaining Inferior Vesical Vessels

Once the limits of dissection are reached along the posterior aspect of the bladder, the lateral attachments of the bladder can be divided. For a non-nerve sparing procedure, this can be done with locking clips or a combination of the bipolar instrument and the monopolar instrument of choice. An endovascular stapler can be used on both sides as well, but we recommend using locking clips as it yielded a more controlled dissection and preserved planes of dissection. It should be remembered that the dissection should be carried caudad through the endopelvic fascia thereby completely mobilizing the bladder from its lateral attachments and the rectum. Often a combination of lateral and posterior dissection is used in an alternating fashion to complete the dissection.

Preservation of the Neurovascular Bundles

In nerve-sparing procedures, the neurovascular bundles are encountered as they project off the posterior–lateral aspects of the prostate down to the anterior surface of the colon. The bundles can be mobilized by releasing lateral fascia anterior to the bundles along the surface of the prostate or vagina. This should be done before ligating the inferior vesical pedicles in order to have them visualized. This is particularly important in cases which energy devices and staplers are employed for vascular ligation. This dissection is connected to the incision anterior to Denonvillier's fascia that has already been performed during creation of the prerectal space. The inferior vesical pedicles and prostate pedicles should be clipped and divided with cold scissors to avoid neurovascular injury. The nerve sparing should be carried down to the genitourinary diaphragm to prevent injury during the apical and urethral dissection.

Mobilization of the Bladder and Completion of the Apical Dissection

The remaining bladder attachments should only be the urachus, anterior attachments, prostate, and urethra. The medial and median umbilical ligaments should be divided as far proximally as possible with electrocautery. The dissection and peritoneal incision is carried lateral to the medial umbilical ligaments caudad to the anterior surface of the bladder. If not already done, the endopelvic fascia should be incised bilaterally. The apical dissection of the prostate or vagina is then completed. At this point the dorsal venous complex can be ligated with a 1 Vicryl suture in a figure of eight fashion. Although an endovascular stapler can be employed for this step, we feel the suture ligation allows for better visualization and identification of the urethra. Furthermore, when a stapler is used, there is likely to be venous ooze into the pelvis once the abdomen is opened for the diversion.

Dissection, Ligation, and Division of the Urethra

It is very important to dissect out a generous urethral stump. This is important even in cases without a planned neobladder. A generous urethral stump allows for easier application of a locking clip or suture ligation to prevent tumor spillage during division. If the previous posterior dissection was adequate, there should be minimal posterior tissue other than some minor remnants of rectourethralis. The urethral catheter is removed by the bedside assistant and a locking clip is placed on the urethra by the bedside assistant or the robotic clip applier. The urethra is divided *distal* to the clip. A frozen section can be taken from the proximal portion of the divided urethra if needed.

Following division of the urethra the specimen is placed in a 15-mm specimen retrieval bag and retracted into the superior aspect of the abdomen. It is very important to ensure that there is excellent hemostasis in the pelvis. Often there is venous ooze from structures such as the dorsal venous complex, urethra, rectourethralis, and neurovascular bundles. Dropping the pneumoperitoneum to 5 mmHg can help identify potential bleeding areas. Strategic placement of "figure-of-eight" sutures and additional maneuvers will prevent postoperative pelvic bleeding. This is a key point as many times this bleeding would otherwise go unnoticed until the diversion is being created and the pneumoperitoneum has been released.

Specimen Extraction

The entire specimen can be entrapped in a 15-mm specimen retrieval bag. It will be extracted though a 5–6-cm infraumbilical or periumbilical incision. Prior to extraction, the tags on the ureters and the ileum should be grasped in a locking grasper by the bedside assistant to allow delivery into and through the extraction incision.

Lessons Learned and Key Points for RARC

- Use a 15-mm port for one of the assistant ports.
- Use a pre-tied suture on the locking clip placed on the ureter to avoid need for tagging.

- Preserve the blood supply from the common iliac to the ureters during dissection if possible.
- Perform meticulous dissection of the vascular pedicles allowing for locking clips to be used for ligation.
- Make a large mesenteric window for easy passage of the left ureter.
- When performing the posterior dissection, carry the dissection as far distally to adequately release any rectal attachments under direct vision to the prostate and bladder. This will allow completion of the cystectomy to be easier and avoid unidentified rectal injuries. Sharp dissection should be used exclusively around the posterior apex of the prostate and rectourethralis to avoid thermal injury to the rectum.
- Be sure to *completely* control the dorsal venous complex and any bleeding sites from the neurovascular bundles and genitourinary diaphragm with suture ligation to avoid venous ooze postoperatively.
- Make the extraction incision *below* the level of the umbilicus and avoid the temptation to try to incorporate one of the port sites such as the camera port. Keeping the incision below the umbilicus makes extracorporeal creation of the diversion much easier.
- Make the extraction incision as large as is needed to facilitate the ureteroileal anastomosis. A few extra centimeters can make a difference when trying to prevent traction and ischemic injury to the ureters. Cutting back on the ureters and working in the pelvis as one would do with an open approach is recommended.

Postoperative Care

A nasogastric tube is not routinely left in place. The patients are maintained on broad-spectrum antibiotics for at least 48 h and can be transitioned to oral regimens based on surgeon preference. Epidural catheters are not used. Intravenous morphine and/or ketorolac are usually adequate for pain management and can be promptly switched to oral narcotics once the patient is tolerating a diet.

It is important to increase patient activity as early as the day of surgery. Patients are encouraged to sit in a chair the same night of surgery. They are ambulated on the first postoperative day. Bisacodyl suppositories may be administered each morning starting on the first postoperative day until bowel function returns. A liquid diet is started once bowel function returns which may be as early as the second or third postoperative day. Daily serum chemistry and hematocrits may be followed until discharge based on surgeon preference. Most patients do not seem to have significant third spacing and will rarely require additional fluid replacement other than standard maintenance fluids. Although postoperative hemorrhage and delayed bowel injury are rare, patients need to be monitored closely for these complications, as the incidence with RARC is unknown.

Ureteral stents and abdominal drains should be managed according to surgeon preference. Currently, the authors remove stents from a urostomy at 7–10 days. Foley catheters are removed from neobladders in 14–21 days. If the stents were not secured to the Foley during creation of the neobladder, then they are removed cystoscopically at the time of foley removal in the office. The decision to perform a cystogram at the time of foley removal is based on surgeon preference and can be decided on an individual case basis.

It should be noted that patients can be discharged home rather quickly which may require leaving drains or stents in place until the first office follow-up. The authors have found that some patients may have a continued leak of lymphatic fluid through a drain site up through the fifth or sixth postoperative day. We believe this is seen because patients are discharged home before their lymphatic channels have completely sealed. Consequently, the abdominal drain may be left in place until their first postoperative follow-up which is on postoperative day 7. If the drain is removed before discharge, then a urostomy appliance can be placed over the drain site to collect the fluid until the incision heals and drainage ceases. We have found this drainage to be self-limiting and uniformly resolves spontaneously as the lymphatic fluid is absorbed intraperitoneally. If there is any concern of a urine leak, the fluid may be sent for creatinine analysis.

Perioperative Outcomes

There have been several large series demonstrating promising perioperative outcomes of patients undergoing RARC [3–6]. Operative times range from 275 to 380 min, blood loss from 270 to 400 cm^3, length of stay from 4.9 to 10 days, with overall and high grade complication rates from 34 to 52 % and 8 to 24 %, respectively. These outcomes are summarized in Table 6.1. RARC has been shown to decrease complications compared to open radical cystectomy in a nonrandomized study [7].

Pathologic Outcomes

Two important pathologic issues that need to be addressed during RARC are incidence of positive surgical margins (PSM) and an adequate pelvic lymph node dissection (PLND). The importance of achieving negative surgical margins during radical cystectomy cannot be overstated as patients with positive soft tissue margins have increased recurrence rates and almost a threefold decrease in survival [8, 9]. The reported rate of PSM for RARC ranges from 0 to 7.6 % [3–5, 10, 11]. Novara et al. provided a benchmark from the open radical cystectomy literature in a multi-institutional series of over 4,000 patients where the PSM rate was 6.3 % [12]. The inclusion of a pelvic lymphadenectomy at the time of cystectomy provides both prognostic information and potential therapeutic benefit [13, 14]. Furthermore, the number of lymph nodes removed has been shown to have prognostic significance by several authors and it is also well established that an extended template will improve lymph node yield [13–16]. The reported lymph node yield for lymphadenectomy during RARC ranges from 17 to 43, with most centers performing an extended template [3–5, 17–19]. In a prospective randomized trial, Nix et al. demonstrated to difference in lymph node yield between robotic and open cystectomy [20]. In a unique study by Davis et al., robotic lymph node dissections had a yield of 93 % compared to open lymphadenectomy when a "second look open dissection" was used following the robotic PLND [18]. The bottom line is that a complete pelvic lymphadenectomy should be performed and is clearly possible with the robotic approach.

Survival Following RARC

Robot-assisted radical cystectomy is in its infancy so no long-term oncological follow-up exists, but there are several reports of short and intermediate-term follow-up that have emerged. Pruthi and Wallen reported short-term cancer outcomes in 50 patients [21]. They had a mean follow-up 13.2 months and experienced an overall and disease-specific survival of 90 and 94 %, respectively. Dasgupta et al. published their RARC experience in 20 patients with >6 months follow-up [22]. This cohort had a mean follow-up of 23 months, with overall and disease-free survival of 95 and 90 %. Martin et al. reported outcomes in series of 80 patients with the longest mean follow-up to date from Mayo Clinic in Arizona [23]. Fifty-nine patients had >6-month follow-up with a mean follow-up of 25 months (range 6–49) The overall survival at 12, 24, and 36 months was 82, 69, and 69 %, respectively, and recurrence free survival at 12, 24, and 36 months was 82, 71, 71 %, respectively (Fig. 6.1—Kaplan Meier curves from Martin paper). The Karolinska Institute found 83 % disease specific survival with a mean follow-up of 25 months [11]. Kauffman et al. report 2-year disease-free, cancer-specific, and overall survival of 74 %, 85 %, and 79 %, respectively [24]. Clearly, oncological outcomes as measured by survival are equivalent in the intermediate-term. Additional data from Mayo Clinic Arizona and University of North Carolina were published on node positive patients having undergone RARC [25]. A total of 275 patients were reviewed with focus on 50 patients with N1 disease. With a mean follow-up of 42 months the oncological outcomes compared favorably to open cohorts reported on in the literature. Nevertheless, long-term follow-up is still eagerly awaited.

Conclusion

Robot-assisted radical cystectomy in the male patient is a feasible and reproducible operation. With appropriate steps and adherence to a standardized technique, results are often superior with regards to recovery in the immediate postoperative period and complications can be kept to a minimum. Intermediate oncological outcomes are favorable and with increasing application, RARC will become a part of the urologist's armamentarium to treat invasive bladder cancer.

Editors' Commentary

Erik P. Castle and Raj S. Pruthi

The chapter seeks to provide a stepwise and reproducible approach to robot-assisted radical cystectomy in the male patient. Hopefully, this description will help guide and launch the surgeon just initiating their robot-assisted radical cystectomy experience to success. Also, we hope that even the more experienced surgeon, already performing RARC, will gain insights, tips, and tricks to perform the procedure in a more effective and efficient manner.

It has been over 8 years since both of us have initiated our experience with RARC. Early, the approach was a careful and even guarded approach studying feasibility, safety, and oncologic integrity with every case. Over the years, and with the ongoing assessment by ourselves and by others (critics and enthusiasts alike), we have witnessed the development of the technique into an increasingly common and appropriate procedure that has served our patients well—all the time preserving the time-tested principles and outcomes of bladder cancer surgery. Today, the careful evidence has demonstrated that RARC has very real benefits and without any suggestion of a compromise to the oncologic outcomes. With a large, multi-institutional, prospective randomized trial well underway, we look forward to the results which will provide the highest levels of evidence-based analysis comparing the open versus robotic approach—putting scientific rigor and patient safety above a rush to novelty, procedural numbers, and marketing. We believe that it is essential to assess this procedure, and any new intervention or technique for that matter, in such a scientifically rigorous manner.

References

1. Parra RO, Andrus CH, Jones JP. Laparoscopic cystectomy: initial report on a new treatment for the retained bladder. J Urol. 1992;148:1140–4.
2. Menon M, Hemal AK, Tewari A, et al. Nerve-sparing robot-assisted radical cystoprostatectomy and urinary diversion. BJU Int. 2003;92:232–6.
3. Kauffman EC, Ng CK, Lee MM, et al. Critical analysis of complications after robotic-assisted radical cystectomy with identification of preoperative and operative risk factors. BJU Int. 2009;105:520–7.
4. Khan MS, Elhage O, Challacombe B, et al. Analysis of early complications of robotic-assisted radical cystectomy using a standarized reporting system. Urology. 2011;77:357–62.
5. Pruthi RS, Nielsen ME, Nix J, et al. Robotic radical cystectomy for bladder cancer: surgical adn pathological outcomes in 100 consecutive cases. J Urol. 2010;183:510–5.
6. Hayn MH, Hellenthal NJ, Hussain A, et al. Defining morbidity of robot-assisted radical cystectomy using a standardized reporting methodology. Eur Urol. 2011;59:213–8.
7. Ng CK, Kauffman EC, Lee MM, et al. A comparison of postoperative complications in open versus robotic cystectomy. Eur Urol. 2010;57:274–82.
8. Dotan ZA, Kavanagh K, Yossepowitch O, et al. Positive surgical margins in soft tissue following radical cystectomy for bladder cancer and cancer specific survival. J Urol. 2007;178:2308–12.
9. Hadjizacharia P, Stein JP, Cai J, Miranda G. The impact of positive soft tissue surgical margins following radical cystectomy for high-grade, invasive bladder cancer. World J Urol. 2009;27:33–8.
10. Hellenthal NJ, Hussain A, Andrews PE, et al. Surgical margin status after robot assisted radical cystectomy: results from the international robotic cystectomy consortium. J Urol. 2010;184:87–91.
11. Schumacher MC, Jonsson MN, Wiklund NP. Robotic cystectomy. Scand J Surg. 2009;98:89–95.
12. Novara G, Svatek RS, Karakiewicz PI, et al. Soft tissue surgical margin status is a powerful predictor of

outcomes after radical cystectomy: a multicenter study of more than 4,400 patients. J Urol. 2010;183: 2165–70.
13. Leissner J, Hohenfellner R, Thuroff JW, Wolf HK. Lymphadenectomy in patients with transitional cell carcinoma of the urinary bladder: significance for staging and prognosis. BJU Int. 2000;85:817–23.
14. Poulsen AL, Horn T, Steven K. Radical cystectomy: extending the limits of pelvic lymph node dissection improves survival for patients with bladder cancer confined to the bladder wall. J Urol. 1998;160: 2015–20.
15. Herr H, Lee C, Chang S, et al. Standardization of radical cystectomy and pelvic lymph node dissection for bladder cancer: a collaborative group report. J Urol. 2004;171:1823–8.
16. Herr HW, Faulkner JR, Grossman HB, et al. Surgical factors influence bladder cancer outcomes: a cooperative group report. J Clin Oncol. 2004;22:2781–9.
17. Hellenthal NJ, Hussain A, Andrews PE, et al. Lymphadenectomy at the time of robot-assisted radical cystectomy: results from the International Robotic Cystectomy Consortium. BJU Int. 2011;107: 642–6.
18. Davis JW, Gaston K, Anderson R, et al. Robot assisted extended pelvic lymphadenectomy at radical cystectomy: lymph node yield compared with second look open dissection. J Urol. 2010;185:79–84.
19. Lavery HJ, Martinez-Suarez HJ, Abaza R. Robotic extended pelvic lymphadenectomy for bladder cancer with increased nodal yield. BJU Int. 2011;107:1802–5.
20. Nix J, Smith A, Kurpad R, et al. Prospective randomized controlled trial of robotic versus open radical cystectomy for bladder cancer: perioperative and pathologic results. Eur Urol. 2010;57:196–201.
21. Pruthi RS, Wallen EM. Is robotic radical cystectomy an appropriate treatment for bladder cancer? Short-term oncologic and clinical follow-up in 50 consecutive patients. Urology. 2008;72:617–22.
22. Dasgupta P, Rimington P, Murphy D, et al. Robotic assisted radical cystectomy: short to medium term oncologic and functional outcomes. Int J Clin Pract. 2008;62:1709–14.
23. Martin AD, Nunez RN, Pacelli A, et al. Robot-assisted radical cystectomy: intermediate survival results at a mean follow-up of 25 months. BJU Int. 2010;105: 1706–9.
24. Kauffman EC, Ng CK, Lee MM, et al. Early oncologic outcomes for bladder urothelial carcinoma patients treated with robotic-assisted radical cystectomy. BJU Int. 2011;107:628–35.
25. Mmeje CO, Nunez-Nateras R, Nielsen ME, et al. Oncologic outcomes for lymph node-positive urothelial carcinoma patients treated with robot assisted radical cystectomy: with mean follow-up of 3.5 years. Urol Oncol. In press 2012.

Robot-Assisted Anterior Pelvic Exenteration for Bladder Cancer in the Female

7

Jeffrey W. Nix and Raj S. Pruthi

Introduction

Radical cystectomy remains one of the most effective oncologic treatments for patients with muscle-invasive bladder cancer and for those with high-grade, recurrent, noninvasive tumors. There continues to be an increasing number of anecdotal reports and case series for minimally invasive approaches to cystectomy. Laparoscopic and robot-assisted techniques have been shown to be viable approaches to cystectomy, demonstrating acceptable surgical and perioperative results [1–5]. A recent multi-institutional analysis encompassing four centers showed acceptable pathologic and perioperative outcomes for a robotic approach to radical cystectomy [6]. Potential benefits of laparoscopic and robotic approaches that have been described include lower surgical blood loss, early return of bowel function, and more rapid postoperative convalescence [3–5]. The majority of these series have reported techniques and outcomes in a predominantly male patient population. The applications of such novel techniques to female cystectomy and anterior exenterative procedures have not been well documented and described. However, given the successful application of robotic techniques in male patients, and given the growing experience of robotic approaches to hysterectomy, salpingo-oophorectomy, and other female pelvic procedures in the gynecologic literature, the stage has been set for the application of robotic approaches to anterior pelvic exenteration for female patients with bladder cancer [7, 8].

Cystectomy in male and female patents is different with regard to the surgical approach. Female patients have a broader pelvis with more ready access to the apical/urethral dissection than the male [9]. On the other hand, female pelvic anatomy may be less familiar to urologic surgeons due to the wealth of surgical experience in male patents, primarily owing to the treatment of prostatic diseases and malignancies. Even with bladder cancer, the preponderance of patients is male by a ratio of 3:1 [10]. Furthermore, the female cystectomy procedure includes exenteration of the anterior pelvic organs including the uterus, fallopian tubes, ovaries, and occasionally part or all of the anterior vaginal wall. Such procedures can be associated with increased blood loss and added morbidity that has been observed in female patients versus male patients in open radical cystectomy series by experienced surgeons [11].

The online version of this chapter (doi:10.1007/978-1-4614-4906-5_7) contains supplementary material, which is available to authorized users.

J.W. Nix, M.D. (✉)
Urologic Oncology Branch, National Cancer Institute, National Institutes of Health, 9000 Rockville Pike, 10 Center Drive, CRC Rm. 1-5940W, Bethesda, MD 20892, USA
e-mail: jeffrey.nix@nih.gov

R.S. Pruthi, M.D., F.A.C.S. (✉)
Department of Urology, The University of North Carolina at Chapel Hill, Chapel Hill, NC, USA
e-mail: rpruthi@med.unc.edu

E.P. Castle and R.S. Pruthi (eds.), *Robotic Surgery of the Bladder*, DOI 10.1007/978-1-4614-4906-5_7,

Herein we describe our technique and experience with robot-assisted radical anterior pelvic exenteration in the female including preoperative preparation, surgical steps, postoperative care while also describing our perioperative and pathologic outcomes of this novel procedure. We describe the stepwise approach to the robot-assisted radical anterior pelvic exenteration for urothelial carcinoma in the female allowing the urologic surgeon to more readily overcome the procedural learning curve.

Methods

Preoperative Evaluation

All patients should undergo appropriate preoperative lab work, imaging studies (chest X-ray, abdominal/pelvic cross-sectional imaging) and endoscopic resection with bimanual examination (i.e., transurethral resection of bladder tumor [TURBT]). Decisions for neoadjuvant chemotherapy should be made at the discretion of the treating medical team. At our institution, neoadjuvant chemotherapy is typically utilized in patients with clinical T3–4 tumors or suspected node positive disease. Overall, indications and preoperative decisions should not be changed by the surgical tool or approach utilized. Bladder cancer is an unforgiving disease and despite the novelty of such minimally invasive procedures and the potential short-term surgical and perioperative benefits, it remains imperative that any such procedure abide to the indications, standards, and principles of the open operation. It is paramount to observe and maintain the oncologic principles of radical cystectomy irrespective of surgical modifications.

Patient Selection

Appropriate patients, especially early in one's learning curve, include those who generally are in good health and performance status. We tend to avoid the robotic approach in patients with severe cardiopulmonary compromise—which is not an uncommon comorbidity due to the high levels of tobacco abuse in this patient population that contributes both to the development of urothelial carcinoma and cardiopulmonary disease. Limitations for patients in poor cardiopulmonary health status is primarily due to the positioning that includes extreme Trendelenburg that may exacerbate ventilatory difficulties and cardiac function.

In one's early experience, prolonged OR times may not be suitable for such patients. We recommend careful patient selection in one's initial experience with robotic anterior pelvic exenteration including patient characteristics as follows:

- Good performance status (independent) [12]
- Non-obese patients (BMI < 30)
- Healthy: age < 70, few comorbidities
- No previous intra-abdominal or pelvic surgery
- No prior chemotherapy or pelvic radiotherapy [13]
- Low volume disease (non-bulky tumors) [13]

Bowel Preparation

Two large prospective randomized trials in elective colorectal surgery, as well as a recent large meta-analysis showed no differeneces in anastamotic leaks, wound infections, fascial dehiscence, or overall morbidity or mortality between patients who received mechanical bowel preparation (MBP) versus no prep [14, 15]. To this end, in all patients undergoing radical cystectomy including those undergoing a robotic approach, we currently no longer perform a mechanical or antibiotic bowel preparation and patients are allowed a regular diet until midnight before surgery. We still use a Fleets® enema the morning of the procedure in order to evacuate the rectum and thereby reduce bowel distension in the deep pelvis.

Intraoperative Considerations

Intraoperative preparation includes shaving the patient from the costal margin to the pubis. The abdomen, perineum, vagina, upper thighs, and perianal area are prepped and draped in the usual sterile fashion. A 20-Fr urethral catheter is inserted. Intraoperative fluids are restricted to 500 ml/h as tolerated by the patient. This minimizes the risk of edema of the face and neck

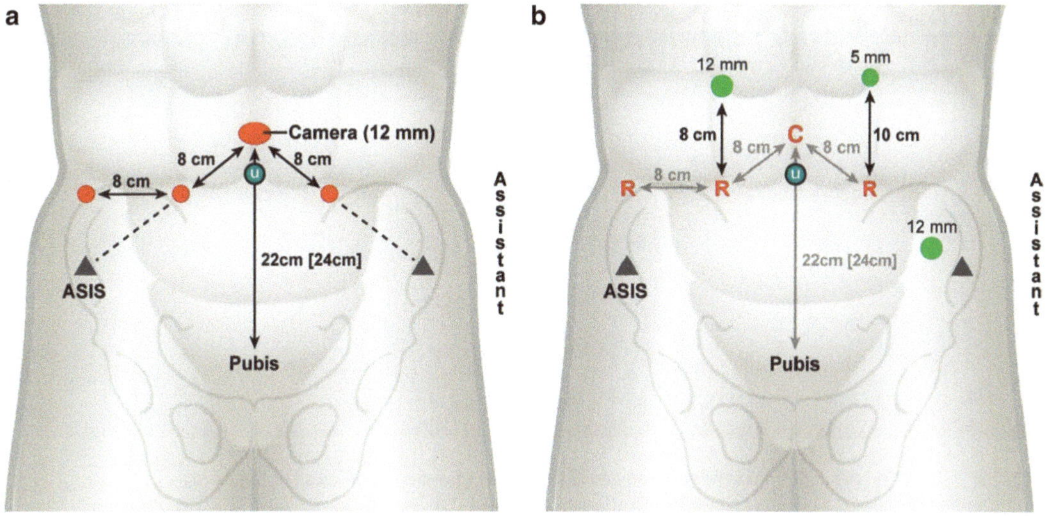

Fig. 7.1 Port placement including robotic ports (*red*) (**a**) and assistant ports (*green*) (**b**)

that can occur due to increased fluids and the steep Trendelenberg position. Multiple studies have also shown that appropriate intraoperative fluid restriction may significantly reduce complications, shorten hospital stay, and time to return of bowel function [16, 17]. A nasogastric or orogastric tube is inserted at the start of the procedure and removed at the end of the case. Occasionally the use of a uterine manipulator is employed and this is placed at the beginning of the case with the patient in the lithotomy position.

Steps of the Procedure

Positioning and Port Placement

Patient Positioning

After positioning, padding, securing, and preparing the patient in the supine position, the table is then placed in a steep Trendelenburg (>20°) position—identical to that of the robotic prostatectomy. For females, we use stirrups and the low lithotomy position with slight hip extension. Great care is taken to adequately pad and support the patient to avoid neuromuscular injury. Sequential compression devices are applied to the legs for DVT prophylaxis. We utilize a bean bag and cross-body taping to secure the patient adequately and test the positioning by tilting the table prior to the skin prep.

Port Placement

Port placement is similar to robotic prostatectomy with the addition of a 12-mm port on the side opposite of the assistant. Figures 7.1a, b and 7.2 demonstrate port placement based on a left-sided assistant. Veress insufflation is achieved through a vertical skin incision above the umbilicus, 22 cm above the symphysis pubis on the deflated abdomen. (In cases in which a more extended lymphadenectomy is anticipated [e.g., para-aortic dissection] or where an intracorporeal diversion is planned, this camera port is placed slightly higher at 24 cm above the symphysis.) The 12-mm camera port is placed here, and the remaining ports are placed under direct vision. Two 8 mm robotic ports are placed 8 cm away from the camera port, along the line from the camera port to the anterior spine of the iliac crest (ASIS) bilaterally. An additional 8 mm robotic port for the fourth arm is placed 8 cm directly lateral to the right sided robotic port. A 12-mm port for retraction and stapling is placed 8 cm cephalad to the robotic port on the right. A 5-mm port is placed 10 cm cephalad to the robotic port on the left. A 12-mm assistant port is placed two fingerbreadths medial and cephalad to the ASIS on the left. The port must be placed at least 8 cm away from the left robotic port and can be moved farther cephalad and lateral if necessary. The

a b

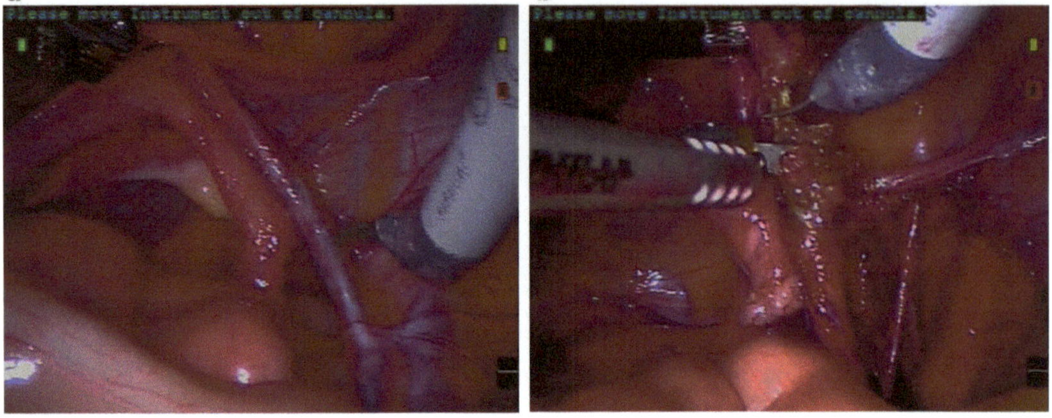

Fig. 7.2 Dissection (**a**) and bipolar fulguration and division (**b**) of ovarian pedicles (IP ligament)

patient is then placed in the steep Trendeleburg position and the robot is docked.

Procedural Steps

See Table 7.1 for list of instruments and accessories.

Divide Ovarian Pedicles (Infundibulopelvic [IP] Ligament)

After any sigmoid adhesions of the left side bladder and pelvis are released sharply, all of the small bowel is vacated from the pelvis. The ovarian pedicles (IP ligaments) are identified on each side superior and lateral to the ovaries themselves (Fig. 7.2a). A window is developed in the broad ligament isolating the ovarian pedicle. They can be ligated with the use of hemolock clips or alternatively fulgurated with the use of bipolar forceps before sharp division (Fig. 7.2b). With the posterior peritoneum overlying the ovarian pedicles incised, this peritoneal incision is extended along the broad ligament lateral to the fallopian tubes in the direction of the uterus and bladder. When the round ligaments are encountered, they are divided with the aid of the bipolar forceps and monopolar scissors. The fundus of the uterus is now freely mobile allowing greater manipulation of the uterus if desired and better visualization of the pelvic structures.

Table 7.1 Instruments and accessories

A. Recommended laparoscopic instruments
• 5 mm endoscopic long suction irrigator (45 mm) • 5 mm endoscopic scissors • 5 mm endoscopic locking grasper • 5 mm endoscopic needle driver (for passing suture) • 10 mm specimen retrieval bag
B. Recommended sutures/clips
• Dorsal vein stitch – 0 Vicryl on CT-2 (6 in.) • Ureteral and terminal ileum tags – 3-0 Vicryl on SH (full length) • Anastomosis stitch (for orthotopic diversion) – 3-0 Vicryl (or Monocryl) suture on RB-1 • Neobladder creation (intracorporeal diversion) – 2-0 Vicryl suture on SH – Stapler with vascular load • Ureteroenteric anastamosis (intracorproeal diversion) – 4-0 Vicryl suture on RB-1 suture • Hem-O-lock® (Weck Closure Systems, RTP, NC) large and extra large clips with endoscopic applier • Endovascular stapler/cutter with 60 mm vascular loads (e.g., Endo-GIA, Covidien, Mansfield, MA)
C. Recommended robotic instruments
• Two large needle drivers • Hot shears (monopolar curved scissors) • Maryland bipolar forceps • Cadiere bipolar graspers • Double fenestrated graspers (intracorporeal diversion)

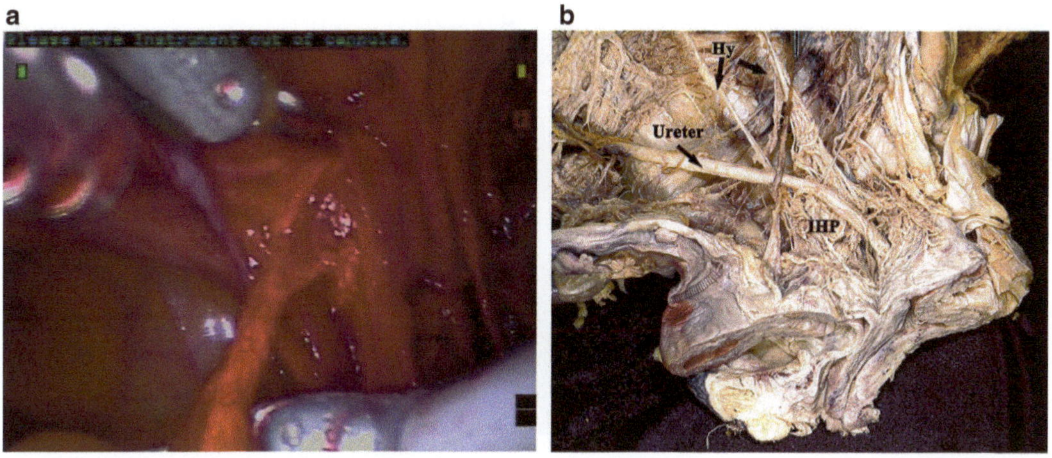

Fig. 7.3 (**a**) identification and dissection of ureters (**b**) Anatomic relationship between distal ureter and inferior hypogastric plexus. Photo used with permission by Keiichi Akita, Professor Clinical Anatomy, Tokyo Medical and Dental University

Isolate Ureters

With the posterior peritoneum incised along the ovaries and fallopian tubes, the medial edge of that incised peritoneum is grasped and lifted. The ureter can be found underlying and somewhat adhered to the posterior peritoneum along this medial leaflet. The ureter is encircled and the ureter is bluntly and sharply dissected distally down towards the level of the bladder (Fig. 7.3a). One should avoid grasping the ureter with the robotic instruments to avoid crush injury and resultant devascularization to the ureter itself. As one approaches the bladder they will encounter the uterine vasculature crossing lateral to medial towards the level of the cervix. Overly aggressive distal dissection in this area can result in bleeding as well as inadvertant damage to pelvic splanchnic nerves supplying portions of the vagina. Careful meticulous dissection in this area will identify the uterine vessels traveling just superficial to the ureter as they branch at the junction of the cervix and the vagina to form ascending and descending perforators to both structures. These uterine vessels (a.k.a the ventral vesicouterine ligament) can be isolated from the dorsally located ureter and transected with electrocautery. The ureter can easily be ligated at this point in most instances with adequate length for subsequent diversion. Hemolock clips (if desired a suture can be secured to the clips for the ureter as a tag for later identification) are used to ligate the ureters and they are divided at this level on each side. The transected ureters are tucked into the upper quadrants away from the pelvic dissection. If extra length on the ureters is desired, careful dissection posterior to the ureter at this level is mandatory, as the surgeon will encounter the vaginal artery and inferior hypogastric nerves. The nerves are located lateral and posterior to the ureter at the level of the uterine artery and ureter crossing in the dorsal vesicouterine ligament [8]. As the ureter enters the bladder, there is an avascular space just posterior to the ureter that can be widened with blunt dissection. Retraction of the ureter lateral and ventral will expose the dorsal vesicouterine ligaments, with its enclosed nerves, and prevent their transection. In general this extra ureteral length is not required. However, knowledge of the anatomy here will prevent transection of these nerves especially when dissecting lateral to the vagina at this level or if partial vaginectomy is required for proper surgical margins of the bladder (Fig. 7.3b).

Posterior Bladder Dissection

The peritoneum is incised between the level of the uterus and vagina (posteriorly) and the bladder (anteriorly): this incision can be made right at the level of the peritoneal reflection. With this lateral ("east to west") incision made, the plane between the bladder and the vagina can be developed bluntly. With the uterine manipulator or a vaginal sponge stick in place, the dissection is carried along the vaginal wall to create an

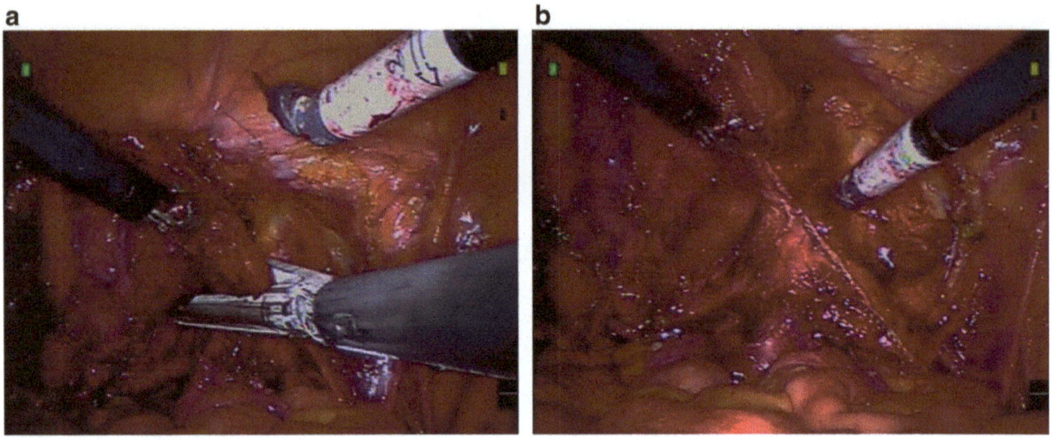

Fig. 7.4 Placement of endovascular stapler to divide pedicles (**a**) and image of divided bladder pedicle (**b**)

adequate wide margin on the level of the posterior bladder wall. In cases where a vaginal-sparing procedure is anticipated, this dissection can be taken down to the level of the bladder neck and urethra preserving the underlying arcus tendinous pelvic fascia (ATPF) The levator fascia, covering the levator ani complex, as it descends medially attaches to the arcus tendinous pelvic fascia (ATPF). The ATPF is composed of the pubocervical fascia, lying between the bladder and the vagina, as well as the rectovaginal septum. These structures are connected to one another as this fascial complex runs laterally to medially [19]. The preservation of this structure is important in nerve-sparing cystectomy as hstiologic studies have identiifed numerous sympthatic and parasympathetic nerve fibers within this mesh-like structure. This fascial plane also acts as a support structure and therfore preservation may decrease occurrence of pelvic organ prolapse and improve voiding patterns in orthotopic diversions [20]. However, as discussed in later sections, this fascial plane is difficult to distinguish as one reaches the level of the proximal urethra, and the muscular component of the anterior vaginal wall can contribute significantly to the posterior urethra at this level. If any aspect of the anterior vaginal wall is to be removed, the vagina can be entered and the anterior vaginal wall taken *en bloc* with the bladder thus creating the plane of dissection within the vagina itself.

Lateral Dissection

The peritoneum is incised just lateral to the medial umbilical ligaments on each side. This incision is carried laterally along side the bladder and extending posteriorly to the previously made peritoneal incisions overlying the ureter and between the bladder and uterus/vagina. (Of note the urachal and medial umbilical attachments are left intact to help suspend the bladder and facilitates the posterior and lateral dissection and the stapling of the bladder pedicles.) Blunt dissection can be used to develop the lateral perivesical space without much difficulty down to the level of the endopelvic fascia. In a non-orthotopic diversion or non-nerve-sparing procedure, the endopelvic fascia can be incised at this point. The lateral vascular pedicles of the bladder including the superior vesical artery can now be readily visualized.

Securing Bladder Pedicles

A laparoscopic endovascular stapler is used to ligate and transect the vascular pedicles to the bladder (Fig. 7.4a, b). Usually a single fire of a 60-mm stapler/cutter is sufficient to secure the bladder pedicles on each side. Alternatively these pedicles can be secured using the bipolar cautery or with the use of hemolock clips and then sharply divided. In cases where the anterior vaginal wall is to be taken *en bloc* with the bladder, the posterior plane of this dissection can be within the

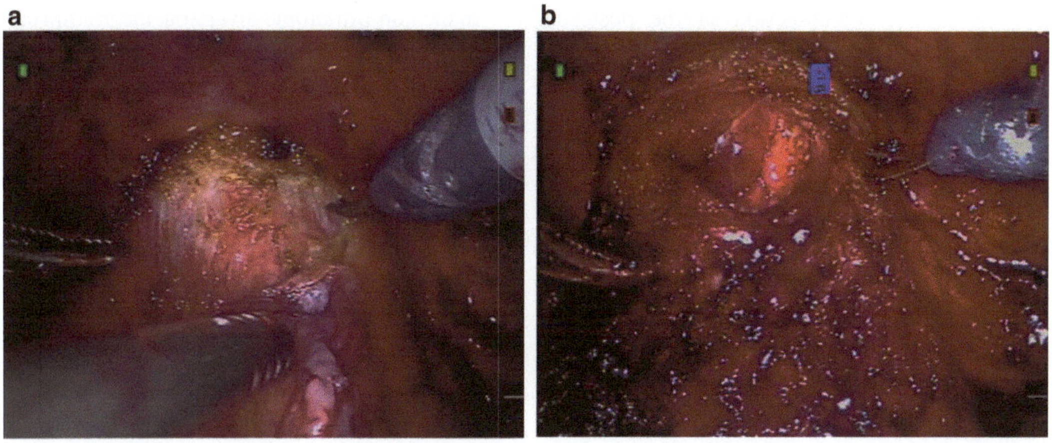

Fig. 7.5 Transection of urethra at the level of the bladder neck (**a**) in an orthotopic diversion. The bladder neck–urethral junction can be visualized and confirmed with catheter movement. Adequate urethral length remains after transection (**b**)

vagina itself—as opposed to between the bladder and vagina in a vaginal-sparing procedure. Vaginal entry can result in loss of pneumoperitoneum. To maintain insufflation pressure a moist laparotomy pad or large occlusive dressing (e.g., Tegaderm dressing, 3M Corp., St Paul, MN) is used to occlude the vaginal outlet and prevent loss of pneumoperitoneum.

Anterior Dissection

With the posterior and lateral dissections complete, attention is then turned anteriorly. The peritoneum is incised anteriorly through the medial umbilical ligament and the urachus thereby "dropping" the bladder. The anterior prevesical space is bluntly developed down to the level of the pubis and exposing the endopelvic fascia on each side. In an orthotopic diversion the endopelvic fascia is left intact to avoid any perturbance of the underlying continence mechanism in the female. In a non-orthotopic diversion the endopelvic fascia is incised, as noted previously, to allow for complete distal dissection of the bladder neck and urethra.

Bladder Neck/Urethral Dissection

The bladder neck is then approached anteriorly. In an orthotopic diversion, great care is made to create this transection precisely at the level of the bladder neck (Fig. 7.5a). Careful and continued evaluation at the location of the bladder neck is performed with the Foley catheter balloon in place to help visualize and identify the bladder neck. For this portion of the procedure the surgeon must carefully consider the competing interests of a sound cancer operation and functional preservation for the best quality of life postsurgically. However the clinican must remember that the foremost concern is for removal of cancerous tissue. Therefore the appropriate disseciton must be a case-by-case decision. In this context it is important to note that a functional and anatomical dissection can be achieved. Several principles are important to consider in regards to functional outcome: the preservation of the ATPF, maximizing urethral length, and preservation of lateral periurethral tissue. The first of these, ATPF preservation has been previously described in the section on posterior bladder dissection.

The contribution that urethral length provides for continence is debated; however, many urologists feel that both urethral length and closing urethral pressure are important considerations in female continence. Animal studies have shown that in a denervated urethra that closing urethral pressure is markedly decreased, therefore urethral length could be increasingly important in this situation [20]. This would argue for transection of the urethra as close to the bladder neck as possible.

However the composition of the posterior urethral wall is varied and has been shown, in cadaveric studies, to include significant contributions from the detrusor muscle in some cases [19]. It is therefore important that the clinician is mindful of this when completing the bladder neck dissection for the orthotopic diversion. Authors have advocated urethral transection as close as 5 mm to the bladder neck to around 1 cm, however, the decision is obviously a balance between sound oncologic principles and functional preservation and must be made at the time of dissection. Also the urethral margin that is performed for frozen section, if orthotopic diversion is desired, should make sure to include a portion of the posterior urethra based on anatomic and histologic studies.

The most common histologic appearance of the posterior urethra shows significant contribution from the anterior vaginal wall [19]. This makes a combined approach to the urethra ideal in our experience. The posterior plane dissection, as described above, significantly aids in delineation of the posterior plane up to the level of the bladder neck and posterior urethra. Then once the bladder is released from its peritoneal attachments the urethra can be isolated with an anterior approach.

The preservation of the lateral peri-urethral tissues is not dissimilar to the dissection that is carried out in the male patient. This tissue contains the perineal membrane, a U-shaped structure at the level of the mid urethra. This supporting structure consisting of collagen and elastic fibers and runs from the anterior mid urethra posterio lateral to the vagina and terminates at the level of the perineal body. This structure is felt to provide support for the urethra and contains in its lateral portion abundant nervous tissue. The cavernous nerves that supply innervation to the vaginal vestibule and vestibular glands runs through the ATPF on the posteriolateral side of the vagina and as it runs more superficial penetrates and runs on the lateral portion of the perineal membrane to supply these structures. Therefore protection of this tissue and medial dissection of the urethra and perineal membrane will aid in sexual preservation for the patient [19].

In the non-orthotopic diversion, the urethra can be dissected quite distally. When a complete urethrectomy is desired, we circumferentially incise the urethra at the beginning of the case before docking the robot. Bovie electrocautery on cutting current can help release the urethra from the vaginal mucosa and allow for a more complete urethrectomy when approached transperitoneally with the robotic dissection. Before transecting or delivering the urethra, we will typically place an extra large hemolock clip on the bladder (specimen) side to avoid any urine spillage.

After urethral transection, some remaining posterior lateral attachments will remain and these can often be divided with blunt and sharp dissection and with the use of monopolar and bipolar cautery. If the anterior vaginal wall has been incised en bloc, the entire bladder and anterior vaginal wall specimen can be removed through the vagina or placed in an impermeable bag.

Specimen Retrieval

In cases of an orthotopic diversion after the bladder neck has been transected at the appropriate level, the Foley catheter is left in place and the remainder of the bladder specimen is completely freed dividing any remaining posterior–lateral attachments. The catheter is clipped with an extra large hemolock (to avoid any urinary spillage and contamination), the Foley is transected, and the cut end is brought into the pelvis (Fig. 7.6a). The specimen is then placed in an impermeable retrievable bag that is moved out of the pelvis (Fig. 7.6b). The pelvis is irrigated, vaginal surface inspected, and hemostasis ensured. A urethral margin is sent for frozen section evaluation.

Vaginal Reconstruction/Hysterectomy/Oophorectomy

This portion of the procedure can either be performed before or after the cystectomy. Blunt and sharp dissection allows for complete freeing up of fallopian tubes and ovaries down to the level of the cervix. The uterus is lifted and the peritoneum is incised circumferentially at the level of the cervix. The lateral tissue at the level of the cervix is fulgurated with the liberal use of the bipolar

a b

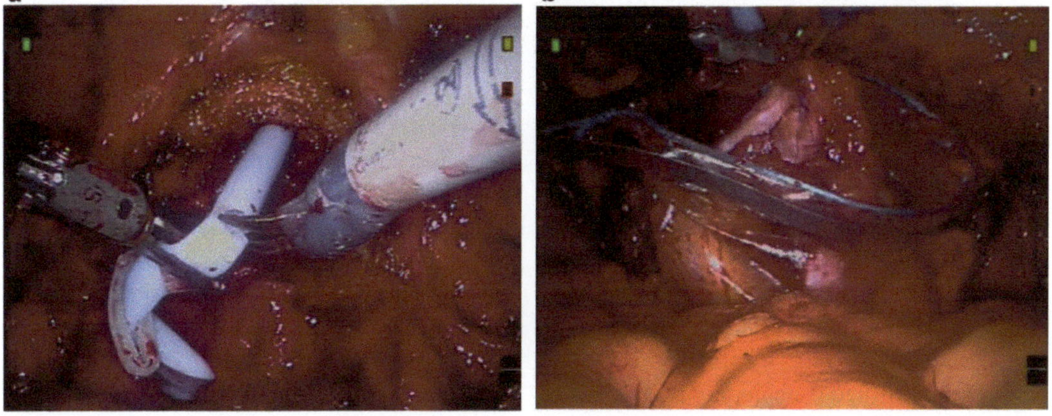

Fig. 7.6 Division of catheter (**a**) and placement of bladder in specimen bag (**b**)

forceps as this is the site of much of the uterine blood supply. The uterus can then be transected at the level of the cervix again with liberal use of monopolar and bipolar cautery. As previously discussed the hypogastric nerves and inferior hypogastric plexus will be located deep to the cardinal ligaments at this level and should not be encountered in a transcervical or supracervical hysterectomy. With the transection complete, the uterus, fallopian tubes, and ovaries are freed and removed out of the pelvis. In a vaginal-sparing procedure, the small os at the level of the cervix remains the only opening into the vagina and this is closed with a figure-of-eight 0 Vicryl suture on a CT2 needle. If the anterior vaginal wall was excised en bloc with the bladder, this defect can be closed in continuity with the reapproximation of the vaginal walls. We typically use a 0 Vicryl suture on a CT2 needle to reconstruct the vagina in a caudad to cephalad (i.e., north to south) manner. Depending on the remaining vaginal anatomy, this can also be done in a transverse manner if appropriate. If orthotopic diversion is desired the surgeon should attempt to prevent overlapping suture lines or plan for interposition of omental tissue if necessary.

Pelvic Lymphadenectomy

The initial surgical step is to identify and expose the external iliac artery and vein. On occasion, these vessels are readily visualized laparoscopically. In some cases, particularly in obese patients, the vessels need to be located and exposed from within the overlying retroperitoneal fat. In such cases, the external iliac artery can be located by noting pulsations along its anticipated course. Blunt dissection (e.g., with the closed scissor tips by the surgeon or with the suction irrigator by the assistant) along the external iliac artery and vein exposes these structures. Blunt and sharp dissection is carried down to the anterior surface of the external iliac artery. The vein can then be found lying immediately adjacent (posterior and medial) to the artery. It is important to dissect into the correct fibroalveolar plane just overlying the artery and the vein. This will allow for easier and more precise dissection of the lymph node packets for the remainder of the procedure. Margins of lymphadenectomy vary according to the discretion of the surgeon, and generally include the obturator nodes, the external iliac nodes, and the common iliac nodes. Para-aortic lymphadenectomy is also possible, particularly with the use of the Da Vinci S and Si systems which allows for more range of motion of the robotic arms. It is important that the surgeon is familiar with the neuroanatomy of the distal aorta at its termination into the common iliac arteries. The superior hypogastric nerve fibers and plexus, containing sympathetic and afferent somatic innervation to pelvic structures, will be located overlying the distal aorta at this level. In patients with significant retroperitoneal fat, these nerve structures may be difficult to visualize and require careful dissection.

The obturator and hypogastric lymph node dissection is begun by locating and developing the medial border of the external iliac vein, thereby exposing the obturator fossa posteriorly. Dissection along the external iliac vein must be done with great care to avoid a venous injury, because the vein is decompressed due to the steep Trendelenberg position. With the medial edge of the external iliac vein identified, the plane between the vein and the obturator packet can be extended to the pubic bone distally. Care must be made to identify the circumflex vein distally and any aberrant branches of the external iliac or obturator veins. Blunt and sharp dissection with the aid of monopolar scissors and fenestrated bipolar graspers—and with the appropriate counter traction placed by the assistant or the surgeon's nondominant hand—can be used to facilitate this dissection by retracting the vein laterally and the obturator node packet medially. Once the dissection off the external iliac vein is complete, the nodal packet can be dissected bluntly off the obturator nerve and vessels posteriorly. In a transperitoneal approach it is not necessary to ligate every lymphatic channel. Monopolar and bipolar cautery can aid in division of smaller lymphatic channels and the use of laparoscopic clips (e.g., Hem-o-lock™ clips) can be used to ligate larger lymphatic channels, pedicles, and vein branches as necessary. The pubic bone and anterior surface of obturator nerve and vessels mark the distal margin of the nodal packet. With the obturator packet freed and divided distally (down to and including the so-called node of Cloquet), it is peeled backed in the cephalad direction to the level of the hypogastric artery—keeping the obturator nerve, medial border of the external iliac vein, and the medial umbilical ligament in clear view. The medial umbilical ligament should be retracted medially to achieve proper exposure for the hypogastric dissection.

The base of the node packet near the internal iliac artery must be dissected with care as the internal iliac artery does not have the same fibroalveolar sheath as the external vessels. Consequently, the nodal tissue can be somewhat adherent with greater need for sharp dissection and coagulation of lymphatic and vascular attachments before division of the cephalad aspect of the packet near the level of the internal iliac artery.

Once the obturator/hypogastric dissection is complete, the extended dissection is undertaken, beginning distally, cephalad to and along the external iliac artery. Again, it is crucial to dissect down to the correct fibroalveolar plane over the artery. While avoiding the circumflex vein distally, all lymphatic tissue is taken between the external iliac vein and artery and laterally on the psoas muscle to the genitofemoral nerve. With this packet divided distally, this lymph tissue is teased and dissected in the cephalad direction with blunt and sharp dissection, occasionally using monopolar and bipolar cautery. Unlike the external iliac vein, it is quite rare to encounter aberrant branches off of the artery, and this dissection is readily performed proximally up to and along the common iliac vessels. One needs to remain cognizant that the ureter will be encountered crossing over the common iliac vessels. If desired, a para-aortic dissection can be accomplished robotically (particularly with the new generation—da Vinci S or Si—robot). If a para-aortic dissection is anticipated and the classic da Vinci platform is used, it may be necessary to place the robotic ports approximately 2 cm superior or cephalad than the typical configuration.

Tagging the Ureters

Before undocking the robot, the ureters are returned to the pelvis. At the distal end of each ureter, a full length 3-0 Vicryl stitch on an SH needle is placed as a tag, and the ends are brought out through the assistant ports on each side. This allows for ready identification and localization of both ureters. A 3-0 Vicryl stitch is placed in the terminal ileum to allow for its ready identification during the urinary diversion. In the case of an orthotopic neobladder, 3-0 Vicryl sutures (on RB-1 needles) are placed at the 5 o'clock and 7 o'clock positions in the urethra and left in the pelvis. These posterior sutures are sometimes the most difficult to place in an open fashion and preplacement under robotic guidance is easier. The robot is then undocked. The robot is not re-docked later for the anastomosis, as this portion of the operation is easily accomplished through the small incision made next.

Urinary Diversion

After the robot is undocked, all ports are removed. The ureteral sutures are kept through their corresponding port sites and tagged. It is important to keep the patient in the Tredelenberg position initially in order to prevent the intestine from descending into the pelvis. A 6–8 cm incision is made midway from umbilicus to the pubis to perform the urinary diversion. Typically, an abdominal wall retractor is not required and minimizing abdominal wall retraction may help reduce post-operative incisional musculoskeletal pain. Through this incision any further mobilization of the ureters can be carried out if needed. For an ileal conduit, the left ureter is tunneled under the sigmoid mesentery. In the case of an orthotopic neobladder where the afferent limb lies on the left side, the right ureter is tunneled underneath the sigmoid mesentery. The terminal ileum is identified with the assistance of the preplaced stitch, and the segment of bowel is harvested. The planned urinary diversion is then performed extracorporeally and the ureteroenteric anastomosis completed. For an orthotopic neobladder, the preplaced posterior urethral stitches are placed in their proper position in the neobladder neck. Anterior anastomotic sutures are placed thereafter. After the anastomotic sutures are placed and tagged, the patient is taken out of the Trendelenberg position.

More recently in certain cases we have performed the urinary diversion intracorporeally—including both ileal conduits and orthotopic ileal neobladders (Fig. 7.7). In such cases, the specimen is extracted through the vagina—either through the anterior vaginotomy in cases in which the anterior vaginal wall is removed or through a separate incision in the posterior vaginal wall in a vaginal-sparing procedure. A posterior incision is used in such cases to avoid the potential for overlapping suture lines in cases of orthotopic neobladder creation.

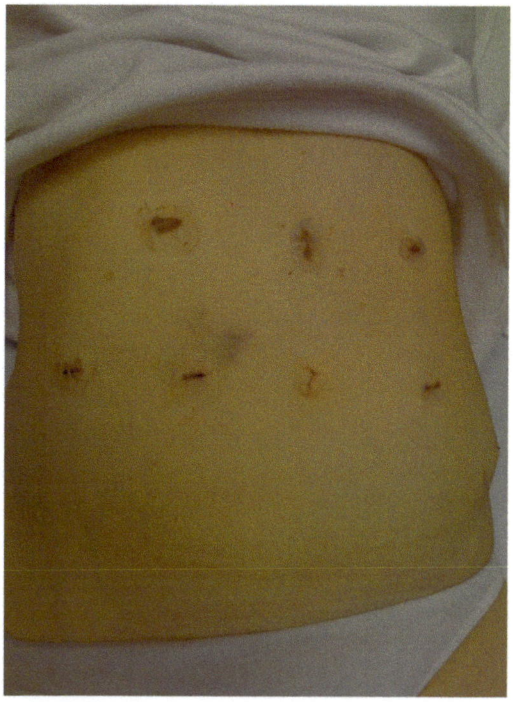

Fig. 7.7 Postoperative picture of female patient who has undergone robotic anterior pelvic exenteration, bilateral pelvic lymphadenectomy, and intracorporeal orthotopic ileal neobladder

A pelvic drain (ten French Jackson–Pratt drain) is placed, and the incisions are closed. Of note, we do not typically reapproximate the fascia on laparoscopic or robotic ports less than or equal to 12 mm.

Postoperative Care

During closure of incisions, fluids are liberalized with the goal of a 1 l bolus of intravenous fluids before leaving the OR. Postoperative care is routine and at the discretion of the surgeon. In our practice we had found no added benefit of leaving the NG tube even overnight and now routinely employ an OG tube intraoperatively that is removed at the end of the case.

After completing the procedure, all patients were taken to the urology inpatient ward and underwent routine postoperative care per our cystectomy care pathway which has previously been reported and which includes the use of

Table 7.2 Cystectomy fast-track program

Preoperative
Counseling/expectations
Outpatient bowel prep (day before surgery)
– Magnesium citrate solution—1 bottle (8 oz) – Fleets® enema – Clear liquid diet
Surgical
– Perioperative antibiotics (seconds or third generation cephalosporin) × 24 h – Removal of OG tube at end of procedure
Postoperative
Prokinetic agents (e.g., metoclopramide 10 mg i.v. q 8 h × 48 h)
Non-narcotic analgesics (e.g., ketorolac 30 mg i.v. q 6 h × 48 h reduce dose to 15 mg i.v. in patients > 65 years)
Early ambulation
Fast-track diet (advanced irrespective of bowel function)
– POD#1—chewing gum initiated (ad lib) otherwise NPO – POD#2—clear liquids—8 oz per 8 h – POD#3—unrestricted clear liquids – POD#4—regular diet

Table 7.3 Perioperative outcomes

	Female ($n=30$)	Male ($n=80$)
Mean age	69.4 years*	63.4 years
Mean BMI	26.3 kg/m^2	27.8 kg/m^2
Mean ASA score	2.8	2.7
Diversion		
Conduit	22	44
Neobladder	8	35
None	0	1
Mean EBL (range)	234 ml	283 ml
Mean OR time (range)	4.4 h*	4.8 h
Post-op		
Mean time to flatus	2.0 days	2.1 days
Mean time to BM	2.7 days	2.8 days
Mean time to discharge	5.1 days	4.7 days
Mean LN yield	18.8	19.1

*$p<0.05$

pro-kinetic agents and non-narcotic analgesics. In addition we employ a "fast-track" program of early diet advancement irrespective of status of flatus or bowel movement (see Table 7.2) [12].

The pelvic drain is typically removed prior to discharge. The patient returns at 10–14 days postoperatively for removal of the ureteral stents. In addition, in the case of an orthotopic neobladder, they will return 17–21 days after surgery for a cystogram and catheter removal. Clinical and oncologic follow-up is thereafter performed in stage-specific manner.

Results

We have performed robot-assisted radical cystectomy in 110 cases and applied it to female patients in 30 procedures. Our experience and perioperative outcomes with robotic anterior pelvic exenteration in the first 30 consecutive female cases are shown in Table 7.3 with comparisons made to 80 male patients also undergoing a robot-assisted radical cystectomy. Female patients were older (69.4 years vs. 63.4 years; $p=0.006$) and had shorter OR time (4.4 h vs. 4.8 h; $p=0.046$) but were not different with regard to other perioperative outcomes. It should be noted that our initial learning curve with robot-assisted radical cystectomy of 20 cases were all male patients and these were included in this comparison.

Pathologic outcomes have also demonstrated an appropriate extirpative procedure in that no patient has a positive margin, and a mean number of lymph nodes removed is 19 (range 9–34) with our standard and extended dissection. Short-term (within 30 days of surgery) complication rate was 23 %. Complications included ileus, a fever of unknown origin, anastamotic urine leak, DVT, acute renal failure, and stent obstruction.

Comment

Despite the novelty of such minimally invasive procedures, several principles and standards must be rigorously evaluated and maintained. First, it remains paramount to observe and maintain the oncologic principles of this operation irrespective of surgical modifications. That is, pathologic endpoints, and consequently oncologic outcomes, must never be compromised with such newer techniques. Second, such procedures should have appropriate perioperative outcomes with regard to operative time, surgical blood loss, and length of hospital stay. Such measures may reflect and impact on patient morbidity and recovery and may also indicate operative difficulty (i.e., the learning curve) for the surgeon. For example, in robotic prostatectomy procedures, operative times have been used as an indirect measure of surgical difficulty and of progress in overcoming the learning curve [22]. Accordingly, novel procedures should not result in insurmountable difficulties or excess morbidities for surgeon or patient alike. Last, any such new procedures should not expose patients to any undue or excessive complications.

In our experience, the oncologic principles and pathologic outcomes appear to be maintained with a robotic approach. In no case has a positive margin observed. In addition, the pelvic lymphadenectomy remains an important aspect of radical cystectomy, and, in our experience, an external iliac and even common iliac lymph node dissection can be readily performed robotically. Indeed, our mean lymph node count of 19 with the robotic approach compares favorably to the mean lymph node count of 16 observed in our open cystectomy experience [5].

Indeed, with regard to perioperative outcomes, the robotic approach to anterior exenteration is associated with a relatively low surgical blood loss. Our low operative blood loss of 234 ml compares favorably to our own open experience and that of other reports in the literature [11, 23]. Indeed, in the report by Lee et al. for open radical cystectomy, blood loss and transfusion requirements in females were significantly higher than that of males [11] In addition, postoperative outcomes including time to flatus, time to bowel movement, and time to hospital discharge are also favorable in our experience.

In our experience, we only attempted robot-assisted radical cystectomy after a wealth of experience and sense of proficiency in both open cystectomy and robotic prostatectomy. And, it is only after an initial robot-assisted radical cystectomy experience of 20 men, did we initiate our robotic series in female patients. It is interesting to note that no differences were observed in the subsequent male series and the concurrent initial female experienc. It appears that a new learning curve for robotic anterior exenteration does not appear to have clinical difficulties or complications with regard to OR time, blood loss, and postoperative convalescence when the female experience is embarked upon after an initial approach in male patients. In other words, transition to proficiency in anterior pelvic exenteration occurred readily with near identical outcomes as the concurrent male experience. It is unclear as to how these outcomes would have differed if female patients were part of that initial learning curve.

In conclusion, in our experience, the robotic anterior exenteration has been readily adapted to the surgical treatment of bladder cancer. The approach appears to achieve the clinical and oncologic goals of radical cystectomy in the female.

Editors' Commentary

Erik P. Castle and Raj S. Pruthi

Cystectomy in male and female patents is different with regard to the surgical approach. Female patients have a broader pelvis with more ready access to the apical/urethral dissection than the male. On the other hand, female pelvic anatomy may be less familiar to urologic surgeons due to the wealth of surgical experience in male patents, primarily owing to the treatment of prostatic diseases and malignancies. Even with bladder cancer, the preponderance of patients are male by a ratio of 3:1. It is therefore not surprising that urologists may be less familiar with female pelvic surgical anatomy, especially with regard to laparoscopic and robotic approaches. Furthermore, the female cystectomy procedure includes exenteration of the anterior pelvic organs including the uterus, fallopian tubes, ovaries, and occasionally part or all of the anterior vaginal wall. Such procedures can be associated with increased blood loss and added morbidity that has been observed in female patients versus male patients in open radical cystectomy series by experienced surgeons.

In our experience, we only attempted the robot-assisted radical cystectomy after a wealth of experience and sense of proficiency in both open cystectomy and robotic prostatectomy.

And, it is only after an initial robotic cystectomy experience of 20 men, did we initiate our robotic series in female patients.

This chapter describes the technique and experience with robot-assisted radical anterior pelvic exenteration in the female including preoperative preparation, surgical steps, postoperative care while also describing our perioperative and pathologic outcomes of this novel procedure. The stepwise approach will hopefully allow the urologic surgeon to more readily overcome the procedural learning curve encountered with robotic surgery in the female patient.

References

1. Cathelineau X, Arroyo C, Rozet F, Barret E, Vallancien G. Laparoscopic assisted radical cystectomy: the montsouris experience after 84 cases. Eur Urol. 2005;47:780.
2. Simonato A, Gregori A, Lissiani A, Bozzola A, Galli S, Gaboardi F. Laparoscopic radical cystoprostatectomy: our experience in a consecutive series of 10 patients with a 3 years follow-Up. Eur Urol. 2005;47:785.
3. Rhee JJ, Lebeau S, Smolkin M, Theodorescu D. Radical cystectomy with ileal conduit diversion: early prospective evaluation of the impact of robotic assistance. BJU Int. 2006;98:1059.
4. Guru KA, Kim HL, Piacente PM, Mohler JL. Robot-assisted radical cystectomy and pelvic lymph node dissection: initial experience at Roswell Park Cancer Institute. Urology. 2007;69:469.
5. Pruthi RS, Wallen EM. Robotic assisted laparoscopic radical cystoprostatectomy: operative and pathological outcomes. J Urol. 2007;178:814.
6. Smith AB, Raynor M, Amling CL, et al. Multi-institutional analysis of robotic radical cystectomy for bladder cancer: perioperative outcomes and complications in 227 patients. J Laparoendosc Adv Surg Tech A. 2012;22(1):17–21.
7. Swan K, Advincula AP. Role of robotic surgery in urogynecologic surgery and radical hysterectomy: how far can we go? Curr Opin Urol. 2011;21(1):78–83.
8. Nezhat C, Saberi NS, Shahmohamady B, Nezhat F. Robotic-assisted laparoscopy in gynecological surgery. JSLS. 2006;10(3):317–20.
9. Stein JP, Skinner DG. Radical cystectomy – technique and outcomes. In: Lerner SP, Schoenberg MP, Sternberg CN, editors. Textbook of bladder cancer. Boca Raton, FL: Taylor and Francis; 2006. p. 445–69. Ref Type: Edited Book.
10. Hall MC, Chang SS, Dalbagni G, et al. Guideline for the management of nonmuscle invasive bladder cancer (stages Ta, T1, and Tis): 2007 update. J Urol. 2007;178:2314.
11. Lee KL, Freiha F, Presti Jr JC, Gill HS. Gender differences in radical cystectomy: complications and blood loss. Urology. 2004;63:1095.
12. Hollenbeck BK, Miller DC, Taub D, et al. Identifying risk factors for potentially avoidable complications following radical cystectomy. J Urol. 2005;174:1231.
13. Orvieto MA, DeCastro GJ, Trinh QD, et al. Oncological and functional outcomes after robot-assisted radical cystectomy: critical review of current status. Urology. 2011;78:977.
14. Matsou A, Vrakas G, Doulgerakis M, Hatzimisios K, Zandes N, Saliangas K. Mechanical bowel preparation before elective colorectal surgery: is it necessary? Tech Coloproctol. 2011;15 Suppl 1:S59.
15. Cao F, Li J, Li F. Mechanical bowel preparation for elective colorectal surgery: updated systematic review and meta-analysis. Int J Colorectal Dis. 2012;27(6):803–10.
16. de Aguilar-Nascimento JE, Diniz BN, Do Carmo AV, Silveira EA, Silva RM. Clinical benefits after the implementation of a protocol of restricted perioperative intravenous crystalloid fluids in major abdominal operations. World J Surg. 2009;33:925.
17. Lobo DN, Bostock KA, Neal KR, Perkins AC, Rowlands BJ, Allison SP. Effect of salt and water balance on recovery of gastrointestinal function after elective colonic resection: a randomised controlled trial. Lancet. 2002;359:1812.
18. Magrina JF, Pawlina W, Kho RM, Magtibay PM. Robotic nerve-sparing radical hysterectomy: feasibility and technique. Gynecol Oncol. 2011;121:605.
19. Hinata N, Murakami G, Abe S, et al. Detailed histological investigation of the female urethra: application to radical cystectomy. J Urol. 2012;187:451.
20. Bhatta DN, Kessler TM, Mills RD, Burkhard F, Studer UE. Nerve-sparing radical cystectomy and orthotopic bladder replacement in female patients. Eur Urol. 2007;52:1006.
21. Pruthi RS, Chun J, Richman M. Reducing time to oral diet and hospital discharge in patients undergoing radical cystectomy using a perioperative care plan. Urology. 2003;62:661.
22. Herrell SD, Smith Jr JA. Robotic-assisted laparoscopic prostatectomy: what is the learning curve? Urology. 2005;66:105.
23. Chang SS, Smith Jr JA, Wells N, Peterson M, Kovach B, Cookson MS. Estimated blood loss and transfusion requirements of radical cystectomy. J Urol. 2001;166:2151.

Variations in Surgical Approach: Partial Cystectomy, Vaginal-Sparing, and Prostate-Sparing

8

Anthony N. Hoang, Ashok K. Hemal, and Piyush K. Agarwal

Introduction

Since its first description in the 1950s by Whitmore and Marshall, radical cystectomy (RC) has been the first-line therapy for the treatment of muscle-invasive bladder cancer as well as refractory cases of high grade, non-muscle-invasive transitional cell carcinoma, or carcinoma in situ (CIS) [1]. According to the surveillance, epidemiology, and end results (SEER) database, more than 70,000 Americans will be diagnosed with bladder cancer in 2012 with approximately 25 % presenting with muscle invasion at diagnosis [2]. Radical cystectomy, considered to be the most effective treatment method for localized muscle-invasive disease, is a highly morbid procedure and has been known to adversely impact both urinary and sexual functions [3–5]. Unlike the incidence rate that increases with age, the rate of radical cystectomy can be as high as 58 % among those patients who are less than 65 years of age, which comprises roughly 30 % of newly diagnosed cases [2]. Standard operation requires complete removal of the bladder in addition to bilateral pelvic lymphadenectomy. In men, the seminal vesicles and prostate are also removed; whereas in women, the uterus, vagina, and bilateral ovaries are also removed as these organs may harbor disease and serve as a source for recurrent tumor. Although removal of the sexual/reproductive organs with the bladder and lymph nodes provides the greatest chance for oncologic cure, it comes with the price of functional morbidities such as infertility, sexual dysfunction, impotence, and urinary incontinence [6]. Even in the best hands with nerve-sparing techniques, the rates of urinary incontinence and erectile dysfunction could be as high as 30 % and 80 %, respectively [7, 8]. Furthermore, urinary diversion poses risks for ileus, rapid colonic transit with diarrhea, malabsorption, metabolic derangements, pyelonephritis, and calculi [3, 4, 9, 10]. Concerns about functional outcomes play an important role in the decision-making process, especially in young patients in whom these quality-of-life issues remain a top priority. To minimize the risk of urinary incontinence and impotence without compromising oncological efficacy, many strategies such as partial cystectomy (PC), vaginal-sparing radical cystectomy (VSRC), and prostate-sparing radical cystectomy (PSRC) have evolved.

A.N. Hoang
Urologic Oncology Branch, National Cancer Institute, National Institute of Health, Bethesda, MD 20892, USA

A.K. Hemal
Wake Forest Baptist Health, Winston-Salem, NC 27157, USA

P.K. Agarwal, M.D. (✉)
Urologic Oncology Branch, National Cancer Institute, National Institute of Health, Bethesda, MD 20892, USA

Urologic Oncology Branch, National Cancer Institute, National Institute of Health, Building 10 – CRC, Room 2-5952, 10 Center Drive, MSC 1210, Bethesda, MD 20892-1210, USA
e-mail: piyush.agarwal@nih.gov

E.P. Castle and R.S. Pruthi (eds.), *Robotic Surgery of the Bladder*, DOI 10.1007/978-1-4614-4906-5_8,

While these approaches may not be appropriate for all patients, many contemporary series have reported superior urinary continence and potency rates in addition to comparable oncological outcomes in carefully selected group of patients. In this chapter, we seek to present the indications and techniques of these surgical variations on robot-assisted cystoprostatectomies and anterior pelvic exenterations.

Preoperative Evaluation

Candidates for PC, VSRC, and PSRC undergo extensive medical evaluation that includes detailed medical history, meticulous physical exam, comprehensive blood work, review of outside pathology by the urologist and GU pathologist, and a restaging workup as described below. Those with comorbidities must receive preoperative medical clearance from their respective specialists. All patients must undergo a restaging workup that consists of the following: (1) a bimanual examination to assess for bladder mobility and the potential presence of clinical T3 disease; (2) an endoscopic resection of any bladder tumors or the tumor bed; and (3) a metastatic workup that includes chest, abdominal, and pelvic cross-sectional imaging and in select settings, a bone scan.

For candidates for PSRC, digital rectal exam (DRE), prostate-specific antigen (PSA) levels, and standard transrectal ultrasound-guided (TRUS) prostate biopsy are warranted to rule out the presence of prostate cancer. Specifically for candidates of PC, special attention during endoscopic evaluation should be given to the tumor size, location, and multifocal status in addition to performing random bladder and prostatic urethral biopsies to rule out concomitant presence of CIS and/or urethral involvement. For candidates of VSRC, of particular importance is the exclusion of gynecologic malignancies such as ovarian or cervical cancers.

Additionally, patients also meet with the anesthesiologist for pre-anesthesia clearance, wound ostomy nurse for conduit care or neobladder self catheterization education, and social workers for any other nonmedical-related issues. Lastly, every patient's case is discussed in a multidisciplinary tumor conference where inputs from medical oncologist, radiation oncologist, pathologist, and radiologist are taken into consideration to determine the patient's best course of treatment.

Patient Preparation

Bowel preparation in minimally invasive surgery is evolving to less intense regimens with increasing surgical experience. Traditional mechanical bowel preparation with large volume polyethylene glycol–electrolyte solution and antibiotic preparation is no longer recommended as there are no significant differences in the rates of anastamotic leakage, abdomino-pelvic abscess, or postoperative ileus between those who received and did not receive it. In fact, there is a significant increase in cardiac events among those who received mechanical bowel preparation [11]. Currently, the authors favor one bottle of magnesium citrate in the afternoon on the day prior to surgery along with a clear liquid-only diet. On the morning of the surgery, a broad-spectrum antibiotic, such as a second-generation cephalosporin (cefoxitin), is administered along with deep vein thrombosis (DVT) prophylaxis in the form of 5,000 U of subcutaneous heparin. Recently, we have been administering alvimopan, a peripherally acting mu-opioid receptor antagonist, which has been shown to expedite the return of bowel function after bowel surgery [12, 13].

Positioning

Prior to prepping and positioning the patient, intraoperative preparation includes shaving of the abdomen ± external genitalia, appropriate padding of all pressure points, properly applying bilateral compressive stockings for DVT prophylaxis, and adequately securing the patient to the table. Using stirrups, positioning involves placing the patient in low lithotomy with the legs apart to accommodate the robot. Next, the abdomen and external genitalia are thoroughly prepped and draped in standard sterile fashion with the exclusion of the anus and perianal area. A 20Fr. foley catheter is inserted and left to gravity drainage. The table is then placed in steep Trendelenburg's position.

Partial Cystectomy (PC)

Indications

Partial cystectomy was initially popularized in the 1950s as a means to achieve comparable oncological control while minimizing the significant morbidities associated with radical cystectomy [14]. Retrospective studies have revealed that between 6 and 10 % of patients with muscle invasive urothelial cancer could benefit from a less radical approach without sacrificing cancer control [15, 16]. Historically, partial cystectomy was perceived to be inadequate due to its high rate of loco-regional recurrence, but this likely resulted from suboptimal patient selection [17]. Several areas of concerns regarding partial cystectomy have been raised. These included the multifocal nature of transitional cell carcinoma and carcinoma-in-situ (CIS), the ability to completely resect the tumor with negative margins, the sufficiency of remaining bladder capacity, and the role of lymphadenectomy [18].

Currently, stringent selection criteria which address the above concerns have reduced the recurrence rate to an acceptable level while optimizing overall survival. Importantly, sexual potency and urinary continence are maximized in the process. Just as the name implies, partial cystectomy involves a full thickness, wide surgical excision of the cancer-involved portion of the bladder along with a healthy margin and the overlying fat. In addition, the regional lymph nodes are also removed, permitting accurate staging. However, this approach should only be limited to patients with the following criteria:

- Functional bladder with good capacity.
- Solitary, primary urothelial tumor at the dome, urachal tumor, or tumor residing in a diverticulum.
- No concomitant carcinoma-in-situ.
- No evidence of lymphadenopathy or metastatic disease.

Steps of the Procedure

After prepping and positioning the patient in low lithotomy position, initial endoscopic evaluation of the bladder is performed. For complicated cases, circumferential delineation of the tumor can be performed with a Collins' knife initially to allow for precise tumor delineation (Cook Medical, Bloomington, IN). In most cases, however, this is not necessary. A flexible cystoscope can be left in the patient's bladder, which allows for a continuous internal picture of the bladder using the tile pro feature on the da Vinci S system™ (Intuitive Surgical, Sunnyvale, CA).

Next, the steps of port placement, establishment of pneumoperitoneum, and bladder takedown are as would be performed during a standard robot-assisted radical cystectomy case and are described in detail in other sections of this book. One important point that should be emphasized is that the bladder should be widely mobilized anteriorly and laterally to allow for at least a 2-cm resection margin and closure without tension. This requires division of obliterated umbilical ligaments and the urachus to completely free its dome of all attachments. Once completely mobilized, the bladder is expanded with fluid to help identify the area of the tumor. The fat that lies directly over the tumor should be removed and sent with the specimen.

With endoscopic guidance from a flexible cystoscope and the bladder fully distended, robot-assisted circumscription of the tumor is performed with cautery marking with at least a 2-cm margin around the tumor (Fig. 8.1). Transillumination of the affected area of the bladder by the cystoscope light facilitates this and the light can easily be seen when the robotic light source is decreased in intensity. Cautery is then used to "cut to the light."

Cautery lines are kept superficial until four 2–0 vicryl stay sutures have been placed lateral to the proposed resection area (Fig. 8.2).

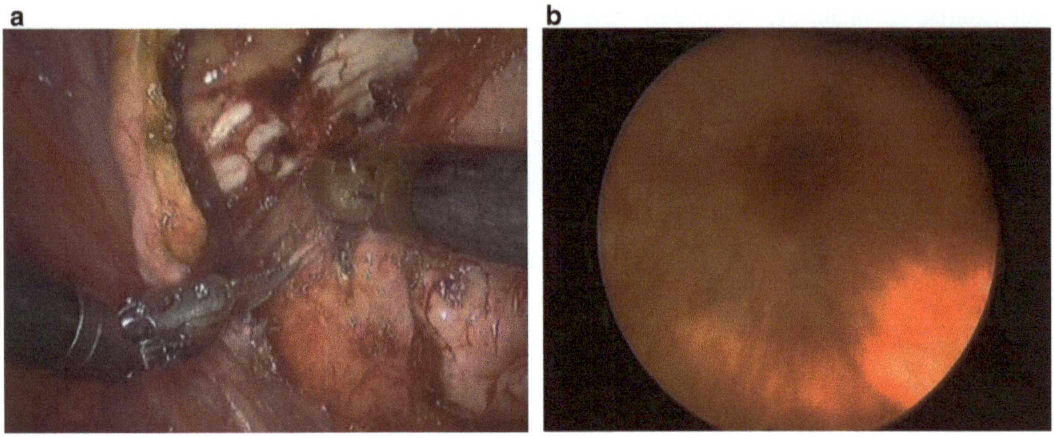

Fig. 8.1 Laparoscopic circumscription (**a**) of the tumor under endoscopic guidance (**b**)

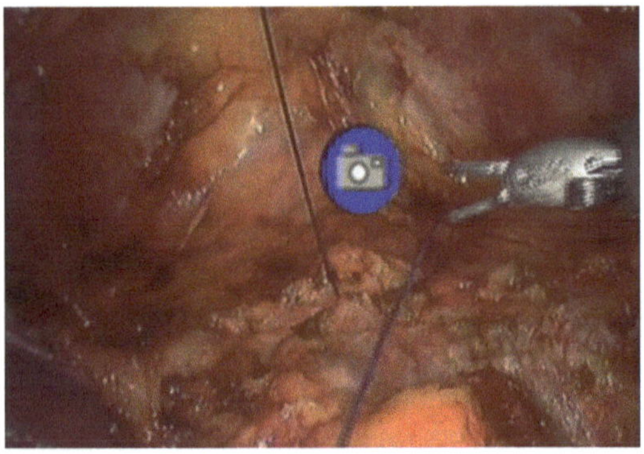

Fig. 8.2 Placement of stay sutures

The bladder is then drained and if possible (e.g., favorable anatomy, lobulated bladder, or bladder diverticulum), a 60-mm Echelon Endopath stapler (Ethicon Endo-surgery, Cincinnati, OH) is brought in through either the left or right 12 mm ports and used to divide the bladder at the proposed lines of resection (Fig. 8.3). If not amenable to the use of a stapler, scissors are used instead to cut sharply along the marked lines of resection with care not to spill bladder fluid/urine into the peritoneum. Pulling up on the stay sutures will facilitate the resection and decrease the risk of fluid spillage into the peritoneal cavity. Multiple specimens are also sent for intraoperative frozen section analysis to ensure negative margins have been achieved. Once negative margins have been confirmed, the specimen is then placed in an Endo-catch bag (Covidien, Mansfield, MA) and removed through an extended port incision at the end of the case.

If the stapler has been used, the remaining suture line on the native bladder is excised while tension is maintained on the stay sutures to prevent any urine spillage and contamination of the peritoneal cavity. This maneuver removes the staples in the suture line that could potentially serve as a nidus for stone formation if left in place. The bladder is emptied completely prior to the resection. Once resected, it is sent for histopathological analysis as the final margin. The bladder is then closed in two watertight layers in a running fashion using 3–0 monocryl/vicryl for the mucosal layer and 2–0 monocryl/vicryl for the outer layer. Moreover, the bladder could be closed in a full thickness, continuous fashion using 2–0 unibarbed V-loc suture (Covidien, Mansfield, MA) [19].

Subsequently, the bladder is tested for any leakage by filling with 250 ml of normal saline while being monitored cystoscopically and laparoscopically (Fig. 8.4). A JP drain is also placed via the 5-mm port.

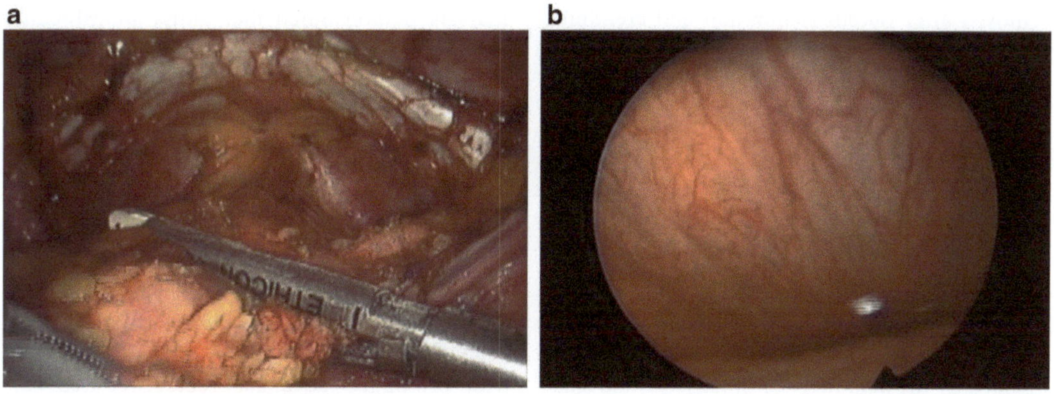

Fig. 8.3 Laparoscopic view (**a**) and endoscopic view (**b**) of bladder resection using Endo-GIA staplers

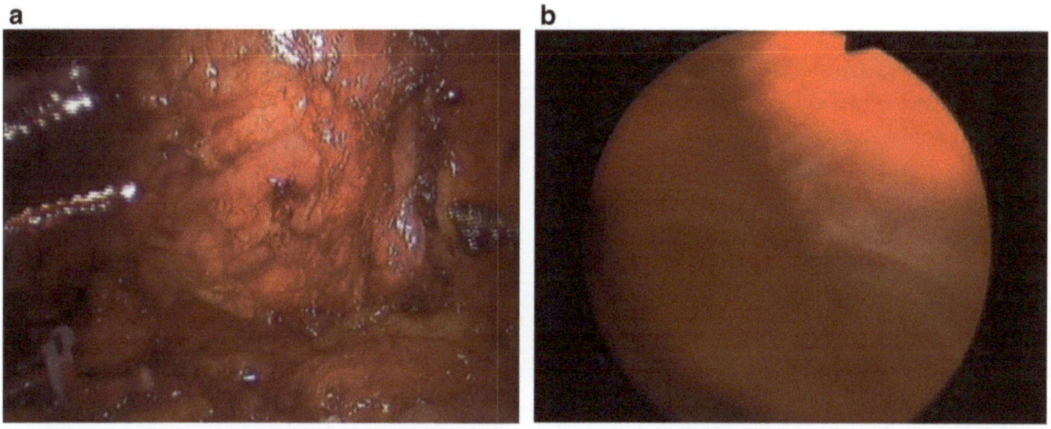

Fig. 8.4 Laparoscopic (**a**) and endoscopic (**b**) monitoring of testing of bladder closure

Finally, bilateral pelvic lymphadenectomy is performed as previously described in other sections of this book.

Postoperative Care and Follow Up

The following standard postoperative care is applied toward all PC, VSRC, and PSRC patients. In our experience, PC patients normally remain hospitalized on average for 1–2 days; while those who undergo VSRC and PSRC remain hospitalized longer (average of 5–6 days). The nasogastric or orogastric tube is typically removed immediately after surgery. Patients are allowed then to chew gum and have ice chips, and their diets are gradually advanced over the course of their hospitalization. Intravenous antibiotic prophylaxis is maintained for at least the first 24 h after surgery, while DVT prophylaxis with subcutaneous heparin is continued after surgery and for the duration of the hospitalization as long as hematocrit levels remain stable. Additionally, patients are encouraged to ambulate as soon as possible, preferably on postoperative day #1. Pain control is initially achieved with ketorolac with IV narcotics for severe breakthrough pain and then quickly converted to oral medications once the patient is tolerating a diet. Daily chemistry and hematocrit levels are routinely checked for the first 48 h and if stable, are then obtained at the surgeon's discretion. JP drain is typically removed after output is minimal and creatinine level of the fluid is consistent with serum creatinine. Urethral foley catheter can be removed in 7–13 days following a normal cystogram.

Follow-up for these patients is dictated by the pathology. Typically, these patients are followed closely every 3–6 months for the first 2 years with history & physical (H&P), voided cytology, labs (CBC, Chemistry, and LFT), and cystoscopic evaluation. Abdominal-pelvic cross-sectional imaging and chest radiographs are dictated by the pathology of the disease and standard NCCN recommendations are followed.

Discussion

Historically, PC had been advocated as a viable alternative to radical cystectomy due to its technical simplicity, decreased perioperative morbidity, and preservation of urinary and sexual functions. However, its popularity was short lived because of its high local rate of recurrence, ranging from 38 to 80 % [20], and low overall 5-year survival [17]. Suboptimal patient selection coupled with advances in surgical techniques associated with radical cystectomy, such as nerve-sparing procedures and continent reservoirs, all contributed to its downfall.

Nevertheless, as society ages and survival from bladder cancer increases, there has been a strong paradigm shift toward improving the quality-of-life issues without sacrificing oncological efficacy. This rekindles the interest in bladder-preserving procedures to be used in the primary setting or as part of a multimodal approach. To avoid the same pitfalls, many experts advocate for stricter selection criteria that include solitary, primary tumors located far away from the ureteral orifices or bladder neck and in an easily resectable area that allows for an adequate resection margin. Additionally, tumor multifocality and the presence of concomitant CIS must be ruled out.

In a retrospective study of 58 patients who had undergone PC from 1995 to 2001, Holzbeierlein et al. reported an overall 5-year survival rate of 69 % at a mean follow up of 33 months and local recurrence rate of only 19 % [16]. Univariate analysis demonstrated that tumor multifocality and the presence of concomitant CIS were significant predictors of recurrence. Similarly, in another retrospective study of 37 patients with a mean follow-up of 72.6 months, Kassouf et al. reported the overall 5-year, disease-specific, and recurrence-free survival rates to be 67 %, 87 %, and 39 %, respectively [21]. On multivariate analysis, higher pathological stage was associated with shorter overall recurrence-free survival; whereas, adjuvant chemotherapy was associated with prolonged advanced recurrence-free survival. In another retrospective study by Fahmy et al. looking at 714 patients with muscle-invasive bladder cancer who had undergone PC from 1983 to 2005 among different institutions, the 5-year overall survival between PC and radical cystectomy groups were similar (49.8 vs. 51 %). At a median of 17.6 months, 23.7 % of these patients recurred and required salvage radical cystectomy [22]. However, these patients had a 50 % increased risk of dying compared to those who underwent radical cystectomy initially.

These selected publications and others all emphasize the importance of optimal patient selection to achieve good oncological control. In carefully selected patients, 5-year overall survival is similar to that of radical cystectomy plus the benefits of decreased morbidity and preservation of urinary and sexual functions. It's worth mentioning that due to the paucity of data, no differences in overall survival, local recurrence rate, and functional outcomes have been demonstrated between different PC approaches [laparoscopic (robotic) versus open]. Rather, the decision to select a specific approach depends on the surgeon's experience and comfort level. However, with the success achieved in robot-assisted prostatectomy, the authors anticipate similar outcomes in robot-assisted PC.

Vaginal-Sparing Radical Cystectomy

Indications

Successes of female radical cystectomy have largely been measured by oncological and urinary outcomes, with little regard to sexual outcomes.

Zippe et al. [23] reported that up to 52 % of female patients experienced sexual dysfunction after RC and that the nature of the dysfunction encompassed both organic and psychosocial domains, such as decreased lubrication, decreased orgasm, lack of sexual desire, and dyspareunia. In a recent review of the literature, Elzevier et al. [24] reported that female sexual dysfunction rate after RC ranged from 20 to 82 % with no difference among the types of urinary diversion. As a result of these data, there has been an increased interest in modifying current surgical techniques to improve sexual outcomes. Anatomic studies have localized the neurovascular bundles to be along the lateral walls of the vagina [25]. Additionally, the removal of the distal urethra is associated with significant devascularization of the clitoris, which could adversely impact sexual arousal and orgasm [26]. Armed with this knowledge, some experts have modified their surgical approaches to include techniques of vaginal-sparing, ovary-sparing, urethral-sparing, neurovascular preserving, and tubular vaginal reconstruction [27–31].

However, the benefits of these organ-sparing approaches must be weighed against the risks of compromising oncologic outcome. Many studies have reported the incidence of urothelial cancer involvement of internal genitalia (vagina, uterus, and ovaries) to be between 2.6 and 5 % and the risk of having concomitant primary genital malignancy to be low as well [32–34]. Therefore, at our center, we only perform vaginal, ovary-sparing, and neurovascular preserving robot-assisted radical cystectomy in those patients who meet the following criteria.

- Good performance status (ECOG≤2) with manual dexterity and willingness to self-catheterize neobladders if needed.
- Non-obese patients (BMI <30) with minimal comorbidities as these could restrict the patient's cardiopulmonary tolerance of the surgery.
- No previous intra-abdominal/pelvic surgeries or prior pelvic radiotherapy.
- Demonstrate T2 disease or better with non-bulky tumors.
- No gynecologic malignancy such as cervical or ovarian cancers.
- Are sexually active with intentions to continue after surgery.

Steps of the Procedures

Port Placement, Establishment of Pneumoperitoneum, Ureteral Mobilization, Posterior Dissection, Control of Round Ligaments, Hysterectomy, and Control of Bladder Pedicles

These steps are as would be performed during anterior pelvic exenteration or female cystectomy and are described in detail in other sections of this book.

Dissection of Vesicovaginal Space

During the posterior dissection step as described in other sections of this book, antegrade dissection through the cul-de-sac allows for the separation of the posterior bladder from the uterus. This dissection plane is carried as far posteriorly as possible, preferably to the junction of the corpus uteri and cervix. The superior portion of the sacro-uterine ligaments along with the round ligaments is transected. However, the cardinal ligaments that attach to the lateral walls of the vagina along with the ovaries are left intact to maintain support to the vagina and to preserve hormonal function, respectively. Next, the bladder is dropped in a standard fashion similar to that of robotic prostatectomy and is described in other section of this book. During this step, the endopelvic fascia is identified and opened to expose the dorsal venous complex (DVC), urethrovesical junction, and lateral walls of urethra. The DVC is controlled using 0-vicryl suture and transected. Using both blunt and sharp dissection, a space between the urethra and the anterior wall of the vagina is created. Control of the bladder pedicles are achieved with Hem-o-lock clips (Teleflex Medical, Research Triangle Park, NC) or a stapler. It's important to know that while the vagina receives its arterial blood supply from multiple sources, vaginal branches from the uterine and inferior vesical arteries are among the important contributors. Additionally, since these branches travel in close proximity to the nerve supply of the vagina and clitoris, it's important to spare them during this step to avoid potential devascularization and denervation.

Using the lateral sulci of the vagina and lateral walls of the urethra as landmarks, dissection of the vesicovaginal space is performed sharply with minimal monopolar coagulation to prevent inadvertent thermal injury to the neurovascular bundles. The authors typically utilize a sponge stick dipped in betadine and inserted into the vaginal vault to help identifying the vaginal apex and anterior vaginal wall during the course of dissection. Hemostasis is obtained with pinpoint monopolar coagulation and suturing. Once the vesicovaginal space is fully developed, the urethra is encountered and transected.

Vaginal Stump Fixation: Variation of the Mansoura Technique

In 2002, Ali-El-Dein et al. [35] introduced the Mansoura modification in hope of preventing postoperative chronic urinary retention or hypercontinence that frequently plagued those who had received a neobladder. The authors demonstrated that by attaching the preserved ends of the round ligaments to the vaginal stump, this effectively fixed and provided support to the vaginal vault as well as prevented posterior and caudal displacement of the neobladder as demonstrated by cystogram. This has resulted in a reported 55 % reduction in the incidence of urinary retention among their patients. Armed with this knowledge, we also perform vaginal stump fixation among all patients who will receive a neobladder. During the standard hysterectomy as described in other section of this book, transection of the round ligaments is made close to its origins in the uterine horns to ensure adequate length for the vaginal fixation. Closure of the vaginal stump is performed horizontally with 2–0 vicryl to prevent narrowing of the vagina. The free ends of the round ligaments are then sutured to both ends of the vaginal apex, in effect suspending and supporting the vagina.

Bilateral Extended Pelvic Lymphadenectomy and Orthotopic Urinary Diversion

These steps are similar to those that have been described in detail in other sections of this book.

Postoperative Care and Follow Up

Postoperative care for VSRC is similar to that of PC except that these patients would have undergone an orthotopic urinary diversion. The ureteral stents of the neobladder are removed at approximately POD #10 and JP drain is maintained to drain any potential extravasation of urine as a result. A pouchogram is performed on POD #14 and if no leakage is noted, both the JP and urethral Foley catheter are removed subsequently. The patient is taught intermittent catheterization and pouch irrigation. Follow-up is similar to that of PC as described above and is also dictated by the pathology. More importantly, patients should continue to follow up with their Ob–gyn for periodic vaginal cytology and gynecologic examination.

Discussion

Standard female exenteration routinely requires the removal of the internal genitalia (vagina, uterus, and ovaries) along with the bladder. However, surgical modifications sparing these internal organs allow for the preservation of fertility and hormonal functions as well as improvement of functional outcomes. Multiple studies have demonstrated the low incidence of recurrence and concomitant urothelial cancer involvement of these organs. In a retrospective review of 609 female radical cystectomy specimens, Ali-el-dein et al. [34] reported the gynecologic organ involvement to be 2.6 % (16/609). Furthermore, no local vaginal recurrence was found at a mean follow-up of 4.3 years. Similarly, Salem et al. and Varkarakis et al. [32, 33] reported the incidence to be 4.4 % and 5.7 %, respectively. Vagina was most commonly involved, with the exception of one uterus. No vaginal recurrence and major sexual problems were encountered at the last follow-up (mean 6 years).

In terms of functional outcomes, it is believed that preservation of the vagina may decrease the risk of neobladder–vagina fistula and improve incontinence by preventing the posterior displacement of the neobladders [35, 36]. Koie et al. [37] reported 80 % (24/30) complete dryness (day and night continence) in those who had undergone vagina-, uterus-, and ovary-sparing radical cystectomy. Likewise, Chang et al. [28] reported 72 % continence rate (daytime and nighttime) in 15 out of 21 patients who had undergone vagina-sparing radical cystectomy. The results of these selected studies demonstrate that successful outcomes can be achieved without compromising oncological control in carefully selected patients.

Prostate-Sparing Radical Cystectomy

Indications

Since its first description, radical cystectomy has gone through various modifications as a means of improving postoperative continence and potency rates. Rossetti et al. [38] first described supra-ampullar cystectomy techniques by sparing the vasa deferentia, seminal vesicles, and prostatic capsule. Spitz et al. [39] reported the first US series of modified radical cystectomies that preserved the vasa deferentia, seminal vesicles, posterior prostate, and most importantly neurovascular bundles in four young men who had non-urothelial malignancy. These and many other series have in common the attempt to minimize dissection near the neurovascular bundles and urinary sphincter. Initially, PSRC was recommended for men without a primary urothelial malignancy. Successful functional outcomes in these patients sparked interest in applying this approach to those patients with primary urothelial malignancies. However, concerns for long-term oncological efficacy of this approach have been questioned. While the exact selection criteria have not been agreed upon, what has been known is that successful oncologic outcomes of PSRC rest mainly with optimal patient selection. Typically, these patients undergo PSRC in conjunction with an orthotopic neobladder. As such, we believe that optimal candidates should include the followings based on the data in the literature, which is discussed in the later section:

- Young, healthy, and potent patients whose potency and fertility remain a priority.
- Good manual dexterity with a willingness to self-catheterize neobladders when needed.
- Demonstrate clinical T2 disease or better without bladder neck, prostatic urethral involvement, or multifocal CIS disease.
- Absence of prostate cancer based on low serum prostate-specific antigen (PSA) levels, negative digital rectal exam (DRE), and negative standard transrectal ultrasound (TRUS)-guided prostate biopsies.

Steps of the Procedures

Standard port placement, pneumoperitoneum establishment, ureteral mobilization, bladder mobilization, control of bladder pedicles, and extended pelvic lymph node dissection are meticulously described in other sections of this book.

Bladder Neck Dissection

After ureteral and posterior bladder mobilizations, the bladder pedicles are carefully controlled as they come off the internal iliac artery using an athermal technique with Hem-o-lock clips (Teleflex Medical, Research Triangle Park, NC) or a stapler to prevent inadvertent thermal injury to the prostatic neurovascular bundles. The dissection is carried towards the prostate base, and only the internal iliac pedicles and superior vesical arteries are clipped and divided while the inferior vesical arteries along with its prostatic branches are spared to promote sexual potency recovery. The bladder is then dropped in a fashion similar to robotic prostate surgery and as described in other chapters of this book. To expose the prostatic–vesical junction in preparation for the bladder neck dissection, one must first develop the lateral pelvic spaces as previously described in

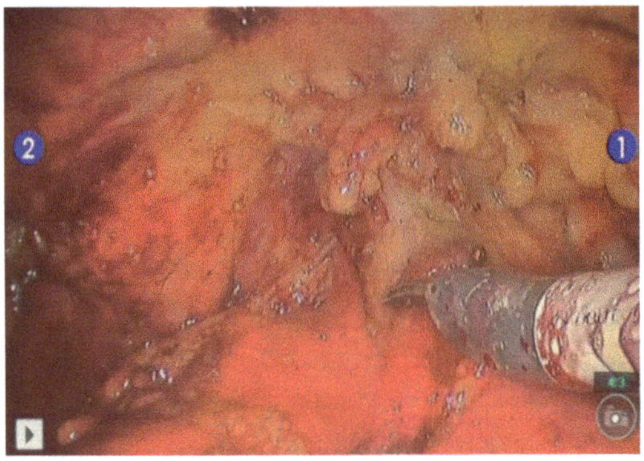

Fig. 8.5 "Defatting" allows for exposure of the urethrovesical junction

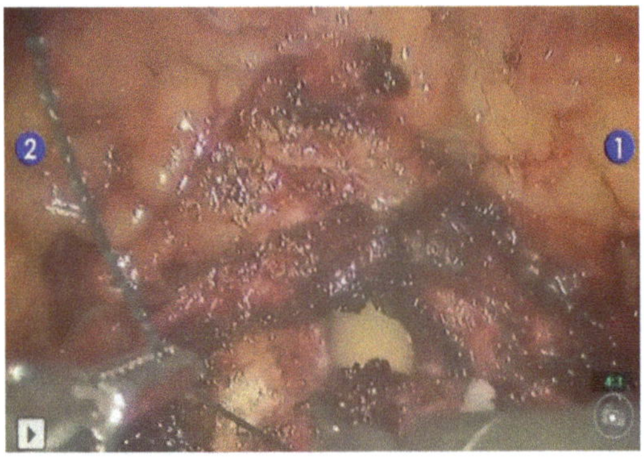

Fig. 8.6 The bladder neck is being ligated to prevent inadvertent spillage as one divides the urethrovesical junction

sections on developing the endopelvic space on either side of the prostate. Minimal to no dissection is done at the apex of the prostate. Once completed, this allows for the identification of levator ani muscles on the lateral pelvic side wall and the lateral and posterior bladder walls medially. "Defatting" of the prostatic–vesical junction can be made with a combination of blunt dissection and point cautery. Occasionally, an accessory pudendal artery is encountered and should be spared. Additionally, once the prostatic–vesical junction is cleanly exposed, the bladder neck is dissected circumferentially (Fig. 8.5) and ligated to prevent tumor spillage as it is being dissected (Fig. 8.6). The bladder is transected at the bladder neck and placed in an Endo-catch bag (Covidien, Mansfield, MA) which will later be removed with an extended midline port incision.

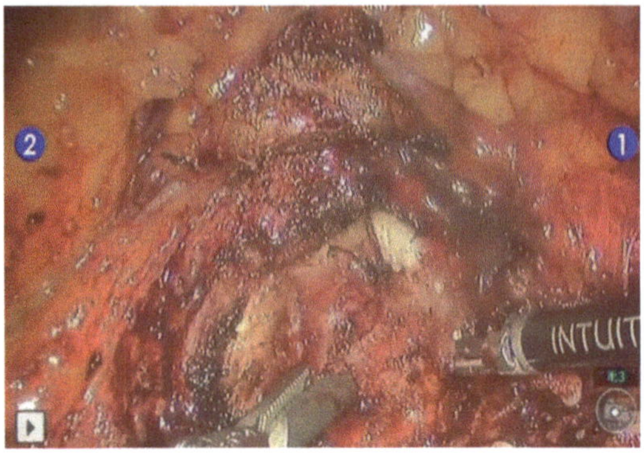

Fig. 8.7 Enucleation of the prostatic adenoma with Harmonic scalpel

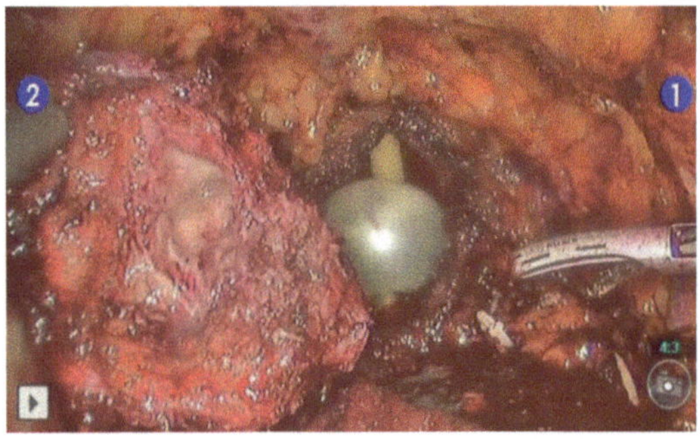

Fig. 8.8 Completed enucleation of prostatic adenoma. Foley inflated in the prostatic capsule to maintain pneumoperitoneum and to tamponade venous oozing

Enucleation of Prostatic Adenoma

Following the specimen removal, attention is directed toward the prostatic adenoma. Using the Harmonic ACE curved shears (Ethicon Endo-surgery, Cincinnati, OH), complete, circumferential enucleation of the prostatic adenoma from its capsule is performed with the urethra divided at the prostatic apex (Figs. 8.7 and 8.8). The device is contained within a special carriage produced by Intuitive Surgical (Sunnyvale, CA) and is utilized through the right robotic port. Vessels up to 5 mm in diameter could be coagulated using this device, allowing for great hemostasis. The Harmonic device allows for relatively bloodless enucleation of the adenoma. Following the removal of the adenoma, a 20Fr. Foley catheter with a 30 cm^3 balloon is inserted and inflated maximally to maintain the pneumoperitoneum and to tamponade any venous oozing.

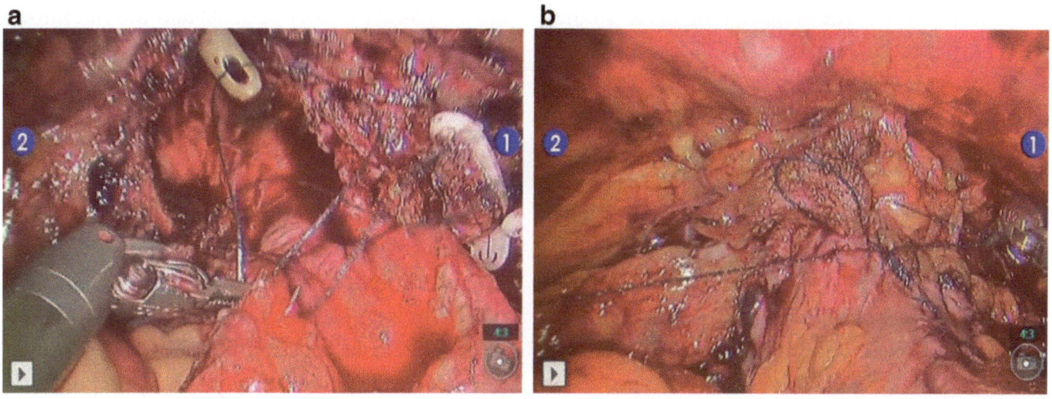

Fig. 8.9 Prostatic capsule–neobladder anastomosis with 3–0 V-loc suture starting at 6 o'clock (**a**) and progressing to 12 o'clock (**b**) using Van Velthoven technique

Urinary Diversion and Urethro-Neobladder Anastomosis

At this point, a 6-cm midline incision extended from the umbilical port is made to remove the bladder and prostatic adenoma. A Studer ileal neobladder urinary diversion is performed extracorporeally through this incision and then placed back within the abdomen after inserting a Foley catheter per the penis that is then tied to the neobladder. The Foley is retracted and used to help guide the neobladder towards the pelvis and towards the prostatic capsule. The fascia around the ports is tightened with sutures and the midline incision is closed around the camera port. Pneumoperitoneum is then reestablished and the patient is placed in reduced Trendelenburg position allowing the neobladder to stay within the pelvis. A watertight prostatic capsule–neobladder anastomosis is executed robotically using a double-armed 3–0 V-loc suture (Covidien, Mansfield, MA) starting at the 6 o'clock position on the prostatic capsule and progressing circumferentially and anteriorly along both sides until the anastomosis is complete (Fig. 8.9) using the Van Velthoven technique. Unlike the classic, urethro-neobladder anastomosis, suturing to the prostatic capsule is less challenging than suturing to the urethral stump due to decreased tension placed on the neobladder in order to make it reach the pelvis. Once completed, a new 20Fr Foley catheter is placed inside the neobladder and tested for watertight anastamosis. A Jackson–Pratt (JP) drain is also placed via a 5-mm port.

Postoperative Care and Follow-Up

Postoperative care is similar to that of PC and VSRC as described above. The ureteral stents of the neobladder are removed at approximately POD #10 while JP drain is kept in to drain any potential extravasation of urine as a result. A pouchogram is performed on POD #14 and if no leakage is noted, both the JP and urethral Foley catheter are removed subsequently. The patient is instructed to perform intermittent catheterization and pouch irrigation as necessary. Follow up is dictated by the pathology. Given that both the prostatic capsule and urethra are preserved and at risk for possible recurrent transitional cell carcinoma and/or prostate cancer, we recommend aggressive follow-up every 3 months for the first 2 years with H&P, voided urine cytology, and blood works (CBC, chemistry, LFTs, and PSA). A DRE is performed every 6 months during these first 2 years. Abdominal-pelvic cross-sectional imaging and chest radiographs are dictated by the pathology of the disease and standard NCCN recommendations are followed.

Discussion

The controversies surrounding PSRC centralize around concerns for prostatic involvement by transitional cell carcinoma (PI-TCC) and occult prostate cancer. In a recent review of literature, Autorino et al. [40] found that the reported PI-TCC incidence varied, from as low as 15 % to as high as 48 %. The majority of these studies were retrospective in nature and CIS was responsible for a significant number of these involved cases. With the application of stricter selection criteria (i.e., no CIS), the incidence of PI-TCC in PSRC was probably lower. Wood et al. [41] retrospectively reviewed 84 radical cystoprostatectomy (RCP) specimens and reported a 43 % incidence of PI-TCC. Among those involved, 94 % exhibited disease in the prostatic urethra with 67 % of these were caused by CIS. Similarly, Richards et al. [42] examined 96 RCP specimens and found that PI-TCC was present in 24 (25 %) patients, including 6 patients with only CIS involvement. Esrig et al. [43] reviewed 489 RCP specimens for PI-TCC and found an overall incidence of 29.2 % (143 patients). Among these, 30 patients had CIS of prostatic urethra and 19 patients had T4 disease where the primary urothelial cancer had extended full thickness through the bladder wall to invade the prostate. Lastly, Nixon et al. [44] found PI-TCC in 30 (15.6 %) out of 192 RCP specimens. Of those patients with CIS of the bladder, 31.3 % (25 of 80) had prostatic involvement.

When looking at risk factors, many studies have found that CIS, multifocal disease, and bladder neck involvement are independent risk factors for PI-TCC. In Nixon et al. [44] series, 34.7 % (25 of 72) of patients with multifocal disease also had concomitant PI-TCC. Multivariate analysis revealed 12- to 15-fold greater risk for PI-TCC when CIS or tumor multifocality was present. Kefer et al. [45] found that none of the 70 patients without CIS, bladder neck involvement, or multifocal disease were found to have PI-TCC. Likewise, Pettus et al. reported only 1 out of 35 patients who did not possess the above risk factors was found to have urothelial involvement of prostatic stroma.

Regarding the incidence of occult prostate cancer on RCP specimens, the reported incidence in the literature also varied widely, ranging from 4 to 60 % [40]. In an attempt to explain these high incidence rates, some authors have attributed them to a higher mean age of bladder cancer patients and the likelihood of diagnostic bias. However, after accounting for the diagnostic bias, Chun et al. and Kurokawa et al. [46, 47] still found a higher incidence of prostate cancer in men with bladder cancer compared to the expected incidence in an age-, sex-, and race-matched general population. Alternatively, some authors have attempted to stratify these occult cancers into clinically significant versus insignificant disease. Revelo et al. reported 50 (41 %) out of 121 specimens had unsuspected prostate cancer but only 24 out of these 50 specimens had clinically significant disease as defined by criteria such as tumor volume ($\geq$0.5 cm^3), Gleason score ($\geq$4 or 5), extracapsular extension, seminal vesicle invasion, lymph node involvement, and positive surgical margins. Similarly, Delongchamps et al. [48] reported the rate of occult prostate cancer on RCP specimens to be 14.2 % (20 out of 141). However, six (30 %) were considered insignificant disease, based on their low grade and microfocal tumor volume.

In summary, the reported incidences of PI-TCC and occult prostate cancer in the literature are highly variable. However, with the application of stricter selection criteria (i.e., no CIS or bladder neck involvement) coupled with surgical prudence (i.e., removal of prostatic urethra/adenoma), the impact of PI-TCC and occult prostate cancer on the patients' overall survival could be minimized.

Conclusion

Results from contemporary series on PC, VSRC, and PSRC are very encouraging. While these surgical variations demonstrate excellent postoperative functional outcomes, concerns raised about their long-term oncological efficacy are valid. It is imperative that any surgical modification must not compromise the primary objective of a good cancer operation in any way. However, in well-selected patients, these surgical variations will play an important role.

Editors' Commentary

Erik P. Castle and Raj S. Pruthi

The authors describe surgical variations and modifications with regard to robotic bladder surgery. A robotic approach is not only feasible for these modifications but also affords a less morbid modification than an open procedure. A great example is a robotic partial cystectomy.

In our practice we have typically performed robotic partial cystectomy to patients with benign conditions (e.g., symptomatic urachal cyst/sinus) or with urachal adenocarcinoma. Urachal adenocarcinoma is a focal condition and not characterized by a polyclonal field defect changes and multiple recurrences characteristic of urothelial carcinomas. As such, we do not typically perform a partial cystectomy (whether open or robotic) for urothelial cancers. However, in urachal cancers and in benign conditions, the robotic partial cystectomy, as described in the chapter, is an excellent which allows for a precise dissection and resection with reduced pain and convalescence. We agree that the use of intraoperative cystoscopy (and with the TilePro multi-input display) can facilitate the accuracy of the dissection—allowing for adequate (but not too wide) margins.

Vaginal-spring and prostate-sparing approaches may also be appropriate in carefully selected patients. The decision to perform such modifications should be driven by the pre and intraoperative oncologic findings and should be done with very careful patient selection. Furthermore, patients must be thoroughly counseled as to the potential risks and benefits of the procedure. Such decisions are irrespective of the surgical approach—whether open or robotic. If a vaginal-sparing or prostate-sparing approach is decided, then the robotic technique remains a viable surgical tool—and the authors describe these approaches skillfully. We commonly perform a vaginal-sparing procedure, barring any oncologic contraindications (discussed in this chapter). Furthermore, we have also performed (albeit uncommonly) a prostate-sparing cystectomy in carefully selected men undergoing the procedure. These men are typically those who are young, potent, and highly motivated to maintain their potency—often to the point of potentially refusing cystectomy. Furthermore, they must meet the careful preoperative analysis to reduce the risk of urothelial carcinoma of the prostate or of prostate cancer [49]. The Montsouris experience with long-term follow-up has given some level of assurance that oncologic outcomes may not be compromised in such carefully selected patients [50].

Acknowledgments Special thanks to Mani Menon, James O. Peabody, Quoc-Dinh Trinh, Jesse Sammon, Shyam Sukumar, Sanjeev Kaul, Sumit De, and Ali Dabaja for the making of prostate-sparing cystectomy video and Manish N. Patel and L. Spencer Krane for the making of partial-cystectomy video.

References

1. Marshall VF, Whitmore Jr WF. Simple cystectomy for cancer of the urinary bladder; 100 consecutive cases; 2 years later. J Urol. 1950;63:232.
2. Fedeli U, Fedewa SA, Ward EM. Treatment of muscle invasive bladder cancer: evidence from the National Cancer Database, 2003 to 2007. J Urol. 2011;185:72.
3. Hautmann RE, de Petriconi RC, Pfeiffer C, Volkmer BG. Radical cystectomy for urothelial carcinoma of the bladder without neoadjuvant or adjuvant therapy: long-term results in 1100 patients. Eur Urol. 2012;61: 1039.
4. Kim SP et al. The implications of hospital acquired adverse events on mortality, length of stay and costs for patients undergoing radical cystectomy for bladder cancer. J Urol. 2012;187:2011–7.
5. Yu HY et al. Comparative analysis of outcomes and costs following open radical cystectomy versus robot-assisted laparoscopic radical cystectomy: results from the US Nationwide Inpatient Sample. Eur Urol. 2012;61(6):1239–44.
6. Hart S et al. Quality of life after radical cystectomy for bladder cancer in patients with an ileal conduit, cutaneous or urethral kock pouch. J Urol. 1999; 162:77.
7. Turner WH, Danuser H, Moehrle K, Studer UE. The effect of nerve sparing cystectomy technique on postoperative continence after orthotopic bladder substitution. J Urol. 1997;158:2118.
8. Schoenberg MP et al. Local recurrence and survival following nerve sparing radical cystoprostatectomy for bladder cancer: 10-year followup. J Urol. 1996; 155:490.

9. Ali-el-Dein B et al. Surgical complications following radical cystectomy and orthotopic neobladders in women. J Urol. 2008;180:206.
10. Parekh DJ, Donat SM. Urinary diversion: options, patient selection, and outcomes. Semin Oncol. 2007; 34:98.
11. Gravante G, Caruso R, Andreani SM, Giordano P. Mechanical bowel preparation for colorectal surgery: a meta-analysis on abdominal and systemic complications on almost 5,000 patients. Int J Colorectal Dis. 2008;23:1145.
12. Becker G, Blum HE. Novel opioid antagonists for opioid-induced bowel dysfunction and postoperative ileus. Lancet. 2009;373:1198.
13. Vaughan-Shaw PG, Fecher IC, Harris S, Knight JS. A meta-analysis of the effectiveness of the opioid receptor antagonist alvimopan in reducing hospital length of stay and time to GI recovery in patients enrolled in a standardized accelerated recovery program after abdominal surgery. Dis Colon Rectum. 2012;55:611.
14. Resnick MI, O'Conor Jr VJ. Segmental resection for carcinoma of the bladder: review of 102 patients. J Urol. 1973;109:1007.
15. Sweeney P, Kursh ED, Resnick MI. Partial cystectomy. Urol Clin North Am. 1992;19:701.
16. Holzbeierlein JM et al. Partial cystectomy: a contemporary review of the Memorial Sloan-Kettering Cancer Center experience and recommendations for patient selection. J Urol. 2004;172:878.
17. Pontes JE, Lopez R. Tumor recurrence following partial cystectomy. Prog Clin Biol Res. 1984;162A:387.
18. Neyyar R, Hemal A. Robotic and laparoscopic partial cystectomy. In: Ghavamian R, editor. Atlas of laparoscopic and robotic urologic oncological surgery. Philadelphia, PA: JP Medical Publishers; 2013. http://www.amazon.com/Laparoscopic-Robotic-Urologic-Oncological-Surgery/dp/9350259583/ref=sr_1_5?s=books&ie=UTF8&qid=1371442261&sr=1-5&keywords=atlas+of+laparoscopic+urologic+surgery#_
19. Shah HN, Nayyar R, Rajamahanty S, Hemal AK. Prospective evaluation of unidirectional barbed suture for various indications in surgeon-controlled robotic reconstructive urologic surgery: Wake Forest University experience. Int Urol Nephrol. 2012;44(3): 775–85.
20. Hollenbeck BK, Taub DA, Dunn RL, Wei JT. Quality of care: partial cystectomy for bladder cancer–a case of inappropriate use? J Urol. Sep, 2005;174:1050.
21. Kassouf W et al. Partial cystectomy for muscle invasive urothelial carcinoma of the bladder: a contemporary review of the M.D. Anderson Cancer Center experience. J Urol. 2006;175:2058.
22. Fahmy N et al. Practice patterns and recurrence after partial cystectomy for bladder cancer. World J Urol. 2010;28:419.
23. Zippe CD et al. Female sexual dysfunction after radical cystectomy: a new outcome measure. Urology. 2004;63:1153.
24. Elzevier HW, Nieuwkamer BB, Pelger RC, Lycklama a Nijeholt AA. Female sexual function and activity following cystectomy and continent urinary tract diversion for benign indications: a clinical pilot study and review of literature. J Sex Med. 2007;4:406–16.
25. Stenzl A, Colleselli K, Bartsch G. Update of urethra-sparing approaches in cystectomy in women. World J Urol. 1997;15:134.
26. Stenzl A et al. Urethra-sparing cystectomy and orthotopic urinary diversion in women with malignant pelvic tumors. Cancer. 2001;92:1864.
27. Hautmann RE, de Petriconi R. Nerve-sparing cystectomy technique in the woman. Urologe A. 1995;34: 221–4.
28. Chang SS, Cole E, Cookson MS, Peterson M, Smith Jr JA. Preservation of the anterior vaginal wall during female radical cystectomy with orthotopic urinary diversion: technique and results. J Urol. 2002;168:1442.
29. Nandipati KC, Bhat A, Zippe CD. Neurovascular preservation in female orthotopic radical cystectomy significantly improves sexual function. Urology. 2006;67:185.
30. Game X et al. Uterus, fallopian tube, ovary and vagina-sparing laparoscopic cystectomy: technical description and results. Eur Urol. 2007;51:441.
31. Menon M, Hemal AK, Tewari A, Shrivastava A, Shoma AM, Abol-Ein H, et al. Robot-assisted radical cystectomy and urinary diversion in female patients: technique with preservation of the uterus and vagina. J Am Coll Surg. 2004;198(3):386–93.
32. Salem H, El-Mazny A. A clinicopathologic study of gynecologic organ involvement at radical cystectomy for bladder cancer. Int J Gynaecol Obstet. 2011; 115:188.
33. Varkarakis IM et al. Pathological review of internal genitalia after anterior exenteration for bladder cancer in women. Evaluating risk factors for female organ involvement. Int Urol Nephrol. 2007;39:1015.
34. Ali-El-Dein B et al. Secondary malignant involvement of gynecologic organs in radical cystectomy specimens in women: Is it mandatory to remove these organs routinely? J Urol. 2004;172:885.
35. Ali-El-Dein B, Gomha M, Ghoneim MA. Critical evaluation of the problem of chronic urinary retention after orthotopic bladder substitution in women. J Urol. 2002;168:587.
36. Bhatta Dhar N, Kessler TM, Mills RD, Burkhard F, Studer UE. Nerve-sparing radical cystectomy and orthotopic bladder replacement in female patients. Eur Urol. 2007;52:1006.
37. Koie T et al. Uterus-, fallopian tube-, ovary-, and vagina-sparing cystectomy followed by U-shaped ileal neobladder construction for female bladder cancer patients: oncological and functional outcomes. Urology. 2010;75:1499.
38. S. Rocca Rossetti, C. Terrone, [Preservation of potency by supra-ampullar cystectomy in patients with bladder neoplasms]. *Archivio italiano di urologia, andrologia : organo ufficiale [di] Societa italiana di ecografia urologica e nefrologica / Associazione ricerche in urologia* **71**, 265 (Sep, 1999).

39. Spitz A, Stein JP, Lieskovsky G, Skinner DG. Orthotopic urinary diversion with preservation of erectile and ejaculatory function in men requiring radical cystectomy for nonurothelial malignancy: a new technique. J Urol. 1999;161:1761.
40. Autorino R et al. Pathology of the prostate in radical cystectomy specimens: a critical review. Surg Oncol. 2009;18:73.
41. Wood Jr DP, Montie JE, Pontes JE, VanderBrug Medendorp S, Levin HS. Transitional cell carcinoma of the prostate in cystoprostatectomy specimens removed for bladder cancer. J Urol. 1989;141:346.
42. Richards KA et al. Developing selection criteria for prostate-sparing cystectomy: a review of cystoprostatectomy specimens. Urology. 2010;75:1116.
43. Esrig D et al. Transitional cell carcinoma involving the prostate with a proposed staging classification for stromal invasion. J Urol. 1996;156:1071.
44. Nixon RG, Chang SS, Lafleur BJ, Smith JJ, Cookson MS. Carcinoma in situ and tumor multifocality predict the risk of prostatic urethral involvement at radical cystectomy in men with transitional cell carcinoma of the bladder. J Urol. 2002;167:502.
45. Kefer JC et al. Risk assessment for occult malignancy in the prostate before radical cystectomy. Urology. 2005;66:1251.
46. Chun TY. Coincidence of bladder and prostate cancer. J Urol. 1997;157:65.
47. Kurokawa K et al. Comparative study on the prevalence of clinically detectable prostate cancer in patients with and without bladder cancer. Urology. 2004;63:268.
48. Delongchamps NB et al. Outcome of patients with fortuitous prostate cancer after radical cystoprostatectomy for bladder cancer. Eur Urol. 2005;48:946.
49. Kefer JC, Campbell SC. Current status of prostate-sparing cystectomy. Urol Oncol. 2008;26(5):486–93.
50. Rozet F, Lesur G, Cathelineau X, Barret E, Smyth G, Soon S, et al. Oncological evaluation of prostate sparing cystectomy: the Montsouris long-term results. J Urol. 2008;179(6):2170–4. discussion 2174–5.

Robot-Assisted Pelvic Lymphadenectomy

9

Kris E. Gaston and John W. Davis

Introduction

Robot-assisted pelvic lymphadenectomy for bladder cancer has developed in the past decade in the setting of fairly established literature from open surgery outcomes that promote the extended template method. The practice pattern of extended versus more limited templates may be inconsistent, but the data from high volume centers certainly point to specific oncologic gains from the former. Therefore, the surgeon setting out to learn this technique should consider three key questions for their learning objectives: (1) What is the background of the extended template? (2) What are the key anatomic considerations for the extended template from the robotic surgery view? And (3) are there remaining concerns about the ability of a robotic surgeon to provide high quality retrieval of lymph nodes at the time of robot-assisted radical cystectomy?

The online version of this chapter (doi:10.1007/978-1-4614-4906-5_9) contains supplementary material, which is available to authorized users.

K.E. Gaston
Department of Urologic Oncology, Carolinas Medical Center, Levine Cancer Institute, Charlotte, NC, USA

J.W. Davis, M.D. (✉)
Urology Director, Urosurgical Prostate Cancer Program, MD Anderson Cancer Center, 1515 Holcombe Blvd., Unit 1373, Houston, TX 77030, USA
e-mail: johndavis@mdanderson.org

Development of the Extended Template Pelvic Lymph Node Dissection at the Time of Radical Cystectomy

Approximately 25 % of patients undergoing surgery for muscle-invasive bladder cancer are found to have lymph node (LN) metastases at the time of surgery [1–6]. The incidence of lymph node positivity increases with increasing tumor stage with a range of 2–5 % in pT1 tumors, 16–22 % in pT2 tumors, 34–51 % in pT3 tumors, and 41–50 % in pT4 tumors [1–9].

Many authors have contributed to the understanding of the lymphatic drainage from the bladder, but this was well summarized by Leadbetter and Cooper [8] who described lymphatic drainage of the bladder to six distinct areas: (1)the lymphatic plexus within the bladder wall, (2) the anterior collated lymph nodes (nodes in the perivesical fat and surrounding the bladder), (3) pelvic collecting trunks–which are the medial lymph nodes of the external iliac and hypogastric lymph nodes, (4) regional pelvic lymph nodes which included the external iliac, hypogastric and sacral lymph nodes, (5) lymphatic trunks to the regional pelvic lymph nodes, and (6) the common iliac lymph nodes.

There has been much controversy over the limits of pelvic lymphadenectomy in regard to adequate bladder cancer surgery. Whitmore and Marshall described the standard lymph node dissection for bladder cancer [9]. In the 1970s, Dretler et al. reported the benefit of lymphadenectomy with

E.P. Castle and R.S. Pruthi (eds.), *Robotic Surgery of the Bladder*, DOI 10.1007/978-1-4614-4906-5_9,

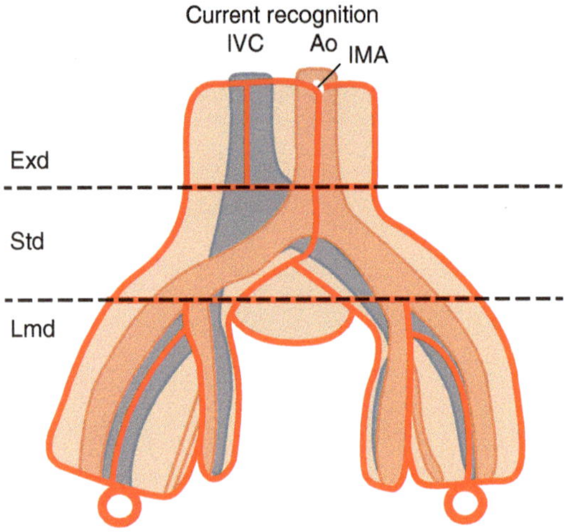

Fig. 9.1 Pelvic node dissection templates—limited (LMD), standard (Std), and extended (Ext)

radical cystectomy and found that survival of node positive patients improved by lymphadenectomy without increasing the morbidity and mortality [10]. Skinner reported in the 1980s a 36 % 5-year survival in patients who underwent a "meticulous" lymph node dissection [3]. A limited pelvic lymphadenectomy traditionally included dissection posteriorly to the obturator nerve, anteriorly to the external iliacs stopping the proximal dissection at the bifurcation of the iliac vessels, and distally to the arcus tendineus of the pubic bone at Cloquet's node. Historically, the standard lymphadenectomy included removal of the lymphatic tissue from the obturator region with the limits of the obturator nerve posteriorly, external iliac vessels up to the common iliac vessels including tissue from the fossa of Marcille cranially, and distally to Cloquet's node at the arcus tendineus of the pubic bone and circumflex vein. Extended pelvic lymph node dissection has varying definitions according to high-volume centers which typically includes the standard dissection in addition to dissection with the cranial limits being the aortic bifurcation plus or minus to the inferior mesenteric artery and inferior vena cava and posteriorly with resection of the hypogastric tissue including presacral lymph nodes (Fig. 9.1). Some authors call the cranial dissection to the IMA and the hypogastric regions a super-extended lymph node dissection [12].

What is considered adequate pelvic lymphadenectomy for bladder cancer and is there a therapeutic benefit in LN positive disease? Smith and Whitmore demonstrated that the obturator and external iliac lymph node regions were the most common sites for lymph node metastases at 74 and 65 %, respectively [11]. Additionally in this study it was found that 19 % of positive lymph nodes were along the common iliac chain. This was one of the first studies indicating that a standard lymph node dissection was likely an inadequate for removal of regionally involved lymph nodes. Leissner et al. performed a study in 447 patients who underwent pelvic lymphadenectomy and found that there was a statistically significant survival advantage in patient who underwent a more extended lymphadenectomy with equal or greater than 16 lymph nodes removed [5]. There was a significant correlation between the number of lymph nodes removed and the 5-year cancer-specific survival in pT1-3 tumors. In a later multicenter study by Leissner et al. that involved 290 patients who underwent radical cystectomy with extended pelvic lymphadenectomy found that approximately 28 % have positive lymph nodes and the percentage of metastases at different sites range from 14.1 % in the right obturator nodes to 2.9 % in the paracaval nodes above the aortic bifurcation [6]. Their analysis found that the incidental LN metastases was 21 % for nodes inferior to the bifurcation of the common iliac artery and 18.6 % at the common iliac and presacral nodes. They also showed that 10 % of primary sites of lymphatic spread were at the common iliac nose, and tumor spread to the contralateral side of the pelvic nodes was also found. They also report reported that 16.5 % of lymph node positive metastases were found between the level of the IMA and the aortic bifurcation suggesting the necessity for dissection of this region especially for the purpose of staging. However, a separate study by Zehnder et al. compared the extended lymphadenectomy data from Skinner's series at the University of Southern California which included superior boundary of the IMA to the

University of Bern with the boundary being the uretero–iliac crossing [12]. The USC group compared to the University of Bern group had a higher number of lymph nodes taken (38 versus 22, $p<0.0001$) and a higher incidence of lymph node metastases (35 versus 28 %, $p=0.02$). However, patient survival and recurrence was almost equivocal between these two large institutions suggesting no additional survival benefit from dissecting more cranial than the level of the ureteroiliac crossing at the common iliacs. Thus, the cranial extent of the dissection remains controversial in regard to survival.

Many authors have made the argument about the increased potential for staging with ePLND in regard to stratification of patient who may need adjuvant chemotherapy after surgery. However, to date there is no level I evidence that strongly supports adjuvant chemotherapy affecting survival in the postoperative setting. However a small retrospective series from Steinberg et al. that demonstrated that patients with lymph node metastases who received chemotherapy lived six times longer than patient who did not receive chemotherapy (48 versus 8 months, $p<0.0001$) [13]. The benefit of adjuvant chemotherapy remains controversial; however, extended staging lymphadenectomy may be important for identifying patients at high risk patients for recurrence. The incidence of patients with nodal positive disease likely increases with a total of number of lymph nodes removed [12]. USC popularized the concept of lymph node density, which was defined as the total number of positive lymph nodes divided by the total number of lymph nodes taken. Lymph node densities greater than 20 % demonstrated an increased risk of death versus patients with a lymph node density less than 20 % (17 versus 43 % 10-year recurrence-free survival) [14]. It has been well established in the literature that the number of lymph nodes that will be reported is dependent on the pathologic processing [15–17]. A number of studies have demonstrated that increased node counts will be reported along with increased positive node detection with the increased number of specimens packet sent [15–17]. There is the potential concern that extended lymph node dissection increases the potential complication rate with radical cystectomy. Brössner et al. performed a prospective study looking at 92 consecutive patients who underwent radical cystectomy with 46 undergoing a standard LND versus 46 undergoing an extended LND. There was no difference in 30-day morbidity between the two groups. The extended lymphadenectomy clearly increases the operative time; however, this is not translated to increase morbidity or mortality in the literature [18]. Nevertheless, the oncologic gains from the extended template must be balanced against the additional time required that may relate to overall anesthetic time and subsequent thromboembolic risk, accumulation of lymphoceles, risk for vascular injury, and temporary or permanent lower extremity edema.

Extended Pelvic Lymph Node Dissection Technique: Making the Transition with Robot-Assisted Platforms

Surgical training for robot-assisted radical cystectomy with extended pelvic lymph node dissection is best rooted in robot-assisted radical prostatectomy [19], first starting with cases that require only a limited node dissection and progressing to an extended template for high risk disease. The latter requires an understanding of the familiar obturator fossa anatomy in which the main task is to retrieve the lymph nodes from under the iliac vein from the distal landmark of the node of Cloquet and proximally to somewhere near the hypogastric artery. Laterally the border is the pelvic sidewall, and inferior is the obturator nerve, which must be preserved. From observing other surgeons and personal experience, it is clear that the distal node of Cloquet is often visible and fairly easy to obtain but likely drains the leg and less often involved with pelvic cancers. However the more proximal tissue in and around the obturator nerve as is passes lateral to the iliac vein is much more difficult to retrieve, and there is tremendous variability in how persistent surgeons are in working for these lymph nodes. These nodes, however, are very close to the hypogastric artery and a common landing site for prostate and bladder cancers.

Expansion of the template to the hypogastric artery zone, as described by Bader et al. [20] requires a more advanced skill set. The obturator fossa is fairly avascular, and the main potential complication is injury to the obturator nerve from blind clipping or errant cutting/coagulating. In the hypogastric template, there are multiple fine arterial/venous branches from the hypogastric and other feeding sources. The surrounding lymph nodes will not lift into the specimen until the vasculature holding them down is controlled with either a bipolar sealant or clip/cut. Furthermore, the exposure of the hypogastric artery requires some work. The peritoneum over the iliac vessels and psoas muscle needs to be divided, and the ureter identified and gently pulled medial—generally in the vicinity of its crossing over the common iliac artery. Within 3–5 cm of the takeoff of the hypogastric artery, the large caliber obliterated artery abruptly turns medial to the bladder. The ureter always passes inferior to this landmark. In prostatectomy, this artery can be preserved, while in cystectomy it must be taken. From this point distally, the hypogastric is a complex structure that dives deep within pelvic spaces, sending out varied patterns of branches medial to the bladder, and distally into the obturator space—some named structures and some not. Dissection along the hypogastric artery at this point occurs for a centimeter or two medially and would stop at the bladder. Lateral to the hypogastric artery, there is ample lymph node tissue present inferior to the obturator nerve all the way to the pelvic sidewall. Again, this region is rich in small caliber vascular branches requiring effective seal. In general, one distinct recommendation for extended pelvic lymphadenectomy for prostate cancer is to limit the lateral/high dissection to the junction between the iliac artery and vein. Thus some external iliac nodes are taken, but the lateral tissue from the artery to the genitofemoral nerve is left alone to decrease the incidence of postoperative lower extremity edema.

Continued evolution of technique from a prostatectomy to radical cystectomy requires expansion of the template. Based upon Bochner et al.'s lymph node mapping study from 2004 [21], we studied our learning curve with this procedure by adopting this template: right and left external iliac, right and left obturator/hypogastric, right and left common iliac, pre-sacral, and para-caval/para-aortic. This map, therefore consists of six paired zones and two midline zones. Initially we performed a protocol with robotic e-PLND to all zones and during the open diversion performed a second look open EPLND. The overall robotic times were a median 117 min (range 89–152) and retrieved a median of 43 nodes (range 19–63). Additional lymph nodes (median 4) were retrieved by second look open, but a majority of zones were completely cleared (67 %) or retrieved non-lymph node tissue (13 %) [22].

Sequence and Exposure

The pelvic lymph nodes can be done first or second. Doing them first leaves the urine drainage intact longer in the case and can setup the pedicles for the cystectomy as second step. The lymph nodes can be organized into 1–2 bags using surgical to separate the different zones. More recently, we have utilized the Anchor Tissue Retrieval System (Anchor Products Company, Addison, IL, USA), which can be reused, however, limiting the extraction to what can fit through a port. We avoid pulling large amounts of unprotected lymph nodes through ports to minimize risk of tumor seeding.

With a lymph node first approach, it is helpful to go ahead and divide the Pouch of Douglas and free up the posterior planes. For a nerve-sparing case, divide/mobilize the seminal vesicles as they will be valuable landmarks for the nerve sparing. To start the nodes, divide the peritoneum over the medial umbilical ligament and then across the iliac vessels and psoas muscle. Leave the midline intact so the bladder is easier to expose at the pedicles—see Video 9.1 and Fig. 9.2.

Instrumentation

The robotic surgeon utilizes the monopolar scissors, bipolar Maryland, and in the third arm the Prograsp or Cautier. The assistants need a

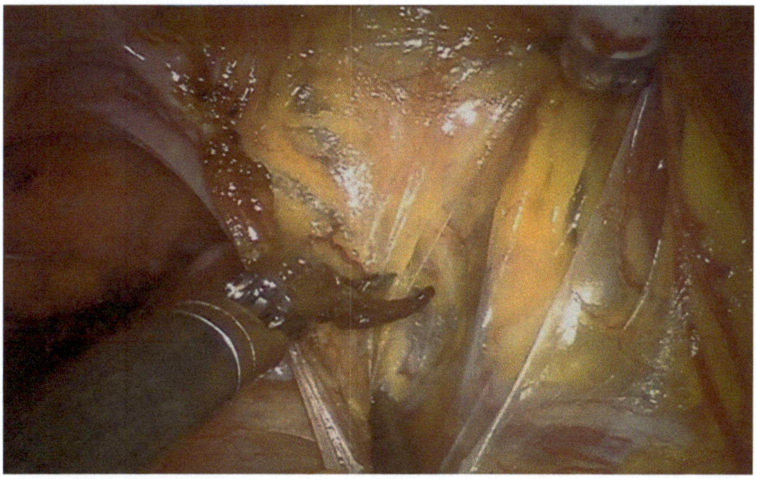

Fig. 9.2 Division of the peritoneum from the medial umbilical ligament and over the iliac vessels permits identification of the ureter and vessels

bowel-friendly grasper such as a laparoscopic Debaky and the suction. The position of the assistant varies by surgeon preference, however, if planning a robotic ileal conduit, the technique presented by Castle [23] calls for a left-sided assistant with two 12-mm port access to allow ideal stapling angles to the bowel.

In terms of dissection style, the monopolar scissors is efficient at dividing tissues and sealing very small vessels <2–3 mm. Vessels any larger require a bipolar and larger than 5 mm may require a clip. Most split/roll lymphatics can be simply divided with cautery, however, the proximal and distal extent of dissection should probably be clipped to decreased lymphatic collection, even though the operation is transperitoneal. Cautery use near the obturator nerve will likely induce a muscular contraction and should be avoided.

Vascular Injury

Any significant effort to clear an entire zone of lymph nodes in the retroperitoneum or pelvis will eventually lead to a vascular injury that needs repair. The iliac vessels are fairly robust and pliable enough to move around for dissection. However an errant use of cautery with the tips pointed into the vessels will likely cause an injury. In general pressure against the vessel to the side wall can control it without needing full circumferential clamping. It is important to recover from the adrenalin surge and carefully articulate repair plans with the staff. Specifically, give very clear instructions as to which instruments will be replaced for suturing and when so as to maintain control of the injury. For small vein lacerations a 3-0 Vicryl figure of eight can work. For an artery, 4-0 prolene figure of eight.

Common locations of injury outside of a cautery injury are near the take off of the external iliac artery/vein—especially lateral common iliac vein.

Extended Pelvic Lymph Node: Zone by Zone Description and Video Illustration

External Iliac Zones

This step is a good starting point for e-PLND. With the monopolar scissors, split the lymphatics down the midpoint of the artery and start another division line with the scissors or bipolar down the far lateral border over the psoas to the genitofemoral nerve. As these two lines are split, the iliac artery/vein becomes more mobile and can be pulled medially to create a sizable groove

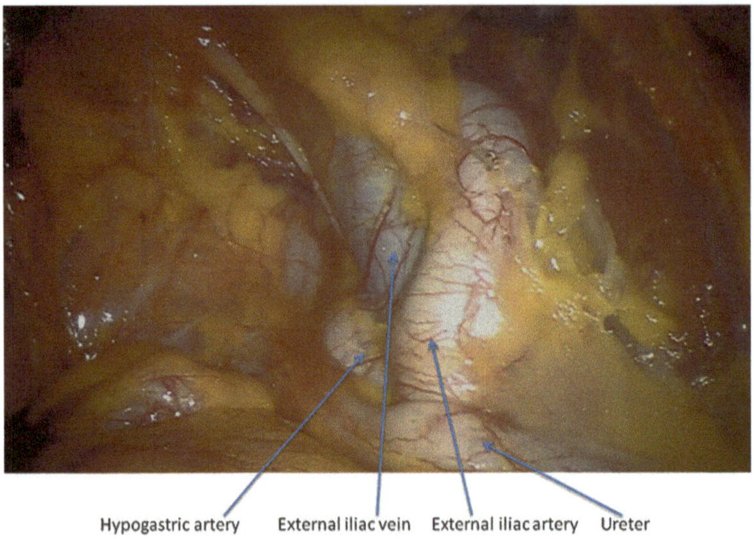

Fig. 9.3 Identification of the ureter and take-off of the hypogastric artery

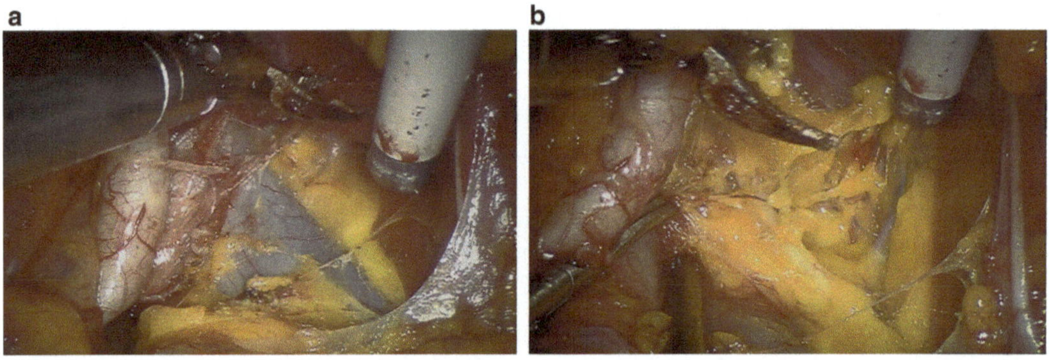

Fig. 9.4 External iliac zone. (**a**) The lymphatics are split down the artery and over the psoas muscle to the genitofemoral nerve. The common iliac vein is encountered (*right side*). (**b**) The right common iliac vein is retracted medially and the obturator nerve is identified. Lymphatics are separated from the many small vessels coming from the pelvic sidewall. On the *left side*, the common iliac vein approaches from a more medial angle and not seen in this space as much

between the vessels and the psoas muscle. Continue the dissection down the sidewall. As the space is cleared you will see the common iliac vein, which can also be retracted medially. Deep to this structure, you will see the obturator nerve as it passes from under the iliac vein to a more lateral position, headed to the sacrum. The lymph nodes are attached to varying micro vessels that often originate from the hypogastric branches but are heading into the pelvic side wall. These micro vessels can be sealed with the tips of the bipolar and the lymphatics mostly mobilized at this step. Doing the dissection in this sequence allows for a large bloc removal when you return from the medial approach through the obturator fossa. Of note, this most proximal nodal tissue that follows the obturator nerve often goes on and on and is difficult to completely clear of lymph and adipose tissue.

Once the groove space developed between the iliac vessels and psoas is cleared, continue to split the tissue in and around the iliac artery, achieving a separation between the artery and vein—Figs. 9.3 and 9.4a, b. This plane is carried back to

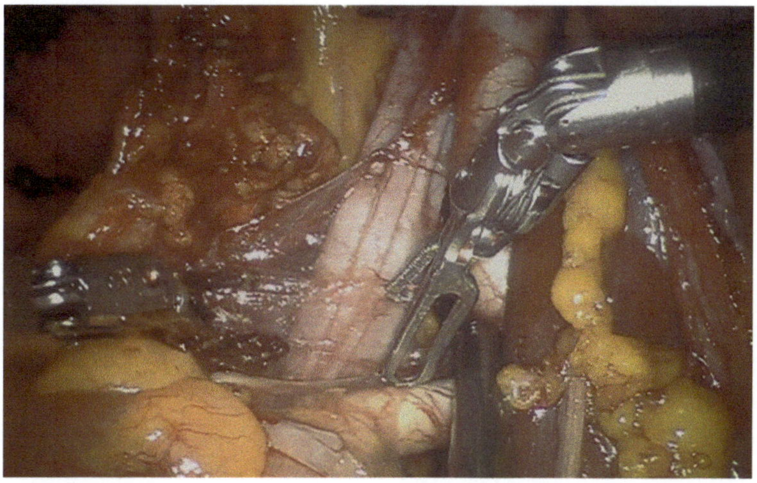

Fig. 9.5 External iliac zone. The dissection split continues in and around the artery creating space between. Once completed, this tissue can be sent as its own zone, and the dissection proceeds with the obturator/hypogastric. The lymphatic tissue seen to the *left* generally falls down and comes out en bloc with the obturator lymphatics

the common iliac artery. These combined nodes can then be extracted at this point. In our pilot study [22], the right external iliac zone took a median 11 min (range 7–20) and yielded a medina 5 nodes (range 2–8). For the left the time was 13 min (range 6–24) and nodal yield 4 (range 0–8). The range of nodes may vary by sequence. If, for example, the obturator packet is dissected first, some of the external nodes can easily be pulled into this bloc of tissue. By the same token, there is no anatomic separation between external iliac and common iliac, and these zone have to be manually separated.

Obturator/Hypogastric Zones

With the ureter mobilized medially, the hypogastric is cleared of tissue from its origin distally. The first major branch encountered will be the obliterated artery, which should be clipped and divided. Then the pattern varies with location and number of send off vessels into the obturator space versus more posteriorly. Often a clear superior vesicle artery is seen quickly and can be divided and clipped. Remaining tissue medially will often be captured in the pedicle dissection. By starting the procedure with the external iliac zone, much of the lateral obturator zone is freed up and comes out en bloc—Fig. 9.5. The tissue around the proximal obturator nerve was also mobilized and the remaining comes out in the obturator zone. Most of this zone can be completely cleared with the exception of the deepest tissue following distal hypogastric and the most proximal tissue along the obturator nerve. Additional tissue around the hypogastric tissue is easy to retrieve when completing the pre-sacral zone.

In our pilot study [22], the right obturator/hypogastric took a median 21 min (range 11–38) and retrieved a median 9 nodes (range 1–18). For the left side, the time was 20 min (range 11–29) and yield 6 (range 4–19). Figure 9.6 shows a post-dissection image of the obturator/hypogastric plane.

Common Iliac Zones and Pre-sacral

Moving higher to the common iliac zones used to be a challenge for the standard model robot due to the size/mobility of the arms. With daVinci S and Si models the access is greater for two reasons: longer instruments allowing higher port placement and greater range of motion by the arm itself. The exposure takes additional division of peritoneum above the location of the ureter crossing. The sigmoid colon generally needs

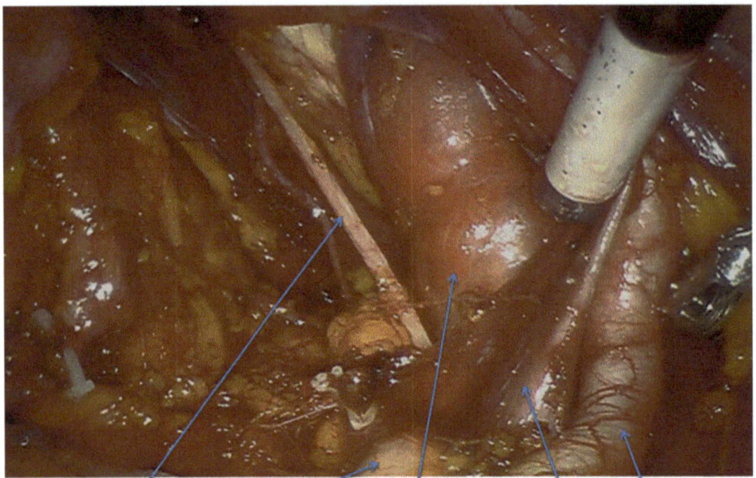

Fig. 9.6 Obturator/hypogastric zone. The obturator space clears easily due to the previous external iliac dissection. The dissection proceeds down the hypogastric artery and then laterally under the obturator nerve to the side wall

specific retraction by an assistant instrument or third robotic instrument. The lymphatics at the takeoff of the external iliac artery can be continued with split dissection to the point of the aortic bifurcation. An additional 3–5 cm of tissue can be split and retrieved in the para-caval right side and para-aortic left side. At some point, the arms lose range of motion. Once the common iliacs are split down the middle, the lateral tissue is mostly sent of designated as common iliacs—left and right. In the space between the common iliac artery, the tissue can be retrieved by retracting the sigmoid colon left and anterior to the abdominal wall. This maneuver with the third robotic arm should allow viewing from the aortic bifurcation to both sides of the common iliac arteries. The tissue between is then retrieved. The left common iliac vein will quickly be seen once lymphatics removed from the crotch of the aorta. Moving distally, the sacral bone is encountered and the tissue connects all the way back to the take off of the hypogastric artery. Moving back to the left side, the colon is push up and right, and the space connected in and around the left common iliac artery. Of note, the spaces around the lateral common iliac artery will often contain very friable common iliac vein branches that are hard to control if avulsed. Ideally, identify them early and seal them properly. Otherwise, packing with surgicel may be required.

Editors' Commentary

Erik P. Castle and Raj S. Pruthi

There are few things that will generate more emotion in the world of urological oncology than the debate regarding the adequacy of a robot-assisted pelvic lymphadenectomy. With the understanding that a complete pelvic lymphadenectomy may be curative in upwards of 30–40 % of cases, it is key that a thorough and complete lymphadenectomy is performed during RARC. The published literature currently supports that the numbers of lymph nodes removed and intermediate oncologic outcomes of RARC are equivalent to the open procedure (see **Chap. 14). In order to achieve this, it is key to adhere to the principles outlined in this chapter. Specific steps such as creating the space lateral to the external iliac vessels often referred to as the "Space of Marcille" as well as meticulous dissection of the lateral aspect of internal iliac artery posterior to the obturator nerve will allow the surgeon to complete a thorough pelvic lymphadenectomy. Extending the proximal extent past the common iliac vessels is based on surgeon preference. The benefits of the pneumoperitoneum will allow for great visualization as venous ooze is kept to a minimum. From a complication standpoint, one consideration is aberrant electrical energy from a compromised sheath on the monopolar scissors which has been described as well as "off screen" vascular injuries by the assistant. Keeping all of these considerations in mind, most surgeons who have undertaken robot-assisted pelvic lymphadenectomy agree that the robot in and of itself is not a deterrent to performing an equivalent and thorough lymphadenectomy. In fact, many believe that they may even be performing a more complete dissection today than they ever did before in their open cases.

References

1. Vazina A, Dugi D, Shariat SF, Evans J, Link R, Lerner SP. Stage specific lymph node metastasis mapping in radical cystectomy specimens. J Urol. 2004;171(5):1830–4.
2. Stein JP, Lieskovsky G, Cote R, Groshen S, Feng AC, Boyd S, et al. Radical cystectomy in the treatment of invasive bladder cancer: long-term results in 1,054 patients. J Clin Oncol. 2001;19(3):666–75.
3. Skinner DG. Management of invasive bladder cancer: a meticulous pelvic node dissection can make a difference. J Urol. 1982;128(1):34–6.
4. Madersbacher S, Hochreiter W, Burkhard F, Thalmann GN, Danuser H, Markwalder R, et al. Radical cystectomy for bladder cancer today–a homogeneous series without neoadjuvant therapy. J Clin Oncol. 2003;21(4):690–6.
5. Leissner J, Hohenfellner R, Thüroff JW, Wolf HK. Lymphadenectomy in patients with transitional cell carcinoma of the urinary bladder; significance for staging and prognosis. BJU Int. 2000;85(7):817–23.
6. Leissner J, Ghoneim MA, Abol-Enein H, Thüroff JW, Franzaring L, Fisch M, et al. Extended radical lymphadenectomy in patients with urothelial bladder cancer: results of a prospective multicenter study. J Urol. 2004;171(1):139–44.
7. Herr HW, Bochner BH, Dalbagni G, Donat SM, Reuter VE, Bajorin DF. Impact of the number of lymph nodes retrieved on outcome in patients with muscle invasive bladder cancer. J Urol. 2002;167(3):1295–8.
8. Leadbetter WF, Cooper JF. Regional gland dissection for carcinoma of the bladder, a technique of one-stage cystectomy, gland dissection and bilateral ureteroenterostomy. J Urol. 1950;63:242–60.
9. Whitmore Jr WF, Marshall VF. Radical total cystectomy for cancer of the bladder: 230 consecutive cases five years later. J Urol. 1962;87:853–68.
10. Dretler SP, Ragsdale BD, Leadbetter WF. The value of pelvic lymphadenectomy in the surgical treatment of bladder cancer. J Urol. 1973;109(3):414–6.
11. Smith Jr JA, Whitmore Jr WF. Regional lymph node metastasis from bladder cancer. J Urol. 1981;126(5):591–3.
12. Zehnder P, Studer UE, Skinner EC, Dorin RP, Cai J, Roth B, et al. Super extended versus extended pelvic lymph node dissection in patients undergoing radical cystectomy for bladder cancer: a comparative study. J Urol. 2011;186(4):1261–8.
13. Gofrit ON, Stadler WM, Zorn KC, Lin S, Silvestre J, Shalhav AL, et al. Adjuvant chemotherapy in lymph node positive bladder cancer. Urol Oncol. 2009;27(2):160–4.
14. Stein JP, Cai J, Groshen S, Skinner DG. Risk factors for patients with pelvic lymph node metastases following radical cystectomy with en bloc pelvic lymphadenectomy: concept of lymph node density. J Urol. 2003;170(1):35–41.
15. Stein JP, Penson DF, Cai J, Miranda G, Skinner EC, Dunn MA, et al. Radical cystectomy with extended lymphadenectomy: evaluating separate package versus en bloc submission for node positive bladder cancer. J Urol. 2007;177(3):876–81. discussion 881–2.
16. Bochner BH, Herr HW, Reuter VE. Impact of separate versus en bloc pelvic lymph node dissection on the number of lymph nodes retrieved in cystectomy specimens. J Urol. 2001;166(6):2295–6.
17. Bochner BH, Cho D, Herr HW, Donat M, Kattan MW, Dalbagni G. Prospectively packaged lymph node dissections with radical cystectomy: evaluation of node count variability and node mapping. J Urol. 2004;172(4 Pt 1):1286–90.
18. Brössner C, Pycha A, Toth A, Mian C, Kuber W. Does extended lymphadenectomy increase the morbidity of radical cystectomy? BJU Int. 2004;93(1):64–6.
19. Hayn MH, Hellenthal NJ, Hussain A, et al. Does previous robot-assisted radical prostatectomy experience affect outcomes of robot-assisted radical cystectomy? Results from the international Robotic Cystectomy Consortium. Urology. 2010;76:1111–6.
20. Bader P, Burkhard FC, Markwalder R, Studer UE. Is a limited lymph node dissection an adequate staging procedure for prostate cancer? J Urol. 2002;168(2):514–8.
21. Bochner BH, Cho D, Herr HW, et al. Prospectively packaged lymph node dissections with radical cystectomy: evaluation of node count variability and node mapping. J Urol. 2004;172:1286.
22. Davis JW, Gaston K, Anderson R, et al. Robot assisted pelvic lymphadenectomy at radical cystectomy: lymph node yield compared with second look open dissection. J Urol. 2011;185:79–84.
23. Castle EP. Robot-assisted ileal conduit. Presented at the Society of Urological Surgeons, May 2012.

Extracorporeal Urinary Diversion

10

Kevin G. Chan and Timothy G. Wilson

Introduction

The purpose of this chapter is to provide a step-by-step approach to the different extracorporeal urinary diversions that may be performed in the setting of robot-assisted radical cystectomy (RARC). Recent reports indicate comparable results to open surgery with regards to intermediate-term oncological outcomes and extent of pelvic lymph node dissection [1, 2]. However, operative times are one of the main obstacles that hinder wide-spread acceptance of RARC. Extracorporeal urinary diversion with RARC provides a method of reconstruction that mirrors that of open surgery with regards to operative times [3]. Complication rates and functional outcomes with extracorporeal urinary diversion also appear comparable to open series [4–6].

We will discuss in detail the extracorporeal techniques of a Studer orthotopic neobladder, Indiana pouch continent cutaneous urinary diversion, and ileal conduit urinary diversion. At our institution, we have performed more than 250 RARCs. All urinary diversions were performed extracorporeally and the majority were continent urinary diversions. We describe our technique that follows a common template, which can be applied to all types of urinary diversion.

We first describe the technique of the Studer orthotopic neobladder. This is the most technically difficult of the three diversions because there are more maneuvers required to adapt it to robotic surgery and because the robot needs to be re-docked. The Indiana pouch and ileal conduit techniques are simpler variations of the same basic template. The port site placement used for the cystectomy portion and referenced later in this chapter has been previously described [7].

Studer Orthotopic Neobladder

The extracorporeal Studer neobladder technique is best described in three stages; steps performed prior to undocking the robot, steps performed while the robot is undocked, and steps performed after the robot is re-docked.

Steps Performed Prior to Undocking the Robot

During the course of the radical cystectomy, there are a number of maneuvers that facilitate the creation of the neobladder. We typically divide our

K.G. Chan (✉) • T.G. Wilson, M.D.
Department of Surgery, Division of Urology and Urologic Oncology, City of Hope National Medical Center, 1500 East Duarte Road, Duarte, CA 91010, USA
e-mail: kchan@coh.org; twilson@coh.org

E.P. Castle and R.S. Pruthi (eds.), *Robotic Surgery of the Bladder*, DOI 10.1007/978-1-4614-4906-5_10,

ureters early in the operation. The ureters are divided between extra large Weck Hem-o-lok® clips. The clips have a pre-tied 8 cm dyed or undyed suture to denote left and right. The clips are placed on the ureter through the right iliac 12 mm bedside assistant's port in a right to left orientation. This allows us to identify any twists in the ureter at the time of the ureteroileal anastomosis. The ureteral sutures are placed aside, out of the operative field, during the completion of the cystectomy.

As the urethra is divided, we place a 9 in. 2-0 Vicryl™ (Ethicon, New Brunswick, NJ) suture, on RB-1 needle, at the 6 o'clock position of the urethra that will be used for the first stitch in the urethral anastomosis. The needle is set aside in the retropubic fat so that it can be easily found when the robot is re-docked for the anastomosis.

Once the cystectomy and lymph node dissection are complete, there are a small number of final steps performed prior to undocking the robot. The left ureter is brought under the sigmoid mesentery by guiding the attached suture with a laparoscopic grasper. An 8-cm silk stitch is placed in the terminal ileum to allow for quick identification though the small midline incision. A 16 Fr red Robinson catheter with an 8-cm silk suture pre-tied to the end is placed in the urethra. The catheter will later be sutured to the neobladder to serve as a handle for the assistant to bring the assembled neobladder down into the pelvis. The two ureteral sutures, the ileal suture, and the red Robinson suture are then placed into the assistant's laparoscopic grasper by the console surgeon. This allows for all four of the components to be readily available for the urinary diversion when the robot is undocked and the midline incision is opened.

Steps Performed After Undocking the Robot

The robot is undocked but kept sterile as it will be used for the urethral anastomosis. Insufflation is turned off and all port sites are kept in place with the exception of the midline port. We keep the patient in Trendelenburg position to keep the small bowel out of the way during the neobladder construction. The midline incision is extended inferiorly 6–8 cm and the specimen is extracted using an Endo Catch™ II 15 mm specimen pouch (Covidien, Mansfield, MA). The use of the specimen bag serves to preserve the intact specimen and to also facilitate using a smaller incision. While the specimen can be removed through a generally smaller incision, 6 cm is approximately the smallest incision that allows us to place the constructed neobladder back into the abdomen.

The laparoscopic grasper holding the sutures on the ureters, ileum, and urethral catheter is brought out through the midline incision. The ureters are placed in their correct anatomic orientation, using both visual and manual evaluation to check for twisting or crisscrossing of the ureters.

The ileum is then brought out through the incision to create the ileal neobladder. For orthotopic diversions, we prefer a low pressure ileal reservoir as described by Studer, however, this technique will also accommodate most other types of orthotopic diversion [8].

Prior to the construction of the reservoir, bowel continuity is restored by means of a stapled anastomosis and the mesenteric trap is closed.

We isolate a 60 cm segment of distal ileum beginning 15 cm proximal to the ileocecal valve. We prefer to discard a 5 cm segment of ileum proximally to afford us better mobility of the neobladder down to the urethra and farther from the bowel anastomosis (Fig. 10.1). The neobladder is constructed in the exact manner as would be done open.

Once the neobladder is complete, we estimate the most dependent portion where we think the urethra will be anastomosed. We place a dyed 0 Vicryl™ figure-of-eight suture at the estimated 6-o'clock portion of the neourethra that will be used as a handle by the console surgeon's fourth arm using a ProGrasp™ forceps (Fig. 10.2). An additional suture is placed in the same position and sutured to the red Robinson catheter that is in the urethra. This acts as an additional handle for the bedside assistant to help bring the neobladder down into the pelvis. An undyed Vicryl™ is placed at the 12-o'clock portion of the neourethra

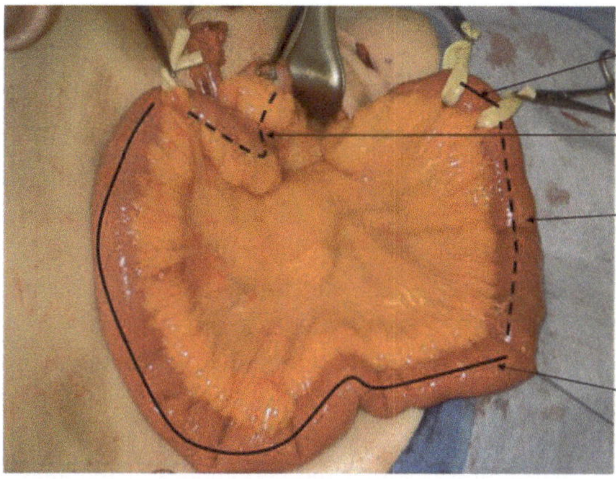

Fig. 10.1 The 6-cm incision provides excellent exposure of small bowel for neobladder reconstruction

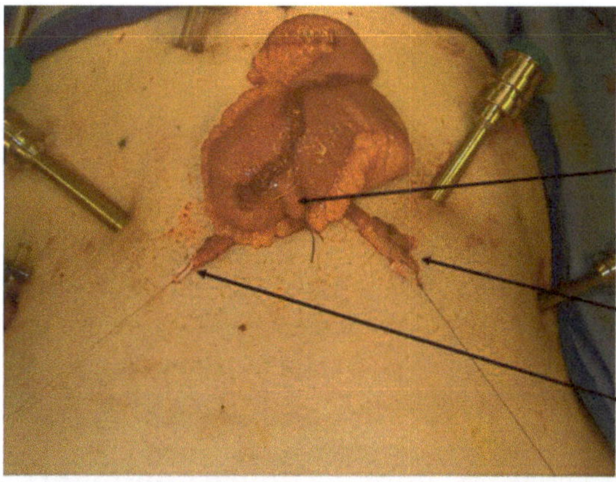

Fig. 10.2 The neobladder is completed with the 6 and 12-o'clock sutures placed at the site of the anticipated neourethra

to give the console surgeon better orientation of the pouch and to provide an additional handle with which to manipulate the pouch.

The neobladder is then placed into the pelvis with only the afferent limb and bilateral ureters exposed at the midline incision (Fig. 10.3). A medium-sized Alexis® Wound Protector/Retractor (Applied Medical, Rancho Santa Margarita, CA) is used to improve exposure for the uretero–ileal anastomoses.

The ureters are once again reinspected to ensure they are oriented in their correct anatomic positions. Each ureter is then spatulated and individually sewn in a Bricker end-to-side fashion with interrupted 4-0 Vicryl™ sutures. Each

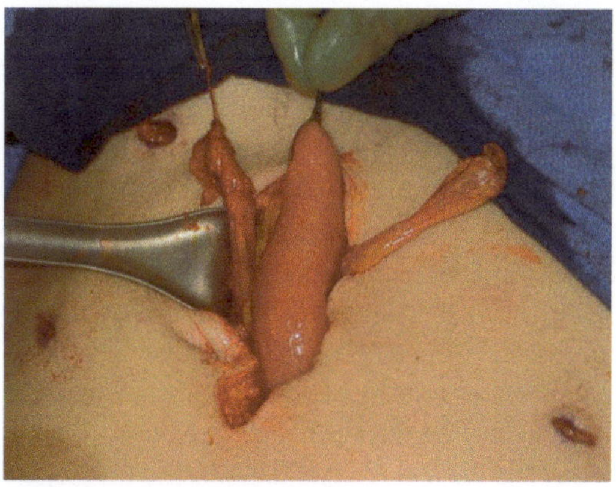

Fig. 10.3 The completed neobladder is placed back into the abdomen, leaving only the ureters and afferent limb exposed for the uretero–ileal anastomoses

uretero–ileal anastomosis is stented with an 8Fr feeding tube that is brought out through an opening in the afferent limb and beside the right paramedian robotic port. The feeding tubes are secured at the afferent limb with a 3-0 plain gut purse string suture.

The midline incision is then closed to the level of the camera port site. We utilize four preplaced interrupted size 1 polypropylene sutures at the superior aspect of the incision where the camera port is replaced. We are then able to tie down one or two of the interrupted sutures with the port in place to ensure an airtight seal for re-insufflation. The use of an AirSeal® Access Port (Surgiquest, Milford, CT) also helps facilitate adequate insufflation after re-docking. The robot is then re-docked.

Steps Performed After Re-docking the Robot

The urethral anastomosis is performed robotically using either a 0 or 30° down lens. We first inspect the uretero–ileal anastomoses to ensure they are lying in their correct orientation.

The redundant sigmoid colon is moved out of the pelvis. The neobladder is then brought down into the pelvis by the console surgeon using the preplaced 6-o'clock Vicryl™ handle and the fourth arm. The assistant can aid in the maneuver by placing gentle traction on the red Robinson catheter that is also attached to the 6-o'clock position of the neobladder.

Occasionally, the neobladder does not completely reach the urethra, creating tension at the anastomosis. Two maneuvers can be employed to decrease this tension. The first is simply perineal pressure. The second is to undock the robot, minimize the Trendelenburg, and re-dock the robot.

The site of the urethral anastomosis on the neobladder is opened using a robotic shear. This site is determined by choosing an area where the opening is well visualized and easy to work with.

Using the 2-0 Vicryl™ suture that was preplaced at the 6-o'clock position of the urethra at the time of the urethral division, we begin the urethral anastomosis by re-approximating the urethral plate with a simple interrupted suture. The anastomosis is then continued and completed by running two interlocked 3-0 V-Loc™ 180 6 in. sutures bilaterally to meet at the 12 o'clock position where the sutures are tied. Special attention is given to cinching down on the V-Loc™ suture after each complete pass through the urethra and neobladder in order to ensure a watertight anastomosis.

The completed anastomosis is tested by irrigating the neobladder with 60–120 ml of normal saline. Any visible area of extravasation from either the neobladder or the anastomosis is reinforced with an additional 3-0 Vicryl™ suture. A new two-way 18F hematuria catheter is placed into the neobladder to gravity drainage.

A closed suction drain is placed through the left paramedian robotic port and placed over the urethral anastomosis and adjacent to our uretero–ileal anastomoses. The drain and stents are secured with sutures. The robot is then undocked. The closure of the midline incision is completed with the preplaced polypropylene sutures. The stents are cut 5 cm from the skin and placed to gravity drainage using a urostomy drainage bag, and the skin incisions are closed.

Indiana Pouch Continent Cutaneous Catheterizable Reservoir

With the Indiana pouch, minimal steps are required prior to undocking the robot. As with the neobladder, the ureteral sutures are secured with a laparoscopic grasper through the right iliac port.

We undock the robot but keep the abdomen insufflated with all ports in place. The Trendelenburg is decreased and the table tilted left as far as possible. Using our existing port placements, we use a conventional laparoscopic technique to mobilize the right colon and hepatic flexure.

The table is then leveled, the ports are removed, the midline camera incision is extended inferiorly 7–8 cm, and the specimen is removed. This incision is larger than the incision made for the neobladder because the pouch tends to be

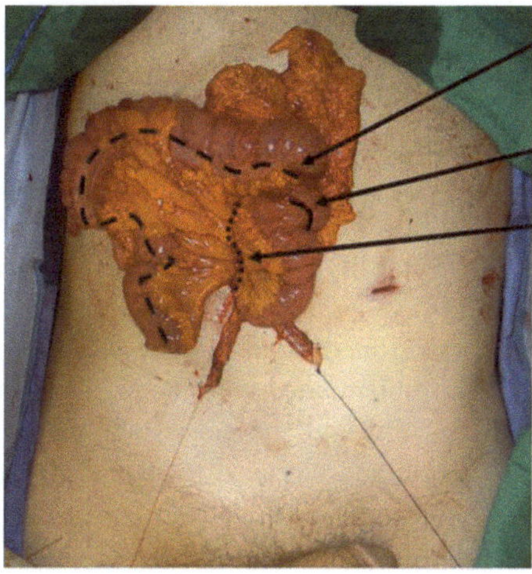

Fig. 10.4 An 8-cm midline incision allows excellent exposure of the right colon and terminal ileum for Indiana pouch construction. Here the ileal–colic anastomosis is completed and the mesenteric trap closed

bigger and this also allows us better exposure for the uretero–colonic anastomoses. In obese patients, the size of this incision may need to be further increased to optimize exposure.

We isolate the 15 cm of proximal ileum along with 31 cm of right colon (Fig. 10.4). The avascular plane of Treves is divided to allow mobility to our stomal segment. Bowel continuity is then reestablished using a side-to-side ileal–colic stapled bowel anastomosis. The mesenteric trap is then closed.

We perform a modified Indiana pouch as described by Ahlering et al. but this technique can be adapted to most continent catheterizable pouches [9]. Once the Indiana pouch is completed, it is replaced into the abdomen with the right-sided suture line oriented downward toward the pelvis. This allows for the most tension free uretero–colonic anastomoses while keeping the mesentery to the Indiana pouch stoma in its correct anatomic position. The ureters are then anastomosed separately, using a Bricker end-to-side, spatulated anastomosis with interrupted 4-0 Vicryl™ sutures. Each ureteral anastomosis is stented with an 8 Fr pediatric feeding tube. The stents are secured at an opening in the Indiana pouch with a 3-0 plain gut suture and brought out through the right iliac port site.

We use a 24 Fr Malecot catheter as a suprapubic catheter that exits out the most superior aspect of the Indiana pouch and is brought out through the assistant's epigastric port site. The suprapubic tube is secured to the anterior abdominal wall in a Stamm fashion. The right paramedian robotic port site is then used as the stoma location, provided it is traversing the rectus abdominis. If the suprapubic port site is too high, it can distract and place tension on the ureteral anastomoses. In this situation, we use the right paramedian robotic port site for the suprapubic tube, and create a separate more inferior opening for the stoma. Once the ileal segment of the Indiana pouch is delivered through the fascia and subcutaneous tissue, it is trimmed at the level of the skin, to minimize redundancy, and matured to the skin with interrupted 3-0 Vicryl™ sutures.

The stents are secured at the skin with a suture and placed to a urostomy gravity drainage bag. The Malecot catheter is placed to gravity drainage and a closed suction drain is placed along the pouch and adjacent to our uretero–colonic anastomoses and brought out through the left paramedian robotic port site. The stoma is dressed with a petroleum dressing and not cannulated until the time of pouch training. The midline incision is then closed.

Ileal Conduit Urinary Diversion

Prior to undocking the robot, as with the neobladder, the ureteral and ileal sutures are secured on a laparoscopic grasper through the right iliac port.

The ports are then removed and the midline camera port site is extended 4–5 cm. This incision can be smaller since it does not have to accommodate a pouch. The specimen is removed and the ureters and ileum are brought out through the incision and oriented.

We isolate our distal ileal segment in the conventional open fashion, discarding an additional 5 cm segment of ileum proximally to give us additional mobility of the afferent aspect of our conduit. Bowel continuity is reestablished with an ileal–ileal, side-to-side stapled anastomosis.

Our uretero–ileal anastomoses are performed using a Bricker end-to-side spatulated anastomosis bilaterally. We mature the stoma and place our closed suction drain into the pelvis and adjacent to our uretero–ileal anastomoses. Our stents are brought out through the stoma and secured with a suture. The midline incision is then closed.

Postoperative Care

Patients are placed on Alvimopan prior to the induction of anesthesia and continued on this postoperatively until first bowel movement. Nasogastric tubes are removed at the end of surgery or on the morning of postoperative day 1. Clear liquid diets are started with the resumption of flatus. Patients are discharged home when tolerating a regular diet. The closed suction drain is typically removed at the time of discharge if outputs stay at or below 200 ml/8 h.

For the continent diversions, a pouchogram is obtained at 3 weeks after surgery and the urinary or suprapubic catheter and stents are removed if no extravasation is identified. A renal ultrasound is obtained 6 weeks after stent removal as a baseline evaluation of the upper tracts.

Advantages and Disadvantages of Extracorporeal Urinary Diversion

The key advantage of extracorporeal urinary diversion compared to the intracorporeal technique is the utilization of open suturing. This results in a shorter learning curve, operative times comparable to open procedures, less time under general anesthesia for the patient, and ultimately less cost. Other advantages include minimizing fecal contamination of the peritoneal cavity and minimizing surgeon fatigue.

The main disadvantage of the extracorporeal urinary diversion is the need for a larger incision (typically ranging from 5 to 8 cm) which can lead to poorer cosmesis and theoretically a higher pain medication requirement. Another potential problem cited with the extracorporeal technique is impaired tissue orientation/positional distortion and the need for considerable mobilization of the ureters, both of which may contribute to ischemia and possible ureteral stricture. Other disadvantages include increased evaporative fluid loss and external bowel manipulation, both of which may contribute to ileus.

Complications and Outcomes

As the technique of RARC matures, we are seeing complication rates at least comparable to open surgery [1, 2, 4]. However, there is a paucity of data looking at functional outcomes with extracorporeal orthotopic and cutaneous continent urinary diversion in the RARC setting. We evaluated 49 patients undergoing an extracorporeal orthotopic Studer neobladder and found a 78 % daytime continence rate at 1 year [6]. In our evaluation of 34 patients undergoing extracorporeal Indiana pouch urinary diversion, 33 (97 %) patients achieved complete continence [5]. While the data is still limited, it appears that both complications and functional outcomes with extracorporeal urinary diversion are comparable to open techniques.

Conclusion

The extracorporeal urinary diversion technique provides an effective and smooth transition from open radical cystectomy to the labor-intensive technique of RARC. We expect that with refinements in technology and surgical technique, complication rates and functional outcomes will continue to improve upon existing open surgical standards.

Editors' Commentary

Erik P. Castle and Raj S. Pruthi

In most cases of radical cystectomy, it is the urinary diversion that is the source of the majority of postoperative complications. This applies to both open and robot assisted approaches. Consequently, the choice and technique of urinary diversion is one of the more critical aspects of the procedure, especially considering that the implications of the potential complications can offset any benefit that a minimally invasive approach may offer. Many experienced RARC surgeons have experimented with various modifications to the steps of extracorporeal urinary diversion, particularly for orthotopic neobladder. The one potential complication that must always be on the surgeon's mind is the potential for uretero–ileal anastomotic stricture. It is this complication that has been observed by surgeons early in their experience. Respecting the vascular supply of the ureters around the common iliacs and minimizing the tension of the left ureter have become two of the most important aspects of extracorporeal urinary diversion. Many of us have even progressed to making the extraction incision much larger that when we first started in order to allow us to work "in the retroperitoneum" in order to be able to do less mobilization of the ureters and cut back on the distal ends. The overall benefits of a minimally invasive surgery are not lost by making the final extraction incision 4–6 cm larger. These are but a few examples of modifications that have been developed throughout the evolution of robot-assisted radical cystectomy and extracorporeal urinary diversion and we expect many more to come as surgeons become more facile with the procedure.

References

1. Challacombe BJ et al. The role of laparoscopic and robotic cystectomy in the management of muscle-invasive bladder cancer with special emphasis on cancer control and complications. Eur Urol. 2011;60(4):767–75.
2. Orvieto MA et al. Oncological and functional outcomes after robot-assisted radical cystectomy: critical review of current status. Urology. 2011;78(5):977–84.
3. Haber GP, Crouzet S, Gill IS. Laparoscopic and robotic assisted radical cystectomy for bladder cancer: a critical analysis. Eur Urol. 2008;54(1):54–62.
4. Yuh BE et al. Standardized analysis of frequency and severity of complications after robot-assisted radical cystectomy. Eur Urol. 2012;62:806–13.
5. Torrey RR et al. Functional outcomes and complications in patients with bladder cancer undergoing robotic-assisted radical cystectomy with extracorporeal Indiana pouch continent cutaneous urinary diversion. Urology. 2012;79(5):1073–8.
6. Linehan J, Whelan CM, Nazmy M, Ruel NH, Menchaca AR, Torrey, RR, Lau CS, Wilson TG, Chan KG. Continence outcomes following robotic-assisted cystectomy with orthotopic urinary diversion, submitted for publication.
7. Josephson DY et al. Robotic-assisted laparoscopic radical cystoprostatectomy and extracorporeal continent urinary diversion: highlight of surgical techniques and outcomes. Int J Med Robot. 2010;6(3):315–23.
8. Studer UE et al. Three years' experience with an ileal low pressure bladder substitute. Br J Urol. 1989;63(1):43–52.
9. Ahlering TE, Weinberg AC, Razor B. Modified Indiana pouch. J Urol. 1991;145(6):1156–8.

Robot-Assisted Intracorporeal Ileal Conduit

11

Magnus Annerstedt and Erik P. Castle

Introduction

Open radical cystectomy with pelvic lymph node dissection and urinary reconstruction is still considered as gold standard treatment in muscle-invasive bladder cancer [1–3]. Despite significant improvements in morbidity and mortality as well as in functional results in recent years, the procedure is associated with substantial early and late complications [4–6]. The adoption of minimally invasive surgery in attempt to reduce morbidity in radical cystectomy started with the first laparoscopic radical cystectomy in 1992 [7]. It was not until the introduction of robot-assisted surgery that larger series were presented [8–16]. When performing robot-assisted radical cystectomy (RARC), most centers perform the extirpative part (cystectomy and lymph node dissection) intracorporeally and the reconstruction of the urinary canal extracorporeally. In an attempt to further reduce morbidity and reduce hospital stay, some centers have developed techniques for intracorporeal urinary diversion [17, 18]. Potential additional benefits are less incisional pain, decreased bowel exposure and risk of wound rupture, preservation of blood flow in the distal ureters due to the intracorporeal anastomosis, and decreased risk of fluid imbalances.

Preparation

There are no specific preoperative preparations necessary other than those for robot-assisted radical cystectomy. The one change that may be employed is placement of the bedside assistant on the left side of the patient. This is particularly important for passing the endovascular stapler during the bowel work. The stoma site is marked preoperatively. As for every minimally invasive procedure, the patient is informed of the risk of conversion to open surgery. In our institutions we do not use any bowel preparation other than "nothing by mouth" the night before surgery. Of course, if there are extenuating circumstances such as a history of radiation, multiple previous surgeries, or a history of problems with constipation, a mechanical preparation can be employed. The patient is in 30° of Trendelenburg throughout the whole procedure. In rare cases, the amount of Trendelenburg may need to be decreased during if the bowel retracts too far proximally in the abdomen.

The online version of this chapter (doi:10.1007/978-1-4614-4906-5_11) contains supplementary material, which is available to authorized users.

M. Annerstedt, M.D. (✉)
Sophiahemmet Hospital, Uro Clinic,
Valhallavagen 91, Box 5605, Stockholm
SE-114 86, Sweden
e-mail: magnus.annerstedt@uroclinic.se

E.P. Castle, M.D., F.A.C.S.
Department of Urology, Mayo Clinic,
5779 East Mayo Blvd., Phoenix, AZ 85054, USA
e-mail: castle.erik@mayo.edu

E.P. Castle and R.S. Pruthi (eds.), *Robotic Surgery of the Bladder*, DOI 10.1007/978-1-4614-4906-5_11,

Instruments and Equipment

Besides the standard robotic instruments for RARC, the Small Grasping Retractor (Intuitive Surgical, Sunnyvale, CA) is very helpful when performing the bowel work. The Cadière Forceps are an alternative but care should be taken not to injure the bowel since they have a higher closing pressure. A 15-mm laparoscopic port is used as the lateral left port allowing the large specimen retrieval bag to pass as well as for the stapling of the bowel. The third robotic metal port can easily be inserted through this port when the third robotic arm is used on the left side. Laparoscopic staplers are used for isolation of the ileal conduit and reestablishment of the bowel continuity. The cartridges should be for small bowel/vasculature. A pre-cut 15 cm or 20 cm suture will be used for measuring the bowel. Two 8 French baby-feeding tubes 55 cm long are used as ureteral stents. Alternatively, standard 90 cm single J urinary diversion stents can be used. They are fixed to the bowel mucosa at the level of the stomal end with absorbable suture. One extra 12 mm laparoscopic port and a laparoscopic Babcock grasper are used to catch the distal part of the conduit through the abdominal wall at the end of the procedure. For a list of instruments and supplies please refer to Table 11.1.

Table 11.1 List of instruments and supplies

Robotic	
	Cadière forceps
	Small grasping retractor
Additional	
	Pre-cut suture (15–20 cm) Endovascular stapler with vascular and small bowel loads—60 mm Laparoscopic babcock 4-0 absorbable monofilament suture 4-0 equivalent barbed suture (*optional*) Urinary diversion stents (Single J) or eight French feeding tubes

Surgical Technique: Step-by-Step

Preparation of the Left Ureter

The left ureter is tunneled under the sigmoid mesentery to the right side (Fig. 11.1). It is important to create a sufficient opening in the mesentery to avoid kinking of the ureter. The left and right ureter are then held together with an extra large Hem-o-Loc® clip (Weck Surgical Instruments, Teleflex Medical, Research Triangle Park, NC). This step makes it easier to find the ureters after the bowel work.

Bowel Identification and Anastomosis

Fifteen to twenty centimeters of the distal ileum are isolated, leaving at least 15 cm to the ileocecal valve. The bowel is divided using a 60-mm laparoscopic stapler with a cartridge for small bowel/vasculature (Fig. 11.2). By using a vascular load (red color) the small vessels of the mesentery are easily controlled along with division of the bowel segment. The assisting surgeon is performing the stapling through the 15-mm port from the left side of the patient. Care is taken to fire the stapler perpendicular to the bowel into the mesentery. In

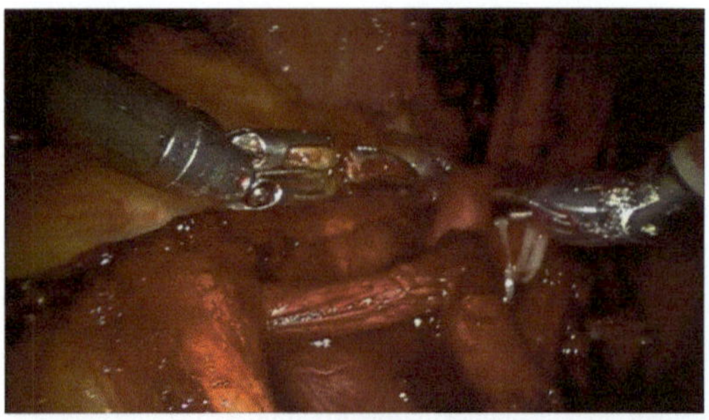

Fig. 11.1 Passing the left ureter through the window in the mesentery

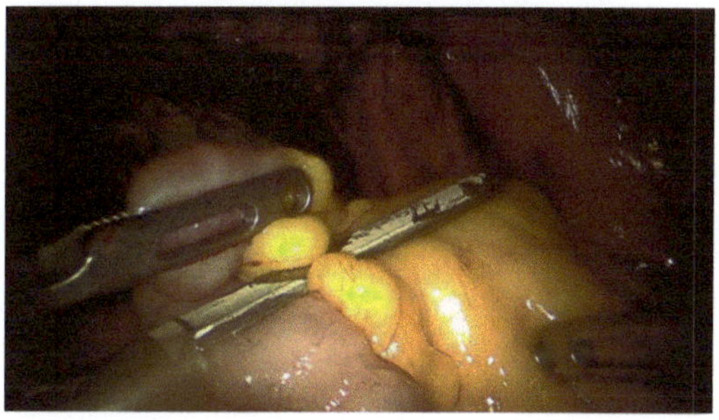

Fig. 11.2 Isolating the bowel segment

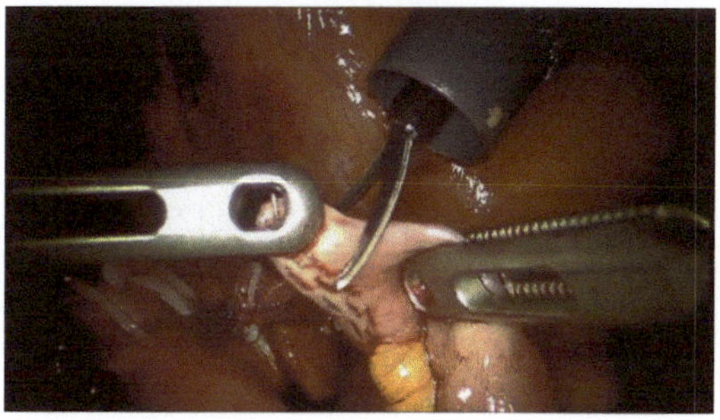

Fig. 11.3 Excising the antimesenteric corners of the staple line in preparation of passing the stapler

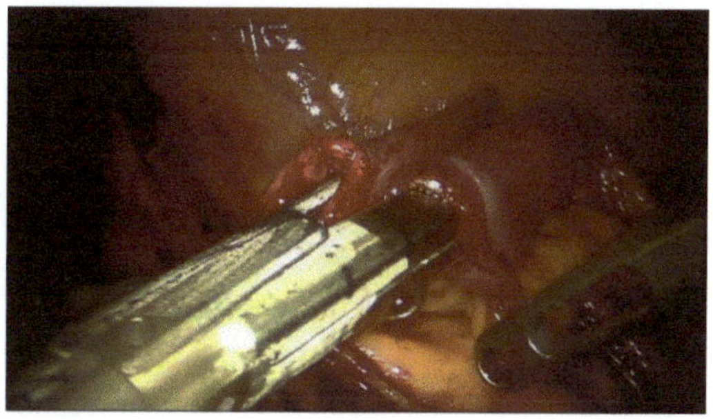

Fig. 11.4 Performing the side-to-side bowel anastomosis

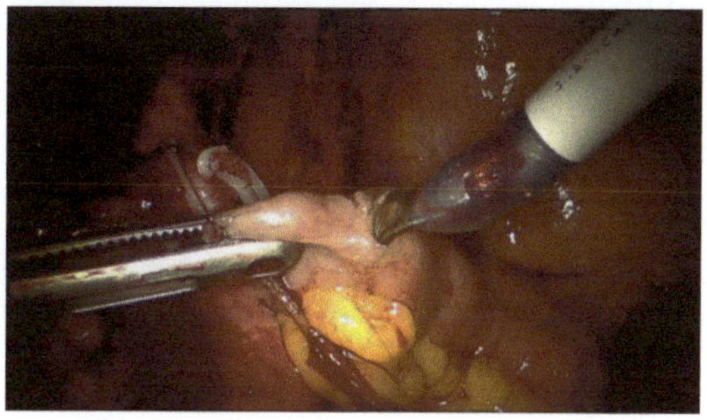

Fig. 11.5 Creating the enterotomy for the anticipated ureteroileal anastomosis

some cases, having tags on the bowel for retraction by the third robotic arm is helpful. It is important to achieve sufficient length at the distal incision in order not to have the bowel anastomosis too close to the stoma. The bowel continuity is restored using the same stapler with a small bowel load (blue color). The stapler is passed through the cut corners on the antimesenteric side of the staple lines of the distal and proximal ends of the ileum (Fig. 11.3). The anastomosis is performed in a "side-to-side" fashion with the antimesenteric part facing each other (Fig. 11.4). An additional transverse firing of the stapler is used to close the open ends of the ileal limbs—similar to what is done in open cases with an open gastrointestinal stapler. It is important to be gentle on the bowel serosa with all of the robotic instruments as inadvertent serosal tears can be encountered with tools such as the robotic needle drivers and robotic graspers.

Ureteroileal Anastomosis

The distal staple line of the conduit is cut away and two separate openings in the proximal part, for the ureteral implantation, are created (Fig. 11.5). At our institution we prefer the separate Nesbit (Bricker) implantation but using the Wallace plate is also an option. The ureters are secured with the third arm and a ProGrasp™ and spatulated approximately 2 cm. The anastomosis between the ureters and the proximal part (butt end for Wallace) of the conduit is carried out using two 4-0 monofilament running sutures, one at each side of the ureter (Fig. 11.6). A slipknot is preferably used when first approximating the ureter and bowel. More recently, barbed sutures have become available. Some surgeons are using the 4-0 equivalents for the ureteroileal anastomoses. Ensuring a watertight anastomosis visually is important since it is difficult to "test" the anastomosis robotically as one would do open.

Before completing the ureteroenteric anastomosis, the baby-feeding tubes (or single J urinary diversion stents) are pushed up to the kidney pelvis and secured at the bowel mucosa with absorbable suture. Two baby-feeding catheters each 55 cm are inserted through the right assistant port and pulled through the ileal segment. The passage of the stents can be challenging and coordination between the assistant and the surgeon is key (Fig. 11.7a, b).

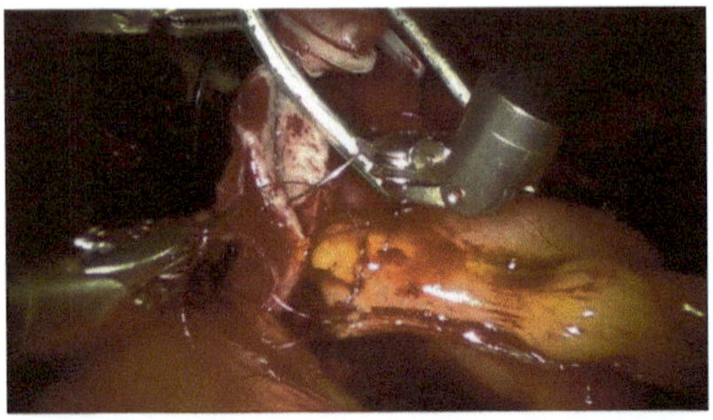

Fig. 11.6 Creating the ureteroenteric anastomosis

The surgeon must be careful to estimate the distance to advance the stents as haptic feedback is not available to know once the kidney is reached. In most cases, passing 20 cm (approximately four lines on marked stents) is sufficient.

Creation of the Stoma

The robot is then undocked with the ports still be in place. A drain is inserted through the second robotic port on the left side. The stoma is then constructed at its appropriately marked location. The skin and underlying fat are removed and the fascia is incised like a cross (cruciate incision). The muscle is separated and a 12-mm laparoscopic port is pushed through peritoneum still having pneumoperitoneum (Fig. 11.8a). A laparoscopic Babcock is used through the laparoscopic port to grab the distal part of the conduit and pull it through the abdominal wall (Fig. 11.8b).

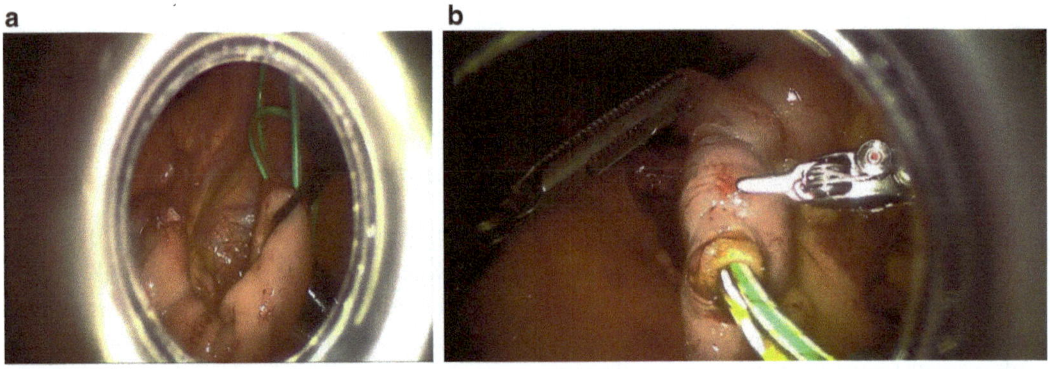

Fig. 11.7 (**a**) Passing the stents; (**b**) pulling through the stents

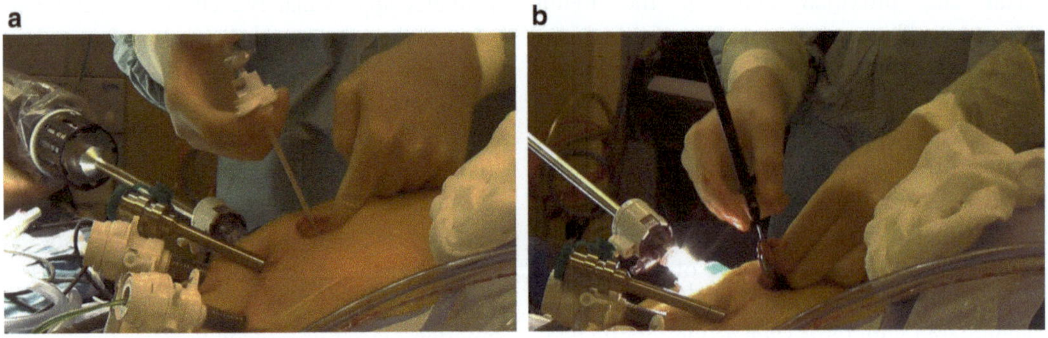

Fig. 11.8 (**a**) Creating the stoma site; (**b**) pulling the conduit through the stoma site with a laparoscopic babcock

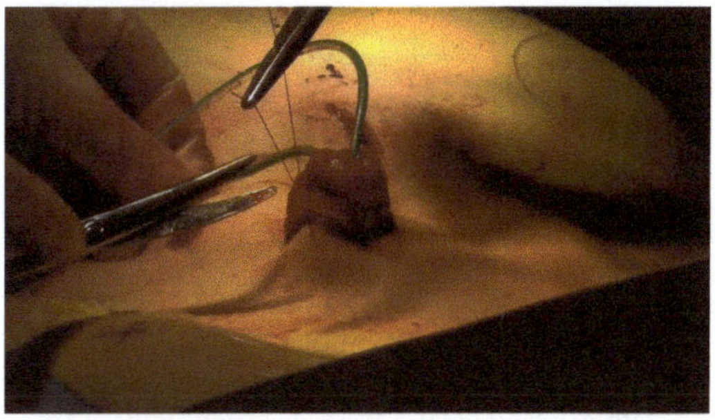

Fig. 11.9 Maturation of the stoma

The stoma is then everted and sutured to the skin (Fig. 11.9). Alternatively, the bowel can be passed to the stoma site through the infraumbilical extraction incision once the bladder is removed.

Results

Some authors have successfully completed total intracorporeal ileal conduit with a mean operative time of 11.5 h [19]. However, a more recent publication reports decreasing operative times [18]. In experienced hands, performing intracorporeal ileal conduits takes approximately 1.5–2 h in addition to the time required for the extirpative part of the procedure. Although results are short term in most reports, the overall consensus is that it is feasible and safe in the hands of surgeons experienced at robot-assisted radical cystectomy.

At our institution we intend to perform every cystectomy robotically with intracorporeal urinary diversion, both ileal conduit and ileal neobladder. Listed in Table 11.2 are unpublished results from our consecutive unselected series of intracorporeal ileal conduit.

Table 11.2 RARC with ileal conduit results (Herlev University Hospital Copenhagen, Denmark—unpublished)

N=69	
Female—18	
Male—51	
Age: 68 (47–81)	
Salvage procedures: 12 (after radiation and/or chemotherapy)	
EBL: 250 ml (50–3,700) no intracorporeal more than 700 ml (including cystectomy and lymph node dissection)	
Conversion to open sugery: 8 pts (11.6 %)	
OR-time: 287 min (155–517) (*skin to skin*)	
Complications according to the Clavien system [20]	
Clavien score	
0	28 pts
1	13 pts
2	10 pts
3a	5 pts
3b	12 pts
4	1 pts
5	0 pts

Conclusion

With time and increased experience, operative times, functional results, and complications will continue to improve. Selection of appropriate urinary diversion following robot-assisted radical cystectomy in the form of intracorporeal or extracorporeal approach needs further studies. At this point in time, intracorporeally performed urinary diversion may be recommended only in the hands of experienced surgeons at high-volume centers.

Editors' Commentary

Erik P. Castle and Raj S. Pruthi

As experience with RARC continues to spread throughout the urologic community, many surgeons who have mastered the cystectomy with extracorporeal diversion are transitioning to intracorporeal diversions. While there may be concern with the added time it may add, there are some significant benefits to an intracorporeal ileal conduit. One of the more important potential benefits is the decreased traction and tension on the ureters during the ureteroileal anastomosis. There have been some anecdotal reports among RARC surgeons during their early experience of ureteroileal strictures. This is likely due to traction and over mobilization of the ureters that is often a consequence early on in experience with extracorporeal diversion. By performing the anastomoses in the retroperitoneum, many feel that this decreases on the risk of stricture.

There are some key points to consider when starting with intracorporeal ileal conduit creation. Firstly, the assistant should be situated on the left side as this provides the best angle for stapling the ileum. Secondly, make the anticipated conduit segment at least 20 cm long as one can always cut back on a long conduit but one too short can pose problems during maturation of the stoma. Thirdly, the surgeon may want to undock the robot and take the patient 15–20° out of extreme Trendelenburg if the bowel is not dropping into the field of view adequately. Finally, passing the diversion stents may be a challenge and we have found that passing the assistant instrument from the anastomosis end to the stomal end to grasp the stent and pull through in order to pass up into the ureter seems to provide the best angle. One should also secure the stent to the stomal end after passing it in order to avoid it falling out when trying to develop the stoma.

References

1. Stein JP, Skinner DG. Radical cystectomy for invasive bladder cancer: long-term results of a standard procedure. World J Urol. 2006;24(3):296–304.
2. Stein JP. Improving outcomes with radical cystectomy for high-grade invasive bladder cancer. World J Urol. 2006;24(5):509–16.
3. Dhar NB, Klein EA, Reuther AM, Thalmann GN, Madersbacher S, Studer UE. Outcome after radical cystectomy with limited or extended pelvic lymph node dissection. J Urol. 2008;179(3):873–8. discussion 878.
4. Konety BR, Allareddy V, Herr H. Complications after radical cystectomy: analysis of population-based data. Urology. 2006;68(1):58–64.
5. Novotny V, Hakenberg OW, Wiessner D, et al. Perioperative complications of radical cystectomy in a contemporary series. Eur Urol. 2007;51(2):397–401. discussion 401–392.
6. Hautmann RE, Volkmer BG, Schumacher MC, Gschwend JE, Studer UE. Long-term results of standard procedures in urology: the ileal neobladder. World J Urol. 2006;24(3):305–14.
7. Parra RO, Andrus CH, Jones JP, Boullier JA. Laparoscopic cystectomy: initial report on a new treatment for the retained bladder. J Urol. 1992;148(4):1140–4.
8. Menon M, Hemal AK, Tewari A, et al. Nerve-sparing robot-assisted radical cystoprostatectomy and urinary diversion. BJU Int. 2003;92(3):232–6.
9. Guru KA, Kim HL, Piacente PM, Mohler JL. Robot-assisted radical cystectomy and pelvic lymph node dissection: initial experience at Roswell Park Cancer Institute. Urology. 2007;69(3):469–74.
10. Murphy DG, Challacombe BJ, Elhage O, et al. Robotic-assisted laparoscopic radical cystectomy with extracorporeal urinary diversion: initial experience. Eur Urol. 2008;54(3):570–80.
11. Wang GJ, Barocas DA, Raman JD, Scherr DS. Robotic vs open radical cystectomy: prospective comparison of perioperative outcomes and pathological measures of early oncological efficacy. BJU Int. 2008;101(1):89–93.
12. Hemal AK, Abol-Enein H, Tewari A, et al. Robotic radical cystectomy and urinary diversion in the management of bladder cancer. Urol Clin North Am. 2004;31(4):719–29. viii.
13. Palmer KJ, Shah K, Samavedi S, Coughlin G, Patel VR. Robot-assisted radical cystectomy. J Endourol. 2008;22(9):2073–7. discussion 2079.
14. Lowentritt BH, Castle EP, Woods M, Davis R, Thomas R. Robot-assisted radical cystectomy in women: technique and initial experience. J Endourol. 2008;22(4):709–12.
15. Khan MS, Shah SS, Hemel A, Rimington P, Dasgupta P. Robotic-assisted radical cystectomy. Int J Med Robot. 2008;4(3):197–201.
16. Pruthi RS, Smith A, Wallen EM. Evaluating the learning curve for robot-assisted laparoscopic radical cystectomy. J Endourol. 2008;22(11):2469–74.
17. Kang SG, Ko YH, Jang HA, et al. Initial experience of robot-assisted radical cystectomy with total intracorporeal urinary diversion: comparison with extracorporeal method. J Laparoendosc Adv Surg Tech A. 2012;22(5):456–62.
18. Jonsson MN, Adding LC, Hosseini A, et al. Robot-assisted radical cystectomy with intracorporeal urinary diversion in patients with transitional cell carcinoma of the bladder. Eur Urol. 2011;60(5):1066–73.
19. Balaji KC, Yohannes P, McBride CL, Oleynikov D, Hemstreet 3rd GP. Feasibility of robot-assisted totally intracorporeal laparoscopic ileal conduit urinary diversion: initial results of a single institutional pilot study. Urology. 2004;63(1):51–5.
20. Clavien PA, Barkun J, de Oliveira ML, et al. The Clavien-Dindo classification of surgical complications: five-year experience. Ann Surg. 2009;250(2):187–96.

Intracorporeal Ileal Neobladder

12

Stavros I. Tyritzis, Alexander Mottrie, Vincenzo Ficarra, and Peter Wiklund

Introduction

We are in the verge of celebrating the tenth anniversary of robot-assisted radical cystectomy (RARC) with urinary diversion (UD) [1] and it seems that this operation is successfully following the footsteps of robot-assisted radical prostatectomy. Even though the EAU Guidelines 2012 still consider this operation as experimental due to the lack of large prospective trials [2], many centers are reaching an adequate number of approximately 50 RARCs per year to be finally considered as centers of excellence, achieving improved postoperative outcomes, including decreased mortality, shorter length of hospital stay, and lower rehospitalization rates [3]. Till 2011, as reported by the database of the International Robot-Assisted Cystectomy Consortium (IRCC), which is a panel of the most experienced surgeon in the field worldwide, approximately 800 RARCs have been performed.

UD with formation of an orthotopic ileal neobladder is probably the most technically challenging procedure in urology. The construction of the reservoir can be performed totally intracorporeally, even though many centers prefer to do this in an extracorporeal way.

The selection of an orthotopic continent reservoir in terms of quality of life (QoL) levels has been discussed over the years. It seems that the ileal neobladder is the preferred choice of the patient when given the option [4]. Two studies have shown a statistically significant difference in QoL in favor of neobladders [5, 6]. Somani et al. in the only prospective cohort study conducted in 2009 concluded that there were no significant QoL differences between the diversion types [7, 8], even though these studies are limited by patient selection and information bias when variables such as body image, symptom tolerance, short or long term follow-up are evaluated. Finally, the EAU Guidelines are giving a level of evidence 2b in the QoL issue, irrespective of the diversion type [2].

In this chapter, we discuss all preoperative, intraoperative, and postoperative matters concerning the construction of an orthotopic ileal neobladder using the DaVinci robotic system.

S.I. Tyritzis, M.D., Ph.D., F.E.B.U. (✉)
Department of Molecular Medicine and Surgery, Section of Urology, Karolinska University Hospital, Karolinska Institutet, Solna, Stockholm 17176, Sweden
e-mail: styritzis@gmail.com

A. Mottrie
Department of Urology, O.L.V. Hospital, Aalst, Belgium

V. Ficarra
Department of Urology, University of Padova, Padova, Italy

P. Wiklund
Department of Urology, Karolinska University Hospital, Stockholm, Sweden

E.P. Castle and R.S. Pruthi (eds.), *Robotic Surgery of the Bladder*, DOI 10.1007/978-1-4614-4906-5_12,

Patient Selection

The inclusion's criteria for robot-assisted formation of an orthotopic ileal neobladder are the same as in open surgery. However, when the patient is not fit for laparoscopic surgery (decreased pulmonary compliance, multiple abdominal adhesions, bulky disease), the operation is contraindicated.

There are absolute and relative contraindications for neobladder formation. The absolute are:

(a) Disease involvement of the urethra distal to the prostate
(b) Compromised renal (serum creatinine >2 mg/dl) and hepatic function
(c) Decreased mental capability and hand dexterity

The relative contraindications are:

(a) Inflammatory bowel disease (Crohn's disease)
(b) Impotent rhabdosphincter, urinary incontinence
(c) History of recurrent urethral strictures
(d) Morbid obesity
(e) Previous abdominal or pelvic irradiation
(f) Severe comorbidities, elderly patients (octogenarians)

Preoperative Care

Pneumatic leg compression system should be used due to risk of decreased vascular perfusion during the procedure. To avoid cardiovascular complications in the patient, anticoagulant treatment is started with low-molecular weight heparin according to the patient's body weight the evening before surgery until the patient is fully mobilized.

Mechanical bowel preparation (osmotic laxative) may be used the day before surgery. Broad-spectrum intravenous antibiotics are administered at the start of the procedure.

Instrumentation

Robotic as well as standard laparoscopic surgical equipment must be supplemented. Table 12.1 is summarizing the necessary instrumentation.

Table 12.1 A summary of the necessary robotic and laparoscopic instrumentation

Robotic (Intuitive Surgical, Sunnyvale, CA, USA)	Laparoscopic
Three 8 mm robotic ports	Two 12 mm ports
Hot Shears™ (Monopolar Curved Scissors)	One 15 mm port
Maryland™ Bipolar Forceps	One 5 mm port
Cadiere™ Forceps	Suction
Large needle driver	Grasper
ProGrasp™ Forceps	Kelly
Basic accessory kit and drapes	Scissors
Intuitive surgical camera head	Ligasure™ (Valleylab, Boulder, CO, USA)
Intuitive surgical 0° and 30° endoscopes	16 mm stapler (Endo-GIA™/ Covidien Corp. Dublin, Ireland)
	Large and small clip appliers (Hem-o-lok®/Weck Closure Systems, Research Triangle Park, NC, USA, Lapra-Ty®/Ethicon Endo-Surgery, CA, USA)
	Three specimen bags
	Ligaloop strings (Braun-Dexon, Spangenberg, Germany)

Patient Positioning

After induction of general endotracheal anesthesia, a nasogastric tube and an 18 Ch Foley urinary catheter are inserted. The patient is placed in lithotomy position with arms adducted and padded. The legs are also abducted and slightly lowered on spreader bars. The table is placed in 25° Trendelenburg position during the RC and PLND. For the urinary diversion the Trendelenburg position is decreased to 10–15°.

Trocar Configuration

Port placement is critical for successful robotic surgery. A six-port technique is used with the camera port placed 5 cm above the umbilicus in the midline (Fig. 12.1). The camera port is placed with the Hasson technique and the other

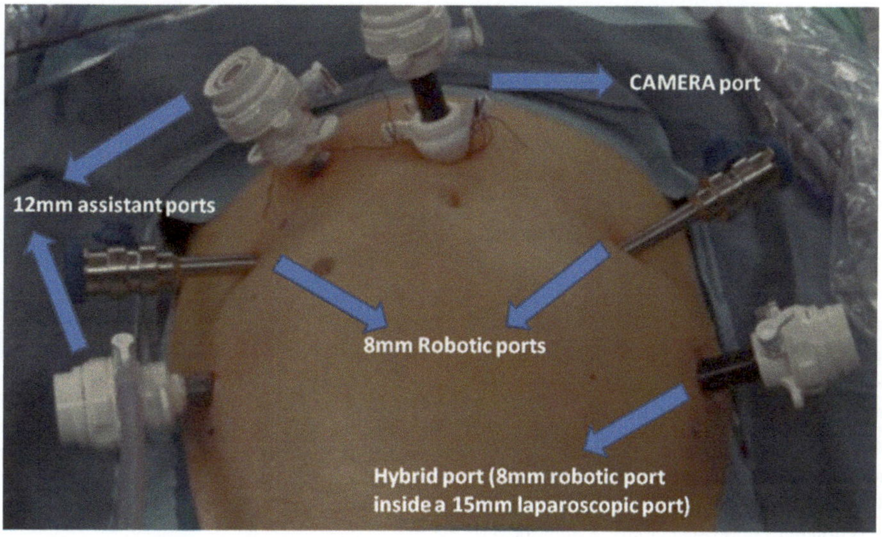

Fig. 12.1 Trocar configuration for robot-assisted radical cystectomy

ports are placed with direct view. During the port placement, a pressure of 18 mmHg can be helpful in creating additional tension on the abdominal wall. Two robotic ports are placed symmetrically in the level of the umbilicus on the left and right side, lateral to the rectus sheath, A third robotic port is placed just above and medial to the left anterior superior iliac spine through a 15-mm port, thereby enabling laparoscopic stapling by the assistant when the third robotic port is temporarily disconnected. This is the so-called hybrid port. Two assistant ports are placed on either side of the right robotic instrument port.

Surgical Technique

It is crucial that the console surgeon follows accurately and always with the same order the steps of the operation in order to have the best results and reduce operating time. The following steps have been refined in our institution many times to achieve the optimum result [9, 10]. All the steps are summarized in Table 12.2. Steps 5–13 concern the urinary diversion with the formation of the ileal orthotopic neobladder.

Entero-Urethral Anastomosis

The patient is placed in reduced 10–15° Trendelenburg position. The 0° lens is used for this initial step. The ileum is sufficiently mobilized in order to reach down to the urethra. Using robotic scissors, a 20 Ch opening (Fig. 12.2) is made to the antimesentric site of the ileum, which is isolated between two Ligaloop strings (Braun-Dexon, Spangenberg, Germany), passed around the intestine. The anastomosis is performed according to the Van Velthoven technique with a two-times 16 cm running 4-0 Quill™ suture, allowing for 10–12 stitches (Fig. 12.3). A needle driver and a Cadiere forceps are used for the above maneuvers. It is important previously to preserve an adequate urethral stump and have a silicone catheter placed.

Isolation of 50 cm Ileum

The orthotopic neobladder is fashioned with the Studer technique from a 50 cm segment of terminal ileum. The intestine is isolated using laparoscopic 60 mm intestinal stapler (Endo-GIA; Covidien Corp., Dublin, Ireland) (Fig. 12.4).

Table 12.2 Robot-assisted radical cystectomy (RARC) with orthotopic ileal neobladder formation "step by step"

1. Dissection of both ureters along the ureterovesical junction
2. Cystoprostatectomy (males)
(a) Posterior dissection of vasa deferentia and seminal vesicles
(b) Enter Retzius space and bladder drop of the right side
(c) Incision of the right endopelvic fascia
(d) Ligation of right vesical pedicles with Ligasure
(e) Intrafascial sparing of the right neurovascular bundle
(f) Repeat (b), (c), (d), (e) on the left side
(g) Closure of the urethrovesical junction with a suture
(h) Apical dissection with preservation of an adequate urethral stump
(i) Completion of cystoprostatectomy or anterior pelvic exenteration (females)
Resection of bladder, urethra, uterus, cervix, ovaries, anterior wall of the vagina (vagina preservation when needed)
3. Extended lymph node dissection
4. Transposition of the left ureter through the sigmoid mesentery
5. Reduction of Trendelenburg tilt to 10–15° from 25°
6. Entero-urethral anastomosis
7. Isolation of 50 cm of distal ileum for Studer neobladder and stapling
8. Detubularization of the ileal segment
9. Suturing of the posterior wall of the pouch
10. Folding of the reservoir
11. Construction of the ureteral Wallace plate, stenting of both ureters through the afferent limp of the Studer pouch
12. Entero-ureteral anastomosis
13. Closure of the remaining reservoir
14. Placing a drain in the small pelvis

The stapler is inserted by the bedside surgeon, using the hybrid 15 mm port. The ileum is stapled 40 cm proximal to the urethro-ileal anastomosis. The continuity of the small bowel is restored by using the same stapler, positioning the distal and proximal end of the ileum side to side with the antimesentery parts facing each other. An additional transverse firing of the Endo-GIA staple is used to secure the open ends of the ileal limbs.

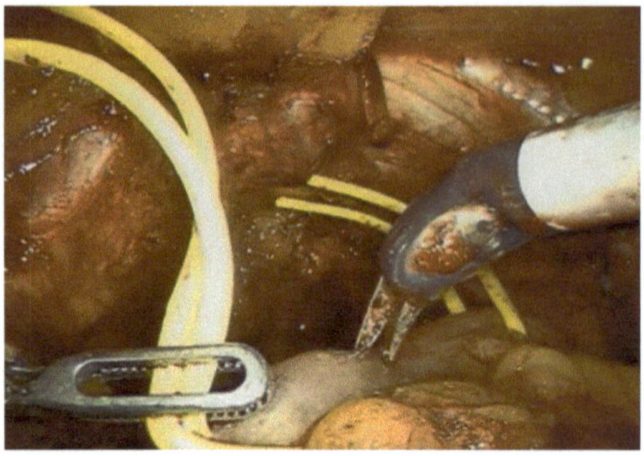

Fig. 12.2 A 20 Ch opening is made using robotic scissors to the respective site for the urethra-ileal anastomosis, which is being mobilized using two Ligaloop strings

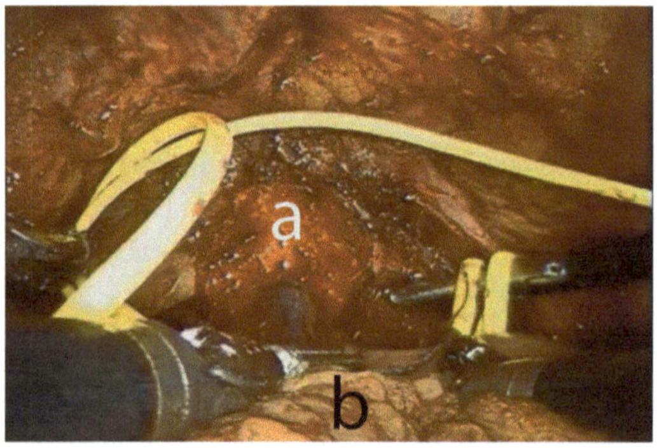

Fig. 12.3 Urethro-ileal anastomosis using the VanVelthoven technique. *a* urethral stump, *b* ileal loop

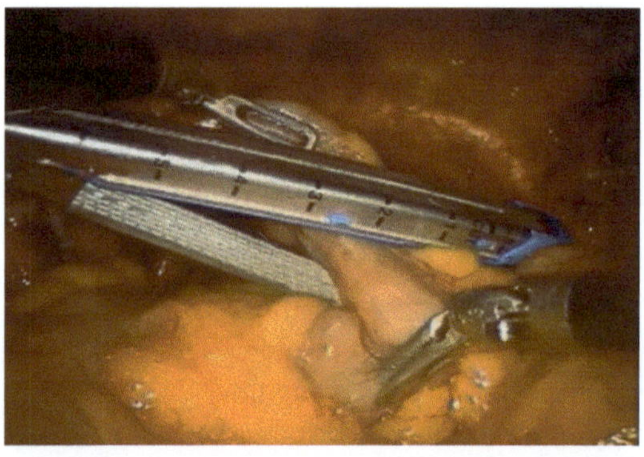

Fig. 12.4 Isolation of 50 cm of ileum for the neobladder. The ruler of the stapler can facilitate measurements. All maneuvers are performed using two Cadiere forceps

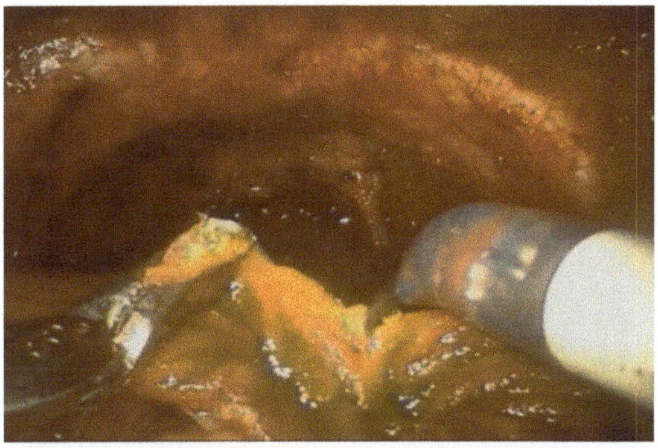

Fig. 12.5 Detubularization of the ileal segment

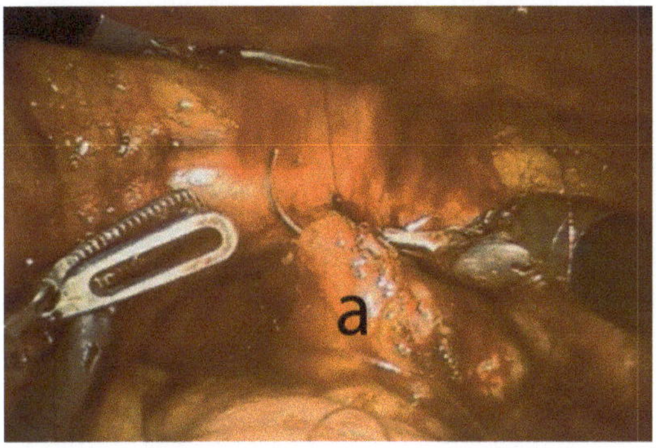

Fig. 12.6 Suturing the posterior wall (*a*) of the reservoir. Observe the stay suture held by the fourth robotic arm

Detubularization

The distal 40 cm of the isolated ileal segment are detubularized along the antimesenteric border with cold scissors (Fig. 12.5), leaving a 10 cm intact proximal isoperistaltic afferent limb.

Formation of Studer Neobladder

The posterior part of the Studer pouch is closed using multiple running sutures (15 cm 3-0 V-Loc™) in a seromuscular fashion, avoiding suturing the mucosa (Fig. 12.6). After the posterior part is sutured, the distal half of the anterior part of the reservoir is sutured, using the same suture. The 0 or 30° lens can be useful for this part of procedure. The proximal half of the anterior part of the reservoir is left open and is closed in the last part of the procedure.

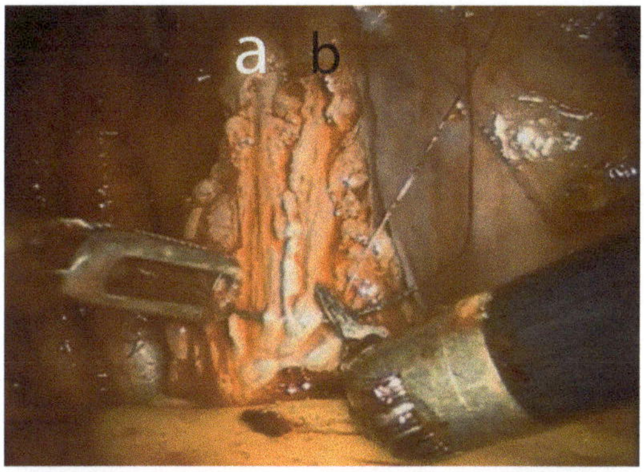

Fig. 12.7 Construction of the Wallace ureteral plate. Left (*a*) and right ureter (*b*) are spatulated 2 cm and tacked in place using a preplaced clip

Uretero-Enteral Anastomosis

The anastomosis between the ureters and the afferent limb is performed using the Wallace technique using a 0 lens (Fig. 12.7). A 3-0 Biosyn® stitch is placed at the distal end of each ureter. The left ureter is transposed to the right side by creating a tunnel under the sigmoid mesentery, just below the inferior rectal artery. The ureters are then spatulated 2 cm. The posterior walls of ureters are sutured side to side, using a 15 cm 4-0 V-Loc™ suture. Before commencing the anastomosis, two single-J 40 cm ureteric stents are introduced via the Seldinger technique through two separate 4 mm incision in the midline just above the pubic symphysis. The stents are pulled through the afferent limb (Fig. 12.8) and pushed up in to the ureters on each side, using the Cadiere forceps. The Wallace plate is sutured to the afferent limb of the Studer reservoir, using a 16 cm 4-0 Quill™ suture. After the uretero-enteral anastomosis is completed, the stents are sutured and fixed to the skin.

Closure of the Studer Reservoir

The remaining part of the reservoir is then closed with a running 3-0 V-Loc™ suture, using a 0° lens (Fig. 12.9). The balloon of the indwelling catheter is filled with 10 cm^3. The neobladder is then filled with 50 cm^3 of saline to check for leakage.

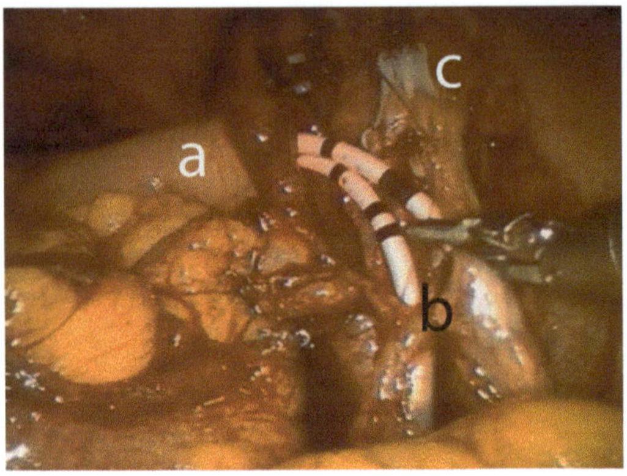

Fig. 12.8 Uretero-ileal anastomosis. Stents are already placed in both ureters using guidewires. The stents are first passed through the afferent limp of the Studer reservoir. (*a*) afferent limp, (*b*) Wallace plate, (*c*) clips at the distal ends of both ureters for obtaining frozen sections

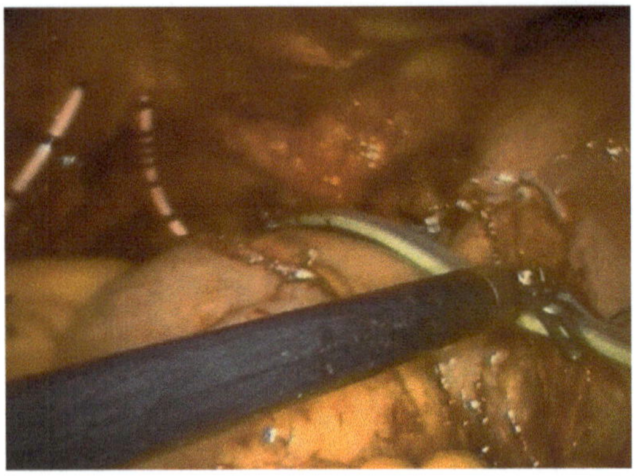

Fig. 12.10 Final intraoperative image. Drain is placed into the small pelvis

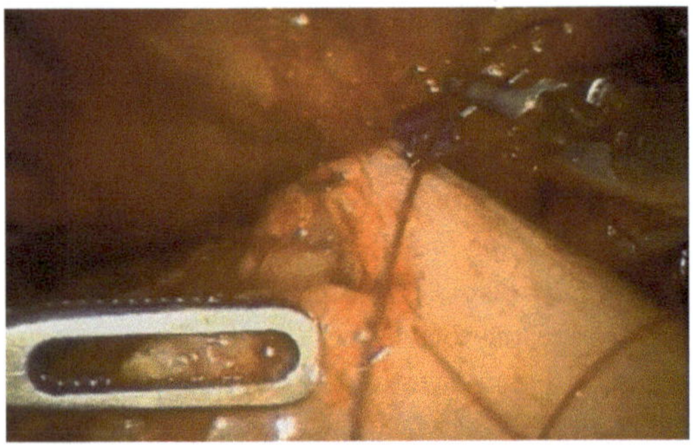

Fig. 12.9 Closure of the remaining anterior part of the pouch

If leakage is observed, extra sutures will have to be considered. A 21 Ch passive drainage is introduced and placed in the small pelvis (Fig. 12.10).

Postoperative Care

Careful manual irrigation of the reservoir has to be performed every 6–8 h to avoid catheter blockage by mucus overproduction. The drain can be removed when the drainage is <200 cm^3. The ureteral stents will be removed 1 week postoperatively. The urethral catheter can be removed approximately 3–4 weeks after the operation, without retrograde cystography. Pain management is achieved with the administration of 10 mg oxicodon b.i.d, 1 g paracetamol q.i.d., and parenteral morphine when required.

The patient is meticulously informed after the removal of the urethral catheter about the method and frequency of urination.

Complications and Management

RARC with neobladder formation remains a high-risk procedure with complications rate ranging from 30 to 50 % [11]. The rate is increasing due to the fact that RARC is being used more often in the elderly population, since the incidence of muscle-invasive bladder cancer peaks in the octogenarians [12]. Recent studies have shown though that even in the elderly patients, results can be similar to the ones of the younger patients [13, 14]. On the other hand, increasing experience, refinement, and standardization of the procedure continuously lowers the complication rates.

Table 12.3 shows the incidence of the short- and long-term complications that are related to the neobladder diversion in general [15–17]. These complications do not differ from the ones occurring in the open procedure. Short-term complications are reported within the first 90 days postoperatively. All complications are graded according to the CLAVIEN classification system, as revised by Dindo [18]. Each respective management is also depicted.

Table 12.3 The incidence of the short- and long-term complications that are related to the neobladder diversion

	Incidence (%)	CLAVIEN grade	Management
Short-term complications			
Urethro-ileal anastomotic leakage	1–5	I	Replacement of catheter, reservoir irrigation
Uretero-ileal anastomotic leakage	2	IIIa	Nephrostomy tube
Intestinal bleeding	1	II	Transfusion
Symptomatic lymphocele	5–10	I–IIIa	Drainage
Intestinal leakage	3	I–IIIb	Conservative-Reoperation
Paralytic ileus	20	II	Conservative
Obstructive ileus	4	IIIb	Reoperation
Mucus overproduction	20	I	Saline irrigation of the reservoir-Mucolytics
Hyperchloremic hypocalemic metabolic acidosis	15	II–IV	Conservative
UTI-Pyelonephritis	5	II	Conservative
Mortality	2–3	V	–
Long-term complications			
Day-time incontinence	5–10	II	Conservative
Night-time incontinence	30–40	II	Conservative
Uretero-ileal stricture	4–7	IIIb	Revision/Laser or ballon dilation-stenting
Urethro-ileal stricture	5	IIIb	Optical urethrotomy-Laser ablation
Hyperchloremic hypocalemic metabolic acidosis	15	II–IV	Conservative
Spontaneous neobladder rupture	1	IIIb	Reoperation
Ureteral reflux	1–2	I	Conservative
Renal failure	5–10	IV	Conservative-Dialysis
Lithiasis of the reservoir	13	IIIb	Lithotripsy
Vitamin B_{12} deficiency	10–12	II	Conservative
Intestinal fistula	1–3	I–IIIb	Conservative-Reoperation
Urethro-vaginal fistula	2	I–IIIb	Conservative-Reoperation
Neobladder–rectal fistula	1–2	I–IIIb	Conservative-Reoperation

It is noticeable that CLAVIEN III complications, which are considered major, exhibit a significant incidence of around 30 % [19]. Of course, the rates represent results of a learning curve.

- Why intracorporeal?

The issue of the superiority of the totally intracorporeal technique for urinary reconstruction over the extracorporeal technique is debatable. Two recent reviews by Haber and Orvieto have suggested that intracorporeal diversion leads to increased operating times and postoperative morbidity [20, 21]. However, these reviews were not dichotomizing diversion to neobladders and ileal conduits. Thus, their suggestions about intracorporeal neobladder formation might be flawed. Till now, there have been only 102 cases published in the literature undergoing intracorporeal formation of an ileal neobladder. Of them, 91 were performed robotically and 11 pure laparoscopically. Of the 91 robotic cases, 36 (40 %) were contributed by Karolinska Institutet. Unpublished data from Karolinska and Herlev would probably increase the total number of cases to more than 150. All the above operations are depicted in Table 12.4 [9, 22–28]. It is evident that no safe conclusions or recommendations can be extracted from these studies. Thus, more prospective studies are awaited.

It has been argued that the intracorporeal approach should only be used if specimen retrieval may be performed without an additional incision. In the female, the specimen may be taken out through an incision in the vaginal wall, and in the male the specimen is extracted through only a 4-cm skin incision at the end of the procedure. This provides not only good cosmetics but might also allow a faster convalescence. The intracorporeal reconstruction is less traumatic

Table 12.4 Published cases undergoing intracorporeal formation of an ileal neobladder

Author	Year	Approach	Patients (*n*)	Operating time (min)	Mean EBL (ml)	Mean hospitalization time (days)	Complication rates
Annerstedt et al.	2012	Robotic	28	320	300	NR	CLAVIEN grade I 14 %, grade II 20 %, grade III 39 % (lymphoceles and leakages), grade IV 2 %, grade V 3 %. Seven conversions due to short mesentery
Kang et al.	2012	Robotic	1	545	500	14	One paralytic ileus
Jonsson et al.	2011	Robotic	36	480	625	9	39 % early, 33 % late
Akbulut et al.	2011	Robotic	12	600	455	10.7	90 days: 26 complications in 8 patients, 1 colonic fistula, 1 death (cardiac arrest at POD 60)
Pruthi et al.	2010	Robotic	12	330	221	5	42 % early
Sala et al.	2006	Robotic	1	720	100	5	NR
Haber et al.	2007	LAP	9	565	788	7.8	12 % during hospital stay, 18 % after discharge
Beechen et al.	2003	Robotic	1	510	200	10	0 %
Gill et al.	2002	LAP	2	630	300	8.5	One gastrointestinal bleeding
Overall			102	522.2	387.7	8.7	

Table 12.5 Two published studies showing continence and potency as two significant functional outcomes

Author	Evaluated patients (*n*)	Day-time continence	Night-time continence	Potency
Jonsson et al.	36 (33 male)	97 %	83 %	16/20 (80 %)
Akbulut et al.	7	85.7 %	71.4 %	55 %

Continence is defined as 0–1 pad use per day and potency as IIEF-5 score >17

for the patient but on the other hand more technically demanding for the surgeon. One major advantage of performing the urinary diversion intracorporeally is that performing the running suture of the anastomosis between the urethra and the ileum minimizes the risk of urinary leakage. There is also less traction on the anastomosis between the reservoir and the urethra using an intracorporeal approach, as an appropriate ileal segment long enough to reach down to the urethra can be used. Moreover the ureters may be cut shorter to reduce the risk of stricture due to ischemia in the distal end of the ureter.

Functional Outcomes

Continence and potency are the two significant functional outcomes directly related to the neobladder. Unfortunately, the number of patients and the follow-up in many series are too low to draw any conclusions or compare them to the gold standard open procedure that is standing the test of time. Only two studies were able to present functional results. Continence is defined as 0–1 pad use per day and potency as IIEF-5 score >17. Table 12.5 shows the extracted data.

Tips n' Tricks

1. No bowel preparation is needed preoperatively. Fast track postoperative protocols are ideal and scientifically proven for avoiding ileus.
2. Preserve as much periureteral tissue as possible during ureteral dissection in order to avoid ischemia.
3. Start first with the anastomosis between the urethra and the chosen intestinal segment, because the anastomosis can be made without tension, and the neobladder will be placed correctly in the small pelvis during the whole procedure. The positioning of the ileal segment for the ileourethral anastomosis can be quite challenging. In cases when the ileal mesentery is applying tension, the surgeon can perform the following:
   (a) Decrease Trendelenburg positioning
   (b) Use Ligaloops for stretching
   (c) Dissect and release the covering peritoneum of the mesentery
   (d) Staple the mesentery further medially.
   (e) Dissect the part of the ileum around the ileocecal valve.
4. Care should be taken during the tunneling of the left ureter behind the colon sigmoid to avoid damaging any vascular structures.
5. Tag both ureters with Hem-o-lok® clip with preplaced Vicryl sutures for ready localization.
6. The suturing of the posterior part of the reservoir requires special attention. Firstly, the use of stay sutures is facilitating the process. Second, the surgeon should be careful not to interfere with the sutures used for the anastomosis to the urethra. It is also easier and safer to start suturing from the distal to the urethra point in order to avoid having an uneven Studer posterior wall of the neobladder, which will be very difficult to compensate.
7. It is important to check for leakage once the neobladder has been created. Extra suturing to secure a watertight reservoir and anastomosis is fundamental to decreasing postoperative complications.

Editors' Commentary

Erik P. Castle and Raj S. Pruthi

Creation of a neobladder can be an overwhelming undertaking whether done open or via a minimally invasive approach. Having a well-established standardized approach is critical to keeping operative time short and in preventing postoperative complications. The authors have a vast collective experience and have performed large numbers of these procedures with good results. One of the early difficulties was the large amount of suturing and finding ways to have the assistant follow and keep tension were key. As technology advances in suture and stapling devices, we may see increased use of this technique. Some have suggested that utilization of the newer "barbed" suture options may help with intracorporeal neobladder creation, particularly early in the learning curve. Some of the advantages described by those experienced in this approach include a watertight neourethrointestinal anastomosis as well as a tension free ureteroileal anastomosis. As experience in RARC increases and spreads throughout the robotic community we may see increased migration to the intracorporeal approach as has been described herein.

References

1. Beecken WD, Wolfram M, Engl T, et al. Robotic-assisted laparoscopic radical cystectomy and intra-abdominal formation of an orthotopic ileal neobladder. Eur Urol. 2003;44:337–9.
2. Stenzl A, Witjes JA, CompÃ©rat E, et al. Guidelines on bladder cancer muscle-invasive and metastatic. Arnhem: European Association of Urology Guidelines; 2012. p. 31.
3. Barbieri CE, Lee B, Cookson MS, et al. Association of procedure volume with radical cystectomy outcomes in a nationwide database. J Urol. 2007;178:1418–21.
4. Saika T, Arata R, Tsushima T, Okayama Urological Research Group, et al. Health-related quality of life after radical cystectomy for bladder cancer in elderly patients with an ileal conduit ureterocutaneostomy, or orthotopic urinary reservoir: a comparative questionnaire survey. Acta Med Okayama. 2007;61:199–203.

5. Philip J, Manikandan R, Venugopal S, et al. Orthotopic neobladder versus ileal conduit urinary diversion after cystectomy - a quality-of-life based comparison. Ann R Coll Surg Engl. 2009;91:565–9.
6. Hobisch A, Tosun K, Kinzl J, et al. Life after cystectomy and orthotopic neobladder versus ileal conduit urinary diversion. Semin Urol Oncol. 2001;19:18–23.
7. Somani BK, Gimlin D, Fayers P, N'dow J. Quality of life and body image for bladder cancer patients undergoing radical cystectomy and urinary diversion—a prospective cohort study with a systematic review of literature. Urology. 2009;74:1138–43.
8. Hayn MH, Stegemann AP, Agarwal PK et al. Pathologic and early oncologic outcomes after robot-assisted radical cystectomy: results from the International Robotic Cystectomy Consortium. AUA 2011 Annual Congress, Washington, DC. Abstract No. 1415.
9. Jonsson MN, Adding LC, Hosseini A, Schumacher MC, Volz D, Nilsson A, et al. Robot-assisted radical cystectomy with intracorporeal urinary diversion in patients with transitional cell carcinoma of the bladder. Eur Urol. 2011;60:1066–73.
10. Hosseini A, Adding C, Nilsson A, Jonsson MN, Wiklund NP. Robotic cystectomy: surgical technique. BJU Int. 2011;108:962–8.
11. Davis JW, Castle EP, Pruthi RS, Ornstein DK, Guru KA. Robot-assisted radical cystectomy: an expert panel review of the current status and future direction. Urol Oncol. 2010;28:480–6.
12. Clark PE, Stein JP, Groshen SG, et al. Radical cystectomy in the elderly: comparison of clinical outcomes between younger and older patients. Cancer. 2005;104:36–43.
13. Guillotreau J, Miocinovic R, Gamé X, Forest S, Malavaud B, Kaouk J, et al. Outcomes of laparoscopic and robotic radical cystectomy in the elderly patients. Urology. 2012;79:585–90.
14. Tyritzis SI, Anastasiou I, Stravodimos KG, Alevizopoulos A, Kollias A, Balangas A, et al. Radical cystectomy over the age of 75 is safe and increases survival. BMC Geriatr. 2012;12:18.
15. Stein JP, Skinner DG. Results of orthotopic urinary diversions, chapter 82. In: Campbell-Walsh textbook of urology, vol. 4. 9th ed. Philadelphia, PA: Saunders.
16. Hautmann RE, de Petriconi RC, Volkmer BG. Lessons learned from 1,000 neobladders: the 90-day complication rate. J Urol. 2010;184:990–4.
17. Hautmann RE, de Petriconi RC, Volkmer BG. 25 years of experience with 1,000 neobladders: long-term complications. J Urol. 2011;185:2207–12.
18. Dindo D, Demartines N, Clavien PA. Classification of surgical complications. A new proposal with evaluation in a cohort of 6336 patients and results of a survey. Ann Surg. 2004;240:205–13.
19. Schumacher MC, Jonsson MN, Hosseini A, Nyberg T, Poulakis V, Pardalidis NP, et al. Surgery-related complications of robot-assisted radical cystectomy with intracorporeal urinary diversion. Urology. 2011;77:871–6.
20. Haber GP, Crouzet S, Gill IS. Laparoscopic and robotic assisted radical cystectomy for bladder cancer: a critical analysis. Eur Urol. 2008;54:54–62.
21. Orvieto MA, DeCastro GJ, Trinh QD, Jeldres C, Katz MH, Patel VR, et al. Oncological and functional outcomes after robot-assisted radical cystectomy: critical review of current status. Urology. 2011;78:977–84.
22. Annerstedt M, Lam G, Steven K. Robot assisted radical cystectomy (RARCx) including extended pelvic lymph node dissection (PLND) and intracorporal urinary diversion as standard procedure. EAU Congress, Paris 2012, abstract no. 709.
23. Kang SG, Ko YH, Jang HA, Kim J, Kim SH, Cheon J, et al. Initial experience of robot-assisted radical cystectomy with total intracorporeal urinary diversion: comparison with extracorporeal method. J Laparoendosc Adv Surg Tech A. 2012;2:456–62.
24. Pruthi RS, Nix J, McRackan D, Hickerson A, Nielsen ME, Raynor M, et al. Robotic-assisted laparoscopic intracorporeal urinary diversion. Eur Urol. 2010;57:1013–21.
25. Akbulut Z, Canda AE, Ozcan MF, Atmaca AF, Ozdemir AT, Balbay MD. Robot-assisted laparoscopic nerve-sparing radical cystoprostatectomy with bilateral extended lymph node dissection and intracorporeal studer pouch construction: outcomes of first 12 cases. J Endourol. 2011;25:1469–79.
26. Haber GP, Campbell SC, Colombo Jr JR, Fergany AF, Aron M, Kaouk J, et al. Perioperative outcomes with laparoscopic radical cystectomy: "Pure laparoscopic" and "open-assisted laparoscopic" approaches. Urology. 2007;70:910–5.
27. Sala LG, Matsunaga GS, Corica FA, Ornstein DK. Robot-assisted laparoscopic radical cystoprostatectomy and totally intracorporeal ileal neobladder. J Endourol. 2006;20:233–6.
28. Gill IS, Kaouk JH, Meraney AM, Desai MM, Ulchaker JC, Klein EA, et al. Laparoscopic radical cystectomy and continent orthotopic ileal neobladder performed completely intracorporeally: the initial experience. J Urol. 2002;168:13–8.

Perioperative Care: The Radical Cystectomy Pathway

13

Raj Kurpad, Eric M. Wallen, and Matthew E. Nielsen

Introduction

Bladder cancer has a significant burden of disease in the USA. As the fourth most common malignancy, there are over 70,000 new diagnoses of bladder cancer each year [1]. The incidence has risen by 40 % since 1975 and a significant proportion, approximately one in four new cases, present at an advanced stage, for which radical cystectomy is the reference standard treatment. Bladder cancer continues to confer significant disease-specific mortality to patients inflicted with the illness [1]. Furthermore, while 75 % of newly diagnosed bladder cancers are non muscle invasive at the time of presentation, 50–75 % of these patients have recurrent disease and 15–30 % progress to muscle-invasive disease [2].

The treatment of bladder cancer encompasses many modalities including endoscopic resection, intravesical therapies, chemotherapy, radiation therapy, and surgery [2–4, 27]. In many instances, given the aggressive nature of the disease, patients are counseled for the need of a cystectomy with urinary diversion [2–4]. While open radical cystectomy with urinary diversion remains the gold standard for treatment of patients with muscle-invasive bladder cancer, robot-assisted surgery has rapidly evolved as an alternative approach, gaining popularity among urologic surgeons [8–11, 26].

Patients are recommended treatment with radical cystectomy and urinary diversion most typically when either muscle-invasive disease is present or when patients have recurrent high-grade T1 and/or CIS disease [2]. Perioperative chemotherapy has a role in many cases, either in the neoadjuvant or adjuvant setting. Neoadjuvant chemotherapy may be particularly desirable among patients with suspected T3 disease and/or evidence of lymphadenopathy on radiographic imaging, in which cases cystectomy may be delayed until after administration of chemotherapy with hopes of debulking tumor burden and potentially treating micrometastatic disease systemically [3, 4]. Factors taken into consideration in preoperative cystectomy counseling include the patient's baseline performance status, which may also influence selection of the approach to surgery, i.e. robot assisted versus open. .

Traditionally, radical cystectomy with urinary diversion has been an incredibly morbid surgery with significant perioperative mortality and morbidity [5, 27]. Advances in surgical technique, anesthetic care, and postoperative management have dramatically reduced the mortality and morbidity associated with cystectomy [5]. Furthermore, the introduction of robot-assisted surgery into the field of urology has also had an impact in the treatment of bladder cancer. While longer term oncologic and survival comparisons are forthcoming, many studies report benefits

R. Kurpad (✉) • E.M. Wallen • M.E. Nielsen, M.D.
Department of Urology, The University of North Carolina at Chapel Hill, Chapel Hill, NC, USA
e-mail: mnielsen@med.unc.edu

E.P. Castle and R.S. Pruthi (eds.), *Robotic Surgery of the Bladder*, DOI 10.1007/978-1-4614-4906-5_13,

utilizing robot-assisted surgery with respect to estimated blood loss, postoperative analgesic usage, and length of stay when compared to the open approach, and intermediate term oncologic outcomes appear comparable [8–11].

Improving Outcomes After Major Abdominal Operations: Lessons from General Surgery

Reducing the mortality and morbidity of radical cystectomy and urinary diversion continues to challenge urologic oncologists today. In contrast to other major urologic oncology procedures, the routine use of intestinal segments for urinary diversion introduces a number of risks and challenges for postoperative recovery. Ileus, bowel obstruction, and other complications consistently rank among the most common and troublesome major complications in series of cystectomy and urinary diversion. Whereas the historical paradigm of bowel surgery was characterized by extreme conservativism, with prolonged nasogastric tube drainage and delayed initiation of enteral feeding until resumption of bowel function was established, standard postoperative care in general surgery has evolved towards earlier introduction of feeding, which in turn appears to be associated with improved outcomes in a variety of contexts [13–21].

A more aggressive approach to postoperative care after colorectal surgery has an established and standardized track record that has been widely adopted. *Enhanced recovery after surgery*, or ERAS, protocols have repeatedly shown improved postoperative outcomes, leading to widespread adoption of these clinical fast-track pathways in that context [13–19]. Key components of ERAS pathways [13] for patients undergoing colorectal surgery include:

1. Minimizing preoperative oral bowel preparation, no longer routine for all patients
2. Preoperative fasting to include NPO for solids 6 h prior and, in some settings, NPO for clear liquids 2 h prior
3. No preanesthetic anxiolytic or analgesic medications
4. Antithrombotic prophylaxis as mandated by local protocols
5. Single dose antimicrobial prophylaxis against both aerobic and anaerobic microorganisms
6. Patients encouraged and informed about utilization of mid-thoracic epidural
7. Minimize surgical incisions
8. Nasogastric tube decompression not be used routinely
9. Intraoperative maintenance of normothermia with infusion of warmed fluids and upper body air-heating cover
10. Oral fluids starting 2 h after surgery on day 0 with a target intake of 800 mL on day 0
11. Goal of discontinuing IV fluids on day 1
12. No routine placement of intra-abdominal drain
13. Urinary catheter drainage until epidural is discontinued
14. Selective use of antiemetics to promote postoperative intake and diminish postoperative nausea
15. Patients encouraged for early mobilization, out of bed at 2 h postoperatively, and every 6 h thereafter
16. Discharge criteria include pain management with oral medications, no need for IV fluids, adequate PO intake, independently mobile or at the same level prior to admission

Over the past decade, there have been many modifications and deviations to the fast-track clinical pathway described above, dependent upon the specific surgery performed, but the basic tenets of minimizing bowel preparations, single dose antibiotic prophylaxis, antithrombotic prophylaxis, minimizing gastric decompression, early reintroduction of oral intake, early mobilization, and maintaining adequate but minimal postoperative analgesia continue to have significant relevance in the postoperative care of patients undergoing a broad spectrum of gastrointestinal operations [13–21].

Benefits of Fast-Track Pathways in the General Surgery Experience

A randomized control trial comparing fast-track protocols after colonic surgery compared to older standard protocols was conducted by researchers in Zurich [13]. Muller et al. reported that utilizing fast-track protocols led to significantly reduced 30 day complications and shorter hospital stays, ultimately driving reduced healthcare costs [13]. This trend was also confirmed in a prospective observational study of more than 900 patients undergoing colonic surgery reported by Gustaffsson et al.; patients with high adherence to the ERAS protocol were found to have a 25 % lower risk of a postoperative complication and 50 % lower risk of postoperative symptoms delaying discharge [14].

In parallel with these clinical and economic benefits, fast-track pathways have also been shown to improve satisfaction of both providers and patients. Postoperative care employing fast-track programs require coordinated efforts between all stakeholders including physicians, nurses, dieticians, nursing assistants, patients, and family caregivers [19–21]. The coordinated efforts of all the individuals involved leads to more robust communication, ultimately enhancing patient care [19–21]. Furthermore, from a nursing perspective, nurses in fact play a larger role in postoperative recovery by encouraging early mobilization and oral intake [20, 21]. As a result, nurses feel more invested as the importance of their roles becomes highlighted in the successful implementation of postoperative fast-track recovery programs [20, 21]. Ultimately, as reflected in survey data, this leads to an overall greater patient satisfaction with their operative experience [21]. In a review of enhanced recovery protocols, authors Khan et al. examined ten studies investigating health-related quality of life (HRQoL) and patient satisfaction, with several studies demonstrating significantly reduced fatigue and pain in the first week after surgery [21]. After the first week of surgery, the authors did not find any statistically significant differences in the results of patient questionnaires [21] leading to the conclusion that these pathways may be particularly critical to improving the quality of life during the early days of the postoperative recovery [21].

Radical Cystectomy: Rationale for Adoption of Fast-Track Pathway

Given the centrality of small or large bowel resection and anastomosis for urinary diversion to the recovery after cystectomy, and the significance of these aspects to the development of complications after cystectomy, implementing the strategies of postoperative care from our colleagues in general surgery is intuitive and lends itself to very similar parallels. While the issues central to gastrointestinal surgery are relatively less relevant in other major urologic oncology procedures such as nephrectomy or prostatectomy, the importance of these issues to the recover after radical cystectomy cannot be underestimated. As such, we strongly believe that the incorporation of insights from the general surgery literature into the postoperative care of patients undergoing radical cystectomy with urinary diversion for the treatment of bladder cancer provides an important avenue to improve outcomes, reduce costs, and enhance the patient's experience and satisfaction.

The UNC Lineberger Experience with Fast-Track Cystectomy Pathway

Our postoperative cystectomy pathway has previously been reported in 362 patients undergoing radical cystectomy from either an open or a robot-assisted approach. Urinary diversions encompassed both ileal conduits and neobladders. The original "fast-track" pathway in our main descriptive report is outlined below:

1. Counseling and expectations of surgery
2. Clear liquid diet the day prior to surgery with a bottle of magnesium citrate and a fleets enema taken the night before. We no longer implement this aspect of the pathway; rather patients are encouraged to eat a regular diet the day prior to surgery and no longer administer a mechanical enema for bowel preparation
3. NPO after midnight the evening prior to surgery
4. Neomycin enema the day of surgery 2 h prior to start of surgery
5. Intraoperative DVT prophylaxis with TED hose and SCDs
6. Perioperative antibiotics with a second or third generation cephalosporin for 24-h coverage
7. Removal of nasogastric or orogastric tube (if placed) at the end of the surgery

8. Postoperative DVT prophylaxis with ambulation, TED, SCDs, and subcutaneous heparin or lovenox at the discretion of the attending surgeon
9. GI ulcer prophylaxis with an H2 blocker
10. Prokinetic agents (metoclopramide 10 mg IV q8 for 48 h)
11. Non-narcotic pain management with toradol 30 mg q6 for 48 h, then celebrex 200 mg BID afterwards for 2 weeks with supplementation with morphine and/or other narcotic PCA as needed
12. Use of toradol as needed if renal function permits
13. Early ambulation with early consultation with physical therapy
14. Diet advanced as follows:
    (a) NPO on postoperative day 1
    (b) 8 oz of clear liquid diet every 8 h on postoperative day 2 (8 q8, irrespective of bowel sounds)
    (c) Unrestricted clear liquid diet on postoperative day 3
    (d) If clear liquid diet tolerated without significant nausea and/or vomiting, regular diet on postoperative day 4

A number of changes have been made to our initial experience which are outlined later in the chapter. However, even our initial experience highlights several significant shifts from the previously accepted norm. Major changes from traditional practice include immediate removal (or lack of placement) of an orogastric or nasogastric tube and the elimination of preoperative bowel preparation as previously described [13–19]. Initial experience of early nasogastric tube removal concomitantly with metoclopramide use was described by Donat et al. where the authors demonstrated that early nasogastric decompression had benefits with regards to earlier return of bowel function as well as fewer complications with atelectasis [22]. However with our series, we noted no benefit with prolonged NG tube decompression and elected to remove it at the end of the surgical operation starting from the 60th case [6]. Non-narcotic pain management was also an innovation to help prevent exacerbating delayed return of bowel function [6].

Table 13.1 Demographics and perioperative outcomes of the 100 most recent patients in the UNC Lineberger fast-track experience

Demographics and perioperative outcomes	
Age	66.9 (33–86)
ASA score	2.7 (2–4)
Mean time to flatus, *d*	2.2
Mean time to BM, *d*	2.9
Mean time to d/c, *d*	5.0
% D/C on POD 4/5	79 %
Overall complication rate	39 %
GI complication rate	16 %
Readmission rate	12 %

Additionally, with the introduction of minimally invasive surgery into the treatment of bladder cancer, particularly with the robot-assisted radical cystectomy, further reduction of narcotic pain requirements has been seen, ultimately facilitating more rapid return of bowel function as well as reducing the length of postoperative hospital stay.

Retrospective analysis of 362 patients with bladder cancers who underwent radical cystectomy with urinary diversion between 2001 and 2008 revealed that patients on the fast-track pathway had shorter time to flatus, bowel movement, and hospital discharge, compared to previously reported literature (see Table 13.1) [6]. Complication and readmission rates were comparable with benchmarks previously reported literature [6].

Patients receiving metoclopramide were less likely to experience nausea and vomiting compared to patients not receiving metoclopramide (see Table 13.2). However, the length of stay in the hospital was not significantly different in the two groups and no direct link made towards the progression to a postoperative ileus [6]. Furthermore, patients chewing gum starting on POD 1 experienced reduced time to flatus as well as time to bowel movement after radical cystectomy (see Table 13.3) [7]. These results are similar to literature published detailing the postoperative care after colorectal surgery [13–19]. Our clinical pathway was not modified on the basis of clinical staging, age, comorbidities, open versus robot-assisted surgery, or diversion type.

Table 13.2 Outcomes of metoclopramide treatment after cystectomy [6]

	Age (years)	Regular diet, *n*	LOS, *d*	GI complications	Ileus	Nausea/vomiting
With metoclopramide	65.8	3.9	5.1	19 %	16 %	3 %
Without metoclopramide	66.7	3.9	5.6	31 %	18 %	12 %
p Value	0.642	0.821	0.330	0.072	0.419	0.011

Table 13.3 Outcomes of gum-chewing on bowel function and length of stay in the hospital [7]

Group	Age (years)	Time to flatus, *d*	Time to BM, *d*	LOS, *d*
Control	66.5	2.9	3.9	5.1
Gum-chewing	64.8	2.4	3.2	4.7
p Value	0.380	<0.001	<0.001	0.067

Complications were classified with regards to the Clavien classification system with major complications defined as grade 3 or higher and minor complications defined as Clavien grade 1 or 2. Major complications included fascial dehiscence, acute renal failure, cardiac ischemia, death, internal herniation, misplaced ureteral stent, and postoperative bleeding, while minor complications encompassed ileus, UTI, arrhythmias, atelectasis, altered mental status, DVT, FUO, urine leak, acute renal insufficiency, clostridium difficile infection, delirium tremens, dehydration, MI, and pneumonia (see Table 13.4) [6].

Table 13.4 Complications in the most recent 100 patients in the UNC Lineberger Pathway experience [6]

Complications	Incidence
Major complications	
Fascial dehiscence	2
Acute renal failure (ARF)	1
Cardiac ischemia	1
Death	1
Internal herniation	1
Misplacement of ureteral stent	1
Postoperative bleed	1
Minor complications	
Ileus/nausea/vomiting	12
UTI	5
Arrhythmias	3
Atelectasis/desaturations	3
Altered mental status	2
Fever of unknown origin	2
DVT	2
Urine leak	2
Acute renal insufficiency	1
C. Diff enterocolitis	1
Delirium tremens	1
Dehydration	1
MI	1
Pneumonia	1

Eliminating Mechanical Bowel Preparation: New Trends

More recently, As the trend for colorectal surgery has been to completely eliminate routine mechanical bowel prep, this issue was similarly explored for patients undergoing radical cystectomy with urinary diversion for bladder cancer. The study by Raynor et al. examined the perioperative outcomes of patients undergoing radical cystectomy with urinary diversion receiving mechanical bowel preparation (our prior standard) compared to those that did not have any bowel preparation [12]. The study examined perioperative outcomes by allowing one of the two cohorts of patients to eat a regular diet the day before surgery and undergo no mechanical bowel preparation the day before surgery, whereas the other cohort underwent traditional bowel preparation consisting of a clear liquid diet the day before surgery as well as a fleets enema the evening prior to surgery. All patients in both cohorts, however, received a neomycin enema 2 h prior to surgery to decrease colonic and pelvic distention intraoperatively. In the cohorts of 37 and 33 patients respectively, there were no differences in gender, age, ASA class, BMI, type of procedure (open vs. robot assisted), or type of diversion (ileal conduit vs. neobladder). The authors found that there was no statistically significant difference in postoperative recovery of bowel function, time to discharge, overall complication rates, or GI complications between the two groups [12]. These data have led us to eliminate preoperative bowel preparation in our patients undergoing radical cystectomy with urinary diversion other than with a neomycin enema 2 h prior to the start of surgery.

The Vanderbilt Cystectomy Pathway Experience

In another series reported by Chang and colleagues from Vanderbilt in 2002, data from 304 patients undergoing radical cystectomy via an open infraumbilical approach with bilateral pelvic lymphadenectomy and urinary diversion involving either an ileal conduit, orthotopic neobladder, or a continent diversion were analyzed. Similar to our experience, patients in this protocol did not routinely have a nasogastric tube placed for gastric decompression. In contrast to our pathway, diets were not advanced until return of bowel function was documented and endorsed by the patient in the form of either flatus or a bowel movement (auscultation of bowel sounds alone was not sufficient). Their perioperative clinical pathway is represented below:

1. Preoperative mechanical bowel preparation prior to arrival to hospital
2. Transfer to regular urology floor after surgery
3. Bloodwork to be drawn on postoperative days 1, 2, and 4
4. Nasogastric tube decompression not routinely performed postoperatively
5. NPO until evidence of bowel function (defined as flatus or a bowel movement) manifests, patients are then advanced to a full liquid diet
6. Patients without evidence of return of bowel function by postoperative day 4 are thought to have an ileus
7. Patients are discharged once they are tolerating a regular diet and have adequate home healthcare instructions and coverage

The Vanderbilt cystectomy pathway experience had similar outcomes to the UNC cystectomy pathway experience and is summarized in Table 13.5.

The study by Chang et al. from Vanderbilt demonstrated a 4.9 % major complication rate, 30.9 % minor complication rate, and a median length of stay of 7 days after radical cystectomy as shown in Table 13.5 [23, 25].

Table 13.5 Demographics, perioperative outcomes, and complications from the Vanderbilt Pathway experience [23]

Demographics	
Men	232 (76.3 %)
Women	72 (23.7 %)
Pathologic stage T0, TIS, and T1	106 (36.4 %)
Pathologic stage T2, T3A, T3B, and T4	185 (63.6 %)
Mean ASA ± SD	2.64 ± 0.54 (median 3)
Diversion type	
Ileal conduit	144 (47.4 %)
Neobladder	145 (47.5 %)
Continent urinary diversion	13 (4.3 %)
Perioperative outcomes	
Mean operative time (minutes)	297.7 ± 85.2
Mean estimated blood loss (mL)	722.3 ± 493.7
Mean length of stay ± SD (days)	8.52 ± 5.06 (median 7)
Major complications	
Cardiovascular accident	2
Return to operating room	7
Sepsis	2
Myocardial infarction	1
Pulmonary embolus	2
Respiratory failure	2
Death	1
Minor complications	
Wound infection	9
Pneumonia	6
Cardiac arrhythmia	3
Angina	3
DVT	2
Pyelonephritis	4
Mental status changes	5
Delirium tremens	1
Acute renal failure	3
Clostridium difficile colitis	1
Pneumothorax	1
Ileus	69
Retained bladder stent	1
Hydronephrosis	2
Intraoperative rectal injury	1
Ureter–intestinal anastomotic leakage	1
Sacral decubitus ulcer	1
Stricture of catheterizable stoma	1

The Vanderbilt series had not come to incorporate robot-assisted surgery into its pathway at that period and it continued to rely on active evidence of return of bowel function prior to initiation of oral intake. However, their series was one of the first to detail the benefits of removing and/or not placing a nasogastric tube in promoting a shorter postoperative length of stay and facilitating quicker return to bowel function. The UNC series makes the change from the Vanderbilt series of introducing a diet in a systematic way regardless of clinical evidence of bowel function [6, 23, 25].

The prevalence of robot-assisted surgery and its part in the treatment of urologic oncology continues to grow rapidly. Fast-track clinical perioperative pathways continue to have a significant role in robot-assisted surgeries. Kaufman et al. from Vanderbilt describe an established clinical pathway for postoperative care after robot-assisted radical prostatectomy, now considered by many to be standard of care [24, 26]. The perioperative pathway described by Kaufman et al. is remarkably similar to the perioperative clinical pathway for open radical retropubic prostatectomies described by Chang et al., also from Vanderbilt. As the major hallmarks (i.e., neurovascular preservation, hemostasis, urethral–bladder neck re-anastomosis and reconstruction, etc.) of both the open and robot-assisted radical prostatectomies are close to being the same, it is not surprising that their respective perioperative pathways are also very similar [24, 26].

Relevance of Fast-Track Pathway to Robot-Assisted Radical Cystectomy

In the case of radical cystectomy, the robot-assisted approach accomplishes all the goals as the open approach, with intermediate-term data supporting at least comparable outcomes with regard to oncologic, perioperative, and quality of life endpoints. In addition to the primary oncological goals shared by the two approaches, optimizing patient recovery is an additional motivation fundamentally underlying the pursuit of robot-assisted radical cystectomy. As such, we believe the potential benefits of fast-track pathways outlined in this chapter are consonant with the values and purposes animating any robot-assisted radical cystectomy (RARC) program.

It is noteworthy that the fast-track pathway experience from our series described in the above section included several years prior to our (early) adoption of RARC, and therefore reflects results in a cohort including a substantial number of open radical cystectomies. Our ongoing experience in a mature RARC program supports consistent benefits in that setting. Given the emphasis of the pathway on issues related to recovery of bowel function, we believe that the benefits of the pathway relate primarily to optimized recovery after urinary diversion, whether performed intracorporeally or extracorporeally.

The contemporary UNC fast-track pathway for robot-assisted radical cystectomy consists of:

1. Counseling and expectations of surgery and recovery—pathway described.
2. No mechanical or oral antibiotic bowel preparation or special diet. Regular diet until midnight before the procedure.
3. Enema 2 h prior to surgery.
4. Perioperative antibiotics with a second or third generation cephalosporin for 24 h coverage—first dose prior to skin incision.
5. Removal of orogastric tube at end of case.
6. Intra and postoperative DVT prophylaxis with ambulation (postoperative), TED, SCDs, and subcutaneous heparin or lovenox.
7. Prokinetic agents (metoclopramide 10 mg IV q8 for 48 h).
8. GI ulcer prophylaxis with an H2 blocker.
9. Non-narcotic pain management with toradol X 48 h, then celecoxib 200 mg BID afterwards for 2 weeks with supplementation with IV or oral narcotics as needed.
10. Early ambulation with early consultation with physical therapy.
11. Discharge planning beginning POD 1 with social work assistance.
12. Diet:
    (a) NPO for POD 1 except for sips and ice chips.
    (b) Introduction of 8 oz of clear, noncarbonated, liquids every 8 h on POD 2—irrespective of bowel function.

   (c) Clear liquid diet on POD 3 with reduction of IVF. Possible advancement to a regular diet in the afternoon if requested.
   (d) Regular diet and discontinuation of IVF on POD 4 with possible discharge in the afternoon.
13. Typically discharged on POD 4 or POD 5.

Reflecting the motivation for the pathway as a vehicle for iterative continuous quality improvement, changes from the original iteration of the pathway described above, and currently in use, include elimination of the preoperative bowel preparation the day prior to surgery, discontinuation of the need for patients to adhere to a clear liquid diet the day before surgery, more consistent advancement of diet postoperatively, and an increased cognizance of limiting postoperative narcotic usage. The elimination of the mechanical bowel preparation not only improves a patient's hydration status before surgery but also decreases a somewhat morbid, and seemingly unnecessary, cleansing of the bowel. The same clinical pathway is utilized regardless of patient demographics, comorbidities, age, sex, or type of diversion. Again, as with the open radical cystectomy, the urinary diversion seems to confer the most morbidity with the robot-assisted radical cystectomy as well. This is despite some experience suggesting potential benefits in earlier return of bowel function, possibly due to reduced insensible losses or other factors by utilizing the robot-assisted approach. Therefore, by standardizing an approach for the introduction of food and liquids to a patient's postoperative care pathway, we believe this strategy may provide a means of substantially minimizing postoperative morbidity.

An important element of this pathway is involvement of the patient and family members as to the expectation, goals, and rationale for each step. In our experience patient satisfaction has increased with a clearly delineated care plan that is understood by patient, family, and care team alike. This plan is described (in verbal and in written form) to the patients at their preoperative visit, and the pathway frequently referenced in the peri and postoperative period.

Conclusions

Clinical pathways contribute enormous value in the treatment of surgical patients. Standardizing a postoperative approach to managing patients who have undergone radical cystectomy, works to not only improve the quality of care provided, as reflected in improved patient outcomes, but also enables cost reduction and higher rates of patient satisfaction. Furthermore, implementation of clinical care pathways can provide a vehicle for a culture of practice within which to apply an evidence-based methodology to postoperative decision-making. Postoperative "fast-track" pathways have been clinically utilized in innumerable general surgery contexts, as well as in the field of urology with noted benefit after prostatectomies, retroperitoneal lymphadenectomies, and partial nephrectomies. Fast-track pathways have also been more recently developed for these same surgeries but specifically intended with the use of robot-assisted technology (i.e., fast-track pathway for patients undergoing robot-assisted prostatectomy). Re-evaluating and evolving clinical pathways will continue to be relevant as newer technologies, approaches, and strategies are developed in the treatment of urologic malignancies.

Editors' Commentary

Erik P. Castle and Raj S. Pruthi

Clinical pathways are an important and potentially powerful tool that may have beneficial affects that include: (1) improvement in quality of care, (2) cost reduction, (3) transparency of treatment, and (4) staff satisfaction with benefits of training and education. Implementation of clinical care pathways and evidence-based fast-track programs have been successfully employed in a wide variety of surgical procedures ranging from colorectal surgery to hepatobiliary surgery to cardiothoracic surgery, just to name a few. To date, application to urologic procedures, however, has been rather limited.

A successful application of a fast-track program has been applied to our patients undergoing radical cystectomy and urinary diversion. The elimination of a mechanical bowel preparation, use of non-narcotic analgesics, and early postoperative diet advancement have been three critical elements of this pathway.

Such a clinical care pathway has the potential to utilize evidence-based modifications to reduce morbidity and improve recovery with regard to early institution of oral diet and early hospital discharge. In addition, such pathways allow for the seamless introduction of guidelines and best practice policies to the perioperative care. Ongoing modification and analysis of this program remain an important aspect of clinical care pathways that provide a ready mechanism by which scientific evidence translates into clinical practice.

Appendix

The Contemporary UNC Fast-Track Pathway for Robot-Assisted Radical Cystectomy

1. Counseling and expectations of surgery and recovery—pathway described.
2. No mechanical or oral antibiotic bowel preparation or special diet. Regular diet until midnight before the procedure.
3. Enema 2 h prior to surgery.
4. Perioperative antibiotics with a second or third generation cephalosporin for 24 h coverage—first dose prior to skin incision.
5. Removal of orogastric tube at end of case.
6. Intra and postoperative DVT prophylaxis with ambulation (postoperative), TED, SCDs, and subcutaneous heparin or lovenox.
7. Prokinetic agents (metoclopramide 10 mg IV q8 for 48 h).
8. GI ulcer prophylaxis with an H2 blocker.
9. Non-narcotic pain management with toradol X 48 h, then celecoxib 200 mg BID afterwards for 2 weeks with supplementation with IV or oral narcotics as needed.
10. Early ambulation with early consultation with physical therapy.
11. Discharge planning beginning POD 1 with social work assistance.
12. Diet:
    (a) NPO for POD 1 except for sips and ice chips.
    (b) Introduction of 8 oz of clear, noncarbonated, liquids every 8 h on POD 2—irrespective of bowel function.
    (c) Clear liquid diet on POD 3 with reduction of IVF. Possible advancement to a regular diet in the afternoon if requested.
    (d) Regular diet and discontinuation of IVF on POD 4 with possible discharge in the afternoon.
13. Typically discharged on POD 4 or POD 5.

References

1. Howlader N, Noone AM, Krapcho M, Neyman N, Aminou R, Altekruse SF, Kosary CL, Ruhl J, Tatalovich Z, Cho H, Mariotto A, Eisner MP, Lewis DR, Chen HS, Feuer EJ, Cronin KA, editors. SEER Cancer Statistics Review, 1975-2009 (Vintage 2009 Populations). Bethesda, MD: National Cancer Institute
2. Hall MC, Chang SS, Dalbagni G, et al. Guideline for the management of nonmuscle invasive bladder cancer (stages Ta, T1, and Tis): 2007 update. J Urol. 2007;178:2314–30.
3. Meeks JJ, Bellmunt J, Bochner BH, Clarke NW, Daneshmand S, Galsky MD, et al. A systematic review of neoadjuvant and adjuvant chemotherapy for muscle-invasive bladder cancer. Eur Urol. 2012;62(3): 523–33.
4. Sonpavde G, Sternberg CN. Neoadjuvant chemotherapy for invasive bladder cancer. Curr Urol Rep. 2012;13(2):136–46.
5. Evans C. Complications of radical cystectomy. In: Teneja SS, Smith RB, Ehrich RM, editors. Complications of urologic surgery: diagnosis, prevention and management. 3rd ed. Philadelphia, PA: WB Saunders; 1999.
6. Pruthi RS, Nielsen ME, Smith AS, Nix J, Schultz H, Wallen EM. Fast track program in patients undergoing radical cystectomy: results of 362 consecutive patients. J Am Coll Surg. Jan 2010;210(1):93–9.
7. Kouba EJ, Wallen EM, Pruthi RS. Gum chewing stimulates bowel motility in patients undergoing radical cystectomy with urinary diversion. Urology. 2007;70(6):1053–6.
8. Pruthi RS, Wallen EM. Robotic-assisted laparoscopic pelvic lymphadenectomy for bladder cancer: a surgical atlas. J Laparoendosc Adv Surg Tech A. 2009;19(1):71–4.

9. Nix J, Smith A, Kurpad R, Nielsen ME, Wallen EM, Pruthi RS. Prospective randomized control trial of robotic versus open radical cystectomy for bladder cancer: perioperative pathologic results. Eur Urol. 2010;57(2):196–201.
10. Pruthi RS, Nielsen ME, Nix J, Smith A, Schultz H, Wallen EM. Robotic radical cystectomy for bladder cancer: surgical and pathological outcomes in 100 consecutive cases. J Urol. 2010;183(2):510–4.
11. Smith AB, Raynor M, Amling CL, Busby JE, Castle E, Davis R, et al. Multi-institutional analysis of robotic radical cystectomy for bladder cancer: perioperative outcomes and complications in 227 patients. J Laparoendosc Adv Surg Tech A. 2012;22(1):17–21.
12. Raynor MC, Lavien G, Nielsen ME, Wallen EM, Pruthi RS. Elimination of preoperative mechanical bowel preparation in patients undergoing cystectomy and urinary diversion. Urol Oncol. 2010;31(1):32–5.
13. Muller S, Zalunardo MP, Hubner M, et al. A fast-track program reduces complications and length of hospital stay after open colonic surgery. Gastroenterology. 2009;136:842–7.
14. Gustafsson UO, Hausel J, Thorell A, Ljungqvist O, Soop M, Nygren J. Adherence to the enhanced recovery after surgery protocol and outcomes after colorectal cancer surgery. Arch Surg. 2011;146(5): 571–7.
15. Faeron KCH, Ljungqvist O, Meyenfeldt MV, Revhaug A, Defong CHC, Lassen K, et al. Enhanced recovery after surgery: a consensus review of clinical care for patients undergoing colonic resection. Clin Nutr. 2005;24:466–77.
16. Pitt HA, Murray KP, Bowman HM, et al. Clinical pathway implementation improves outcomes for complex biliary surgery. Surgery. 1999;126:751–6. discussion 756–758.
17. Ronellenfitsch U, Rossner E, Jakob J, et al. Clinical pathways in surgery—should we introduce them into clinical routine? A review article. Langenbecks Arch Surg. 2008;393:449–57.
18. Kehlet H, Wilmore DW. Evidence-based surgical care and the evolution of fast-track surgery. Ann Surg. 2008;248:189–98.
19. Mohn AC, Bernardshaw SV, Ristesund SM, Hovde Hansen PE, Rokke O. Enhanced recovery after colorectal surgery – results from a prospective observational two-center study. Scand J Surg. 2009;98:155–9.
20. Sjetne IS, Krogstad U, Odegard S, Engh ME. Improving quality by introducing enhanced recovery after surgery in a gynecological department: consequences for ward nursing practice. Qual Saf Health Care. 2009;18(3):236–40.
21. Khan S, Wilson T, Ahmed J, Owais A, MacFie J. Quality of life and patient satisfaction with enhanced recovery protocols. Colorectal Dis. Dec 2010;12(12): 1175–82.
22. Donat SM, Slaton JW, Pisters LL, Swanson DA. Early nasogastric tube removal combined with metoclopramide after radical cystectomy and urinary diversion. J Urol. 1999;162:1599–602.
23. Chang SS, Baumgartner RG, Wells N, et al. Causes of increased hospital stay after radical cystectomy in a clinical pathway setting. J Urol. 2002;167:208–11.
24. Chang SS, Cole E, Smith Jr JA, et al. Safely reducing length of stay after open radical retropubic prostatectomy under the guidance of a clinical care pathway. Cancer. 2005;104:747–51.
25. Chang SS, Cookson MS, Baumgartner RG, et al. Analysis of early complications after radical cystectomy: results of a collaborative care pathways. J Urol. 2002;167:2012–6.
26. Kaufman MR, Baumgartner RG, Anderson LW, Smith Jr JA, Chang SS, Herell SD, et al. The evidence-based pathway for perioperative management of open and robotically assisted laparoscopic radical prostatectomy. BJU Int. 2007;99(5):1103–8.
27. Stein JP, Lieskovsky G, Cote R, et al. Radical cystectomy in the treatment of invasive bladder cancer: long-term results in 1,054 patients. J Clin Oncol. 2001;19:666–75.

Oncologic Outcomes

14

Dipen Parekh, G. Andy Ransford,
and George S. Kallingal

Introduction

When appraising a new technique in surgery, several elements are important to evaluate including cost, complications, cosmesis, and a host of perioperative factors. However, for bladder cancer, oncologic efficacy is paramount. Residual cancer or incomplete resection can render a much worse prognosis for the patient and may greatly decrease the chance of cancer-specific survival [1]. Open radical cystectomy (ORC) with or without neoadjuvant chemotherapy has been the time-tested gold standard for the extirpation of bladder cancer. Any surgical technique convened to address bladder cancer must offer similar oncologic efficacy to open radical cystectomy. In this chapter we will examine the current status of oncologic efficacy of robot-assisted radical cystectomy (RARC). In evaluating RARC, several factors are important to bear in mind. First, the oncologic efficacy of RARC is gauged entirely by the extirpative portion. The reconstructive phase of this procedure (ileal conduit, neobladder, etc.) certainly has impact on morbidity, cost, cosmesis, and complications but does not directly impact cancer-related survival and hence will not be discussed in this chapter. Moreover, robotic technology is not making its debut in Urology. Compared to series looking at early robotic prostatectomy, the RARC data consists mainly of surgeons who have experience with robotic technology, including robotic prostatectomy and often robotic pelvic lymph node dissection. As such, technical and technique driven difficulties have been largely been assessed and to some degrees, addressed. In this chapter, we will look at specific markers of oncologic efficacy, namely cancer-specific survival, cancer-free recurrence, as well as surrogates of oncologic efficacy: positive surgical margins and lymph node status. We will also evaluate the current literature with regards to long term follow-up, comparison of ORC with RARC, and assess other factors influencing oncologic efficacy.

D. Parekh
Department of Urology, University of Texas Health Sciences Center at San Antonio, San Antonio, TX, USA

G.A. Ransford, MD
University of Miami, Miller School of Medicine, Miami, FL, US

G.S. Kallingal, M.D., M.P.H. (✉)
Department of Urology, Martin Army Community Hospital, 7950 Martin Loop, Fort Benning, GA 31909, USA
e-mail: kallingalmd@gmail.com

Cancer-Specific Survival, Cancer Recurrence, and Overall Survival

Ideally, oncologic efficacy would be determined with data on cancer recurrence and cancer-specific survival with a large patient database, long-term follow-up and minimal bias. However, with the limitations introduced by the nature of research, the disease process, the availability of

E.P. Castle and R.S. Pruthi (eds.), *Robotic Surgery of the Bladder*, DOI 10.1007/978-1-4614-4906-5_14,

data, and patient factors, we are left with an assortment of studies, from which we can infer oncologic efficacy. Although cancer-specific survival and cancer recurrence represent perhaps the most important measure of oncologic efficacy, medium- and long-term follow-up is critical is defining these metrics. RARC, however, is still a relatively new technique and long-term data is lacking at present; nevertheless, the relevant literature is growing rapidly and relevant medium-term follow-up is being reported.

Pruthi et al. reported 21.2-month follow-up on his first 100 consecutives cases of RARC. In his series, he had 0 positive surgical margins and retrieved an average of 19 lymph nodes [2]. In that time period, 15 % of patients had evidence of recurrence. Distant metastasis was the most common in 11 %, with local recurrence alone in 2 %, and local plus distant metastasis in another 2 %. Six patients died of bladder cancer during follow-up, yielding a cancer-specific survival of 94 %. Three patients died of other causes yielding an overall survival of 91 %.

Mmeje et al. reported on 139 patients who underwent RARC with nearly 3 years of follow-up (35.9 months) [3]. At that time point, 39 patients had recurrence, 27 died of bladder cancer, and 5 died of other causes. This yields a recurrence-free survival of 80 %, and cancer-specific survival of 71 %, and an overall survival of 68 %. As expected, patients with organ confined disease fared better than those with advanced disease (pT3, pT4 or lymph node positive). In concert, these studies indicate comparable results to ORC with medium-term time follow-up. What remains to be seen is whether these metrics will hold in the long term.

Surgical Margin Status

Surgical Margin status is the most utilized immediate surrogate for oncologic efficacy for bladder cancer surgery. Surgical margins status is extremely useful as it provides instantaneous information and does not require long-term follow-up. Several studies have elucidated the relationship between a positive surgical margin and bladder cancer outcomes. Dotan et al. assessed the impact of a positive surgical margin in a large ORC series at MSKCC. They assessed 1,589 patients and found a PSM in 67 (4.2 %) patients [1]. A PSM was statistically more likely in females, patients with higher pathologic stage, vascular invasion, and lymph node positivity. In addition, patients with extravesical disease carried a 9 % PSM rate, versus 0 % with locally confined disease. This highlights the importance of clinical staging in affecting pathologic outcomes. What the authors ultimately found was that a PSM conferred an increased risk of both local recurrence and metastatic disease. 3.6 % of patients experienced local recurrence with median time to recurrence at 16 months. Five-year freedom from local recurrence was seen in 94 % of patients with negative surgical margins versus 79 % of patients with PSM. Three hundred and fifty-eight patients developed metastatic disease with a median time of 21 months from cystectomy. At 5 years, the freedom from metastasis was 68 % in patients with a negative surgical margin versus 26 % in patients with a PSM. With regard to cancer-specific survival, the authors found that patients with a negative surgical margin had a 72 % CSS at 5 years versus 36 % CSS at 3 years. Overall, patients with a PSM had a dismal median survival of 1.8 years.

A larger, multi-institutional retrospective database shows similar results. Novara et al. combined data at 12 major academic centers and assessed 4,410 patients who underwent radical cystectomy. In that large cohort, the PSM rate was 6.3 % [4]. They found similar rates of cancer free recurrence (62.8 % with negative surgical margin vs. 21.6 % with PSM) and similar data on CSS with 5-year survival at 69 % in patients with negative surgical margin and 26.4 % in patients with PSM. These two articles establish that surgical margin status is a legitimate surrogate for oncologic efficacy and that a PSM confers a much higher risk of recurrence and cancer-specific mortality. Since this relationship underlies a biological etiology, it can be applied equally to ORC and RARC.

For surgical margin status, RARC must meet the oncologic standards of an open radical cystectomy. Oncologic standards often vary by time

Table 14.1 Oncologic outcome variables: surgical margin status

Journal	Subjects	Follow-up	Organ confined disease (%)	Extra-vesical disease (%)	PSM (%)
Pruthi et al. [2]	100	21.2	67 (67)	33 (33)	0 (0)
Guru et al. [6]	67	n/a	29 (43.3)	38 (56.7)	6 (8.9)
Kang et al. [7]	104	12	73 (70.1)	31 (29.9)	5 (4.8)
Hellenthal et al. [8]	513	n/a	337 (65.7)	176 (34.3)	35 (6.8)
Richards et al. [9]	60	n/a	38 (63.3)	22 (36.6)	6 (10)

and place; however, in 2004, Herr et al. analyzed 1,091 cystectomy patients and reported widely cited oncologic standards for radical cystectomy. For all patients, the overall PSM rate should be less than 10 %. For patients with bulky T3–4 disease, a PSM rate should be less than 15 % and for patients undergoing a salvage radical cystectomy, the PSM rate should be less than 20 %. They also made recommendations for the lymph node dissection and recommended that 70–80 % of patients should undergo a standard pelvic lymph node dissection (or more) and at least 10–14 nodes should be harvested [5].

Pathologic data from RARC trials has been maturing in recent years. In Table 14.1, we list the five largest recent trials assessing oncologic outcomes. In total, over 800 patients underwent RARC in this series and the overall PSM rate was 6.16 %. The largest series comes from the International Robotic Cystectomy Consortium (IRCC). The IRCC includes surgeons from 15 centers in the USA, Spain, UK, Belgium, and Sweden and includes data from 513 patients. The authors found an overall 6.8 % PSM rate. Pathologic stage was significantly associated with PSM. Patients with pT2 or less disease had 1.5 % rate of PSM, compared to 8.89 % in pT3 patients and 39.1 % in pT4 patients. This translates to a 6- and 40-fold increase in PSM in patients with pT3 and pT4 disease, respectively, compared to those patients with organ-confined disease. Hence, a PSM was statistically much more likely with advanced tumor stage. In this study, increasing age and positive lymph nodes also predicted a positive surgical margin. Importantly, institutional case volume and sequential case number did not correlate with surgical margin status, indicating that the learning curve did not play a significant role in the quality of extirpation. In a single institution setting, Pruthi et al. confirms similar findings. In their report of 100 patients undergoing RARC, they found zero cases of PSM. In a very large Korean study, Kang et al. reported 104 patients undergoing RARC with a PSM rate of 4.8 %. At 1-year follow-up, they report a cancer-specific survival rate of 96.2 %. In total, the data from Table 14.1 give us a diverse impression of the PSM rate in RARC. It includes very large multi-institutional data, single surgeon data, international data and data from programs in a young learning environment. Collectively, the data set from Table 14.1 suggests that RARC meets the standards of oncologic efficacy with an acceptable PSM rate, well within the recommended 10 % standard.

The critical factor in achieving negative surgical margins is wide resection where the tumor may encroach. Unfortunately, precisely where the tumor encroaches is usually not known until the final pathologic specimen is analyzed. However, the quality of surgical extirpation may play a role. Dotan et al. found 0 PSM in patients with organ confined disease, where as those with extravesical disease had 9 % PSM rate [1]. Hence, for open radical cystectomy, a positive surgical margin is rarely due to surgeon error but more likely from the extension of disease. Furthermore, they found that the most common locations for a PSM in men were in the periprostatic tissues and seminal vesicles in 37 %, followed by the lateral walls in 29 %. Whereas in women, the PSM were more likely in the periurethral and vagina in 38 % and lateral walls in 28 %. It is not yet known whether the robotic PSM are in similar locations. In the next few years, it will be critical to assess this data in the robotic patient population.

Lymph Node Status

The second most important surrogate for oncologic efficacy is lymph node status. The most common site of bladder cancer metastasis is the pelvic lymph nodes, and removal of these lymph nodes provides improved surgical staging and possibility of therapeutic benefit. Leissner et al. found significantly improved survival in 447 patients when more lymph nodes were removed [10] in open radical cystectomies. In that study a mean of 14 lymph nodes were removed. Patients with >15 nodes removed had better 5-year recurrence free survival (65 % vs. 51 %), less loco-regional metastasis (17 % vs. 27 %), and less distant metastasis (17 % vs. 10.5 %). This translates to an increased cancer-specific survival, regardless of stage and regardless of lymph node positivity. Although the limits of pelvic lymphadenectomy have been debated, it is suggested by some groups that an extended pelvic lymphadenectomy (above the iliac bifurcation) can improve staging and survival [11–13].

In addition to providing oncologic information, a lymph node dissection is a reflection of surgical skill and completeness of extirpation. It has been unequivocally demonstrated that an adequate lymph node dissection can be performed robotically. Table 14.2 lists five large studies involving 768 patients who underwent RARC with robotic lymphadenectomy. In this series, an average of 18 nodes per patients was harvested robotically. This easily meets the 10–14 lymph node standards set for ORC mentioned above by Herr et al. [12].

Table 14.2 Oncologic outcome variables: lymph node status

	Pts	Number lymph nodes	Pts with positive LNs	Extended LND
Pruthi et al. [2]	100	19 (18–40)	20 (20 %)	n/a
Guru et al. [6]	67	18 (6–43)	n/a	100 %
Kang et al. [7]	104	18 (5–61)	10 (9.6 %)	31.7 %
Hellenthal et al. [8]	437	17 (0–68)	80 (18 %)	n/a
Richards et al. [9]	60	17 (5–34)	18 (30 %)	n/a

Multiple factors play a role in pathologic analysis including handling of specimens and quality of pathologic review [14], which vary from institution to institution; however, the comparative studies mentioned below (Nix et al. and Styn et al.) show similar lymph node counts between ORC and RARC in single center environments, obviating differences in pathologic review within a single institution.

Direct Comparison of Open and Robot-Assisted Radical Cystectomy

Comparative trials are often regarded as superior to studies focusing only on one modality. So, how does RARC directly compare to ORC? Styn et al. performed a matched comparison of 68 patients undergoing RARC with 306 patients who underwent ORC at the University of Michigan [15]. They found no statistically significant differences in oncologic outcomes measures. PSM rates were 16 % vs. 11 % and mean lymph nodes removed were 14.3 and 15.2, in the RARC and ORC cohort, respectively. There were no mortalities in the RARC group at 30 and 90 days with a median follow-up of 8 months. More compelling, Nix et al. performed a prospective, randomized controlled trial comparing RARC with ORC in 42 patients at the University of North Carolina [16]. They had 0 PSMs in both groups and similar lymph node counts (19 in RARC group versus 18 in the ORC group). Furthermore, a prospective, randomized, controlled trial comparing RARC to ORC at the University of Texas Health Science Center San Antonio also shows no significant difference in PSM (5 % vs. 5 %) and lymph node yield (23 vs. 11) in 40 patients [17]. In concert, these studies demonstrate that the reported oncologic success of RARC hold up even in direct comparison to ORC. At present, there is a prospective, randomized, multi-institutional trial underway in the USA comparing ORC vs. RARC. In a few years, data from this trial will allow us to compare oncologic outcomes between the two approaches.

How does the quality of a robotic lymph node dissection compare to an open dissection? Davis et al. looked at 11 patients who underwent a robot-assisted radical cystectomy with pelvic lymph node dissection followed by a second look open pelvic lymph node dissection via mini-laparatomy [18]. They found a robotic yield of 43 mean lymph nodes (range 19–63) while open second look yielded only a mean of four lymph nodes (range 0–8). In 80 % of these patients, no additional lymph nodes were found despite open dissection. This study suggests that robotic lymph node dissection can be performed with a completeness approaching that of open surgery.

The Learning Curve

As with any new procedure, especially one that involves a relatively new technology such as the da Vinci robotic system, there is a period of time during which the inexperience of the surgeon makes the operation more difficult. This is commonly referred to as the learning curve. Some surgeons would say that they passed the learning curve once they felt comfortable performing a procedure. Given the subjective nature of what "comfortable" means to various surgeons, there are attempts to look at more objective metrics to measure the learning curve of an operation and to establish its effect, if any, on oncologic efficacy.

Given the infancy of RARC, the long-term oncologic outcomes of ORC vs. RARC have yet to be firmly established. Moreover, determining long-term oncologic outcomes in early vs. late learning curve cases also remains to be established. In the meantime, however, there has been literature published regarding operative and postoperative complications, oncologic outcomes, and survival. Pruthi et al. retrospectively reviewed their first 50 patients undergoing RARC, dividing them into quintiles, and analyzing metrics such as estimated blood loss (EBL), total OR time, margin status, number of lymph nodes removed, and complication rate [19]. They noted differences in EBL and operative time, but positive margin rate and lymph node yield were not significantly different over the course of the learning curve, when evaluated by quintile and by halves.

In contrast to Pruthi et al.'s single-site experience, Hayn et al. examined data from the International Robotic Cystectomy Consortium [20]. After identifying 496 patients who underwent RARC by 21 different surgeons at 14 institutions between 2003 and 2009, learning curves were defined for metrics such as operative time, lymph node yield (LNY), EBL, and margin positivity. After grouping surgeons by case volume (<30, 30–50, >50), the median overall operative times were 441, 368, and 307 min, respectively ($P<0.0001$). Using mixed statistical models, the learning curve for operative time revealed that after 21 cases, an overall operative time of 390 min (6.5 h) could be achieved. The extent and number of pelvic lymph node dissection is a highly debated topic. In the present study, the mean yield was 18 nodes, with 23 % having positive lymph nodes—a figure comparable to a large open cystectomy series [5, 21, 22]. Herr et al. recommended 10–14 lymph nodes as standard for pelvic lymph node dissection [5], while Ghoneim suggested a cut-off of 20 nodes [21]. In the present study by Hayn et al., after applying statistical modeling, the learning curves show clear improvement in lymph node yield (LNY) with an increased case number of 30 patients needed to obtain 20 nodes. Furthermore, median LNY increased by 73 % between surgeons who had done <30 cases and >50 cases ($P<0.0001$). Regarding positive surgical margins (PSM), the learning curves did show an improved PSM rate with increased experience. To achieve a PSM rate of <5 %, they estimated the surgeon would need to have performed 30 cases. Otherwise, there was no significant difference in metrics such as length of stay, rate of intraoperative transfusion, or positive surgical margin rate.

In a more focused, single-site study by Hayn et al., they sought to determine the outcome of 164 consecutive RARC performed by a single surgeon [23]. When divided into groups of 50, 50, and 64 patients, they found that mean operative time was significantly different between the first (180 min) and third groups (136 min) ($P<0.001$). Also, median LN yield (16) increased from the first group to the third group (24), however, it is important to note that the increase may partially have been due to a change in the LND boundaries. After the initial 50 cases, 100 % of PLNDs were extended to the aortic bifurcation, whereas only 80 % went to the bifurcation in the first 50 cases. There was no significant difference in EBL or positive surgical margins seen in this study.

Lastly, Richards et al. reported on 60 prospective RARC cases, divided into tertiles, performed at a single medical center from January 2008 to March 2010 [9]. Similar to other studies, there was no difference in EBL, hospital stay length, or LN yield. In concert, these studies suggest that lymph node yield tends to be influenced by the learning curve, however, positive surgical margins tend to be consistent. Variability in lymph node yield may be reflective of individual surgeon preferences with regards to extent of lymph node dissection that is debatable at present, rather than any limitation imposed by the robotic approach.

Elderly Patients

Given that bladder cancer is a disease frequently encountered in the elderly, with a median age of diagnosis at 70 years old, RARC must be shown to have oncologic equivalence in this population. In a study by Guillotreau et al., 146 patients undergoing laparoscopic or RARC were identified [24]. They divided the patients into those younger than 70 and those 70 or older. The oncologic variables for those two groups were remarkably similar. The PSM rate was 5.6 % and 5.4 %, and the lymph node yield was 12.4 versus 11.6, respectively. Similarly, tumor stage, number of positive lymph nodes, and overall follow-up were also not significantly different. Coward et al. retrospectively examined 99 patients who underwent RARC at a single institution after dividing them by age greater or less than 70 years old [25]. In those groups, lymph node yield and PSM rate were statistically similar. These data indicate that age, by itself, does not seem to render a worse prognosis for patients electing robot-assisted radical cystectomy.

Conclusions

As a rapidly accepted technology, RARC is gaining ground as a viable alternative to ORC. The true markers of oncologic success (cancer-specific survival and cancer-free recurrence) take time and are not yet available to definitely establish the oncologic equivalence of RARC and ORC. Nevertheless, intermediate- and short-term oncologic outcomes with RARC are reassuring. Medium-term studies are showing satisfactory cancer-specific survival and cancer-free recurrence. The PSM rate for RARC seems to be firmly equivalent to ORC and lymph node yields are comparable as well. Furthermore, these data seem to be holding true not only for retrospective analysis studies, but in direct comparative studies as well. In the upcoming months, data from a large randomized, controlled, multi-institutional study directly comparing RARC with ORC should be released which may help establish oncologic equivalence. Certainly, the near future will bring more randomized trials, longer reported follow-ups, and intriguing analyses of RARC. In the interim, however, we have a growing collection of studies supporting the oncologic efficacy of RARC in a variety of patients.

Editors' Commentary

Erik P. Castle and Raj S. Pruthi

In this chapter, the authors present collective data from several large RARC series showing comparable rates of positive surgical margins and similar lymph node yields—both that serve as short-term surrogates for oncologic efficacy. They also examine several head to head comparisons of RARC compared to open radical cystectomy, again showing similar oncologic outcomes. Medium-term studies (up to 3 years of follow-up) are also demonstrating satisfactory cancer-specific recurrence and survival. Such early evidence holds promise for the ability of the robotic approach to achieve oncologic equivalence to the open technique. Indeed, many who have performed robot-assisted radical cystectomy will attest to the experience that the procedure itself does not necessarily compromise visualization, access, or technical extirpation of the bladder or surrounding tissues and organs, nor does it limit ones ability to thoroughly remove lymph nodes up to the most proximal extents.

Most who care for patients with bladder cancer understand that the ultimate goal of radical cystectomy is oncologic success—irrespective of operative technique. The oncologic efficacy is indeed paramount and any iatrogenic compromise to cancer outcomes is simply unacceptable. In this disease we have essentially no salvage regimens to rescue the patient who may suffer from recurrence due to a suboptimal surgical procedure by open or robotic techniques. As such, careful evaluation of the oncologic integrity of this operation is essential if this procedure is to be continued and adopted in a widespread manner. Surgeons performing this procedure (robotic or open, for that matter) should be well aware of their own oncologic outcomes to ensure they maintain the highest standards of surgical care for the bladder cancer patient.

References

1. Dotan ZA, Kavanagh K, Yossepowitch O, Kaag M, Olgac S, Donat M, et al. Positive surgical margins in soft tissue following radical cystectomy for bladder cancer and cancer specific survival. J Urol. 2007;178(6):2308–12. discussion 13.
2. Pruthi RS, Nielsen ME, Nix J, Smith A, Schultz H, Wallen EM. Robotic radical cystectomy for bladder cancer: surgical and pathological outcomes in 100 consecutive cases. J Urol. 2010;183(2):510–4.
3. Mmeje CO, Nunez-Nateras R, Pruthi RS, Nielsen ME, Wallen EM, Humphreys MR, Castle EP. Robotic radical cystectomy: medium-term oncologic follow-up. J Clin Oncol. 2011;29 Suppl 7:abstr 288.
4. Novara G, Svatek RS, Karakiewicz PI, Skinner E, Ficarra V, Fradet Y, et al. Soft tissue surgical margin status is a powerful predictor of outcomes after radical cystectomy: a multicenter study of more than 4,400 patients. J Urol. 2010;183(6):2165–70.
5. Herr H, Lee C, Chang S, Lerner S. Standardization of radical cystectomy and pelvic lymph node dissection for bladder cancer: a collaborative group report. J Urol. 2004;171(5):1823–8. discussion 7–8.
6. Guru KA, Sternberg K, Wilding GE, Tan W, Butt ZM, Mohler JL, et al. The lymph node yield during robot-assisted radical cystectomy. BJU Int. 2008;102(2):231–4. discussion 4.
7. Kang SG, Kang SH, Lee YG, Rha KH, Jeong BC, Ko YH, et al. Robot-assisted radical cystectomy and pelvic lymph node dissection: a multi-institutional study from Korea. J Endourol. 2010;24(9):1435–40.
8. Hellenthal NJ, Hussain A, Andrews PE, Carpentier P, Castle E, Dasgupta P, et al. Surgical margin status after robot assisted radical cystectomy: results from the International Robotic Cystectomy Consortium. J Urol. 2010;184(1):87–91.
9. Richards KA, Kader K, Pettus JA, Smith JJ, Hemal AK. Does initial learning curve compromise outcomes for robot-assisted radical cystectomy? A critical evaluation of the first 60 cases while establishing a robotics program. J Endourol. 2011;25(9):1553–8.
10. Leissner J, Ghoneim MA, Abol-Enein H, Thuroff JW, Franzaring L, Fisch M, et al. Extended radical lymphadenectomy in patients with urothelial bladder cancer: results of a prospective multicenter study. J Urol. 2004;171(1):139–44.
11. Leissner J, Hohenfellner R, Thuroff JW, Wolf HK. Lymphadenectomy in patients with transitional cell carcinoma of the urinary bladder; significance for staging and prognosis. BJU Int. 2000;85(7):817–23.
12. Herr HW, Bochner BH, Dalbagni G, Donat SM, Reuter VE, Bajorin DF. Impact of the number of lymph nodes retrieved on outcome in patients with muscle invasive bladder cancer. J Urol. 2002;167(3):1295–8.
13. Poulsen AL, Horn T, Steven K. Radical cystectomy: extending the limits of pelvic lymph node dissection improves survival for patients with bladder cancer confined to the bladder wall. J Urol. 1998;160(6 Pt 1):2015–9. discussion 20.
14. Bochner BH, Herr HW, Reuter VE. Impact of separate versus en bloc pelvic lymph node dissection on the number of lymph nodes retrieved in cystectomy specimens. J Urol. 2001;166(6):2295–6.
15. Styn NR, Montgomery JS, Wood DP, Hafez KS, Lee CT, Tallman C, et al. Matched comparison of robotic-assisted and open radical cystectomy. Urology. 2012;79(6):1303–9.
16. Nix J, Smith A, Kurpad R, Nielsen ME, Wallen EM, Pruthi RS. Prospective randomized controlled trial of robotic versus open radical cystectomy for bladder cancer: perioperative and pathologic results. Eur Urol. 2010;57(2):196–201.
17. Parekh DJ, Messer J, FItzgerald J, Ercole B, Svatek R. Perioperative outcomes and oncologic efficacy from a pilot prospective randomized clinical trial of open versus robotic assisted radical cystectomy. J Urol. 2013;189(2):474–9.
18. Davis JW, Gaston K, Anderson R, Dinney CP, Grossman HB, Munsell MF, et al. Robot assisted extended pelvic lymphadenectomy at radical cystec-

tomy: lymph node yield compared with second look open dissection. J Urol. 2011;185(1):79–83.
19. Pruthi RS, Smith A, Wallen EM. Evaluating the learning curve for robot-assisted laparoscopic radical cystectomy. J Endourol. 2008;22(11):2469–74.
20. Hayn MH, Hussain A, Mansour AM, Andrews PE, Carpentier P, Castle E, et al. The learning curve of robot-assisted radical cystectomy: results from the International Robotic Cystectomy Consortium. Eur Urol. 2010;58(2):197–202.
21. Ghoneim MA, Abdel-Latif M, el-Mekresh M, Abol-Enein H, Mosbah A, Ashamallah A, et al. Radical cystectomy for carcinoma of the bladder: 2,720 consecutive cases 5 years later. J Urol. 2008;180(1):121–7.
22. Stein JP, Lieskovsky G, Cote R, Groshen S, Feng AC, Boyd S, et al. Radical cystectomy in the treatment of invasive bladder cancer: long-term results in 1,054 patients. J Clin Oncol. 2001;19(3):666–75.
23. Hayn MH, Hellenthal NJ, Seixas-Mikelus SA, Mansour AM, Stegemann A, Hussain A, et al. Is patient outcome compromised during the initial experience with robot-assisted radical cystectomy? Results of 164 consecutive cases. BJU Int. 2011;108(6):882–7.
24. Guillotreau J, Miocinovic R, Game X, Forest S, Malavaud B, Kaouk J, et al. Outcomes of laparoscopic and robotic radical cystectomy in the elderly patients. Urology. 2012;79(3):585–90.
25. Coward RM, Smith A, Raynor M, Nielsen M, Wallen EM, Pruthi RS. Feasibility and outcomes of robotic-assisted laparoscopic radical cystectomy for bladder cancer in older patients. Urology. 2011;77(5):1111–4.

15 Perioperative Outcomes and Complications of Robot-Assisted Cystectomy

Daniel A. Barocas and Mark L. Gonzalgo

Introduction

The main impetus for the development of minimally invasive surgery is to reduce surgical morbidity. Therefore, many early investigations of the effects of new minimally invasive techniques focus on perioperative outcomes and surgical complications.

In this chapter, we report on the peer-reviewed literature on robot-assisted cystectomy (RARC), with respect to perioperative outcomes and complications.

Methodology

A literature search was performed for various permutations, using the terms "robot," "cystectomy," "outcome," and "complication." Articles published before April 2012 were included. The references of each article identified were then searched for additional papers on these topics. Once we identified all of the papers that addressed each topic, we narrowed our search to include one paper (the most recent, largest number of patients, or most complete with respect to the outcome of interest) from each institution. We excluded other publications from the same institution, and excluded review articles, in order to avoid double counting of cases.

Overall, we identified 22 unique series [1–22] representing 967 patients, of which six series contained at least 50 robotic cystectomies [2, 3, 7, 10, 11, 13] from a single institution (529 patients). Most institutions reported case series of robot-assisted cystectomies, without a comparison group. However, there were five unique cohort studies containing both open and robot-assisted cystectomies [5, 20, 21, 23, 24] and one randomized trial comparing open with robot-assisted cystectomy [25]. In addition, there were several studies specifically comparing subgroups of RARC patients: one each by age 70 and over vs. under 70 [26], intracorporeal vs. extracorporeal diversion [27], high vs. low cardiac risk index [28], and flat vs. bulky index tumor [29]. Many other case series had subgroup analyses within them for specific outcomes. Where it is illustrative to compare the open and robotic groups or subgroups of robotic patients, we report these comparative studies in addition to the case series, even if they may contain overlapping patient cohorts. We highlight the results of the one randomized trial, since this study design has the lowest risk of bias.

D.A. Barocas, M.D., M.P.H.
Department of Urologic Surgery, Center for Surgical Quality and Outcomes Research, Vanderbilt University Medical Center, Nashville, TN, USA

M.L. Gonzalgo, M.D., Ph.D. (✉)
Department of Urology, Sylvester Comprehensive Cancer Center, University of Miami Miller School of Medicine, Miami, FL, USA
e-mail: mgonzalgo@gmail.com

E.P. Castle and R.S. Pruthi (eds.), *Robotic Surgery of the Bladder*, DOI 10.1007/978-1-4614-4906-5_15,

Perioperative Outcomes

Each of the perioperative outcomes reported in the literature provides a means of assessing the quality or value of the intervention. Perioperative outcomes for the series with at least 50 patients and for the cohort studies and randomized trial comparing open with robot-assisted radical cystectomy are shown in Tables 15.1 and 15.2, respectively.

Operative Time

Operative time is an important perioperative parameter because of its impact on cost and complications. Operative time is the primary driver of operative cost and the longer operative time associated with robotic surgery is the main source of cost difference between the open and robotic approaches [5]. A cost analysis by Martin et al. demonstrated that operative time had a greater impact on perioperative costs than any other parameter. On sensitivity analysis, an operative time greater than 361 min was associated with a higher total perioperative cost for robot-assisted cystectomy compared to open cystectomy.

Longer operative time is also associated with perioperative complications, length of stay, and interval to return of bowel function in many procedures, including laparoscopic colorectal surgery [30], though these associations have not been demonstrated conclusively in open or robot-assisted cystectomy [13, 31]. Still, an expeditious operation is desirable, since many cystectomy patients have comorbidities that make them vulnerable to the side effects and complications associated with a prolonged anesthesia and operative time. Longer operative time also limits the productivity of the operative surgeon and other resources.

Operative time may be influenced by surgeon experience, so it may be most appropriate to assess after the "learning curve" flattens. Nonetheless, most case series include the initial cases, so the mean operative time may appear longer than expected, and some of the difference between open and robotic operative times may be exaggerated. Operative time may also be influenced by the extent of lymphadenectomy, diversion type (continent vs. conduit), surgical approach to the diversion (intracorporeal vs. extracorporeal), gender, pelvic anatomy, prior surgery, efficiency of the operative assistant and other operating room staff, and a variety of other factors.

Among the 22 unique case series, 19 reported total operative time [1–8, 10–13, 15–21], and the range of reported means and medians was quite wide: 261–697 min. In series with at least 50 patients [2, 3, 7, 10, 11, 13], the range of means and medians was somewhat narrower: 261–492 min. Five of the six studies reported the mean operative time [2, 3, 7, 10, 11], permitting the calculation of a weighted mean over these 373 cases: 340 min or 5 h 40 min.

Several studies addressed the effect of the learning curve on operative time and, in general, operative time decreases as experience increases. In one example, Richards et al. found that the mean operative time decreased over the course of their first 60 cases, from 524 min for the first 20, to 503 for the second 20, and 449 for the last 20, $p=0.059$ [3]. Similarly, Wang et al. found a reduction in mean operative duration of 112 min between the first 16 cases and the second 16 ($p=0.007$) [32].

As with the open procedure, continent diversion prolongs operative time. In two of the larger case series, Kauffman and Khan each showed approximately a 2-h difference in mean operative time between conduit and continent diversion [7, 11].

Some robotic surgeons have experimented with intracorporeal diversion (see Chap. 11). Intracorporeal urinary diversion was associated with increased operative time of approximately 1 h (mean 318 min vs. 252 min, $p<0.001$) in one study which included 10 intracorporeal and 20 extracorporeal diversions [27]. Another study showed no significant difference, but had higher operative times overall (median 372 vs. 384) among 24 intracorporeal and 132 extracorporeal diversions [13].

Most studies comparing open with RARC find that RARC is associated with longer operative time. In the available comparative studies, the

Table 15.1 Robot-assisted radical cystectomy case series with at least 50 patients: perioperative outcomes

First author, year	Hayn, 2011 [13]	Treiyer, 2011 [2]	Richards, 2011 [3]	Khan, 2011 [7]	Pruthi, 2010 [10]	Kauffman, 2010 [11]
Institution	Roswell Park	U. Saarland, Germany	Wake Forest	Guy's Hospital, U.K.	UNC Chapel Hill	NYP—Cornell
Number of pts	156	84	60	50	100	79
Gender, *n* (%)						
Male	125 (80)	70 (83)	48 (80)	44 (88)	73 (73)	62 (78)
Female	31 (20)	14 (17)	12 (20)	6 (12)	27 (27)	17 (22)
Diversion						
Continent cutaneous		0	2	0		8
Orthotopic neobladder	11 continent	22	3	5	38	25
Ileal conduit	145	62	55	45	61	46
OR time (min)						
Mean (median)	(378)	261	492	361	276	378 (360)
Range (IQR)	(300–426)	243–618	290–700	240–600		
Blood loss (mL)						
Mean (median)	(400)	298	483	340	271 (250)	460 (400)
Range (IQR)	(250–700)	50–2,000		100–1,150		
Transfusion rate	16 %			4 %		
Time to bowel activity (days)						
Flatus, mean		2.12			2.1	
Bowel movement, mean		2.87			2.8	

Table 15.2 Studies comparing open and robot-assisted radical cystectomy: perioperative outcomes

First author, year	Martin et al. [5]			Nix, 2010 [25]			Ng, 2010 [23]			Pruthi, 2007 [24]			Rhee, 2006 [20]			Galich, 2006 [21]		
Institution	Mayo Clinic Arizona			UNC Chapel Hill			NYP—Cornell			UNC Chapel Hill			University of Virginia			U. Nebraska		
	Robotic	Open	*p* value	Robotic	Open	*p* value	Robotic	Open	*p* value	Robotic	Open	*p* value	Robotic	Open	*p* value	Robotic	Open	*p* value
Number of pts	19	14		21	20		83	104		20	24		7	23		13	24	
OR time (min)																		
Mean (median)	(280)	(320)	NR	252 (252)	211 (204)	<0.05	375	357	NS	366	222	<0.05	638	507	<0.05	(697)	(395)	<0.05
Range (IQR)	192–390	211–408								258–432	156–300					240–828	300–664	
Blood loss (mL)																		
Mean (median)	(255)	(696)	NR	258 (200)	575 (600)	<0.05	460	1,172	<0.05	313	588	<0.05	479	1,109	<0.05	(500)	(1,250)	<0.05
Range (IQR)	50–700	200–1,400								100–700	200–1,100					100–1,000	300–10,200	
Transfusion																		
Mean units per patient							1.42	3.65	<0.05				1.6	2.7	NS			
Transfusion rate													57 %	87 %	NS	54 %	75 %	NS
Time to bowel activity (days)																		
Flatus, mean				2.3 (2)	3.2 (3)	<0.05				2.1	2.9	<0.05						
Bowel movement, mean				3.2 (3)	4.3 (4)	<0.05				2.8	3.8	<0.05						
Length of stay																		
Mean (median)	(5)	(10)	NR	5.1 (4)	6 (6)	NS	(5.5)	(8)	<0.05	4.4	5.3	<0.05	11	13	NS	(8)	(10)	<0.05
Range (IQR)	4–11	5–31					3–28	3–60								4–23	6–35	

difference in mean operative time ranged between 18 and 302 min [5, 20, 21, 23–25], but it seemed to narrow in the more recent series in which the RARC experience is greater. For example in the randomized trial, Nix et al. found a difference of only 41 min between the open ($n = 20$) and robotic approaches ($n = 21$) (211 min vs. 252, $p < 0.001$). In a prospective nonrandomized study, Ng et al. found no significant difference in mean operating room time between the open ($n = 104$) and robotic ($n = 83$) approaches (357 min vs. 375, $p = 0.29$). Another study showed that the difference in operative time between the robotic and open approaches was significant only among patients undergoing continent diversion and not for those in whom a conduit was performed [32].

Clearly, there is quite a bit of variation in operative time between institutions. This may be driven by differences in measurement (e.g., skin-to-skin operative time vs. total time spent in the room), amount of time spent teaching, surgeon experience with robotics in general and RARC in particular, efficiency of the operating assistant and operating room staff, or other factors. The fact that open and robotic times vary in proportion across institutions suggests that "systemic" factors are at play, such as differences in measurement and the overall pace of work in the operating room, and they do not seem to be specific to the procedure itself.

In summary, operative duration is an important parameter because of its clear influence on the economic viability of robot-assisted radical cystectomy and because of its potential impact on postoperative complications. While operative times are longer in RARC compared to the open approach, the difference is decreasing as robotic experience is increasing. As one would anticipate, continent diversion and intracorporeal diversion prolong operative time in RARC, while surgeon and institutional experience tend to decrease it.

Blood Loss and Transfusion

Blood loss and transfusion have important implications for the quality of radical cystectomy, since they are strongly associated with postoperative complications [31, 33, 34] although this has not been conclusively demonstrated in RARC [13]. They may also influence convalescence time, time to functional recovery (e.g., ability to perform activities of daily living), and quality of life measures (e.g., sense of well-being). Perioperative blood transfusion is also associated with a higher risk of cancer recurrence and disease-specific mortality in diseases such as colorectal cancer [35] and may be associated with increased overall mortality after cystectomy [36]. Blood loss and transfusion also increase costs associated with surgery [37]. For these reasons, operative blood loss and transfusion are useful clinical indicators for comparing the effectiveness of alternative surgical approaches to radical cystectomy for bladder cancer.

All 22 studies reported a mean, a median and/or a range of estimated blood loss (EBL) [1–22]. The means and medians ranged from 160 to 615 cm^3, with most clustered between 200 and 500. Five of the six studies with 50 or more RARC patients reported the mean EBL [2, 3, 7, 10, 11], permitting the calculation of a weighted mean over these 373 cases: 360 cm^3.

Each of the studies that compared open with robot-assisted radical cystectomy showed a clinically and statistically significantly lower EBL in the robotic group [5, 20, 21, 23–25]. While there were substantial differences across institutions, within each institution, the mean EBL was approximately twice as much in the open group compared to the robotic. The mean EBL for the robotic group ranged from 255 to 500 cm^3, while the mean for the open group ranged from 575 to 1,250. In the randomized trial the open patients had an average EBL of 564 cm^3 compared to 273 cm^3 for the RARC patients ($p < 0.001$) [25].

Few publications include data on the use of blood products. In two small comparative studies, Rhee reported use of blood transfusion in four out of seven robotic cases (57 %) compared with 20 out of 23 open cases (87 %) and Galich et al. reported a 54 % transfusion rate in their first 13 robotic cases, compared to 75 % in 24 contemporaneous open cystectomies [20, 21]. More recently, Hayn et al. logged a 16 %

transfusion rate among 156 patients undergoing RARC and Khan had only two transfusions in 50 patients (4 %) [7, 13]. Wang et al. demonstrated the difference in transfusion usage between the open and robotic groups by showing the mean number of units per patient: 0.5 units per RARC patient vs. 2 units per open cystectomy patient, $p=0.007$ [32].

Much like the total operative time data, there are large discrepancies across institutions, but consistent comparisons between the open and robotic approaches within institutions. One can expect, on average, about twice as much blood loss during an open case than a robotic one. While the transfusion data are sparse, they seem to parallel the EBL data in favoring the robotic approach. These differences could have significant implications for comparisons of cost, complications, recovery metrics, and potentially even cancer recurrence between the open and robotic approaches.

Return of Bowel Function

One of the most salient postoperative milestones is the return of bowel function. The timing of its return influences the patient's sense of well being and quality of life. Some researchers have focused on the role of nutritional status in driving cystectomy outcomes [38]. In this light, the timing of return of bowel function may herald the patient's emergence from the perioperative catabolic state and may, in turn, affect the pace of functional recovery. In the USA, it also signals the patient's readiness for discharge. Because the interval to return of bowel function influences length of stay, and length of stay is one of the primary drivers of cost, the return of bowel function has important implications for cost.

Studies from two institutions (UNC Chapel Hill, and University of Saarland, Germany) and one consortium (Korea) included data on time to return of bowel function [2, 10, 12, 24–27]. The single institution studies from the USA and Germany reported a mean of 2.1 days between surgery and flatus, and 2.8–2.9 days to the first bowel movement. The Korean multicenter consortium found an average of 3.4 days to flatus.

One prospective cohort study and one randomized trial (both from the same institution) compared these outcome metrics between open and robotic cohorts. In the cohort study, the average number of days to flatus was 2.1 for the robotic group and 2.9 for the open group ($p<0.001$) and time to first bowel movement was 2.8 days compared with 3.8, respectively ($p<0.001$) [24]. The results of the randomized trial were similar (median 2.3 vs. 3.2 days, $p=0.0013$ for flatus and 3.2 vs. 4.3 days, $p=0.0008$ for bowel movement) [25]. This difference was associated with a statistically significantly lower length of stay in the nonrandomized study (mean 4.4 vs. 5.3 days, $p=0.007$), but not for the randomized trial (median 5.1 vs. 6.0 days, $p=0.2837$).

Thus, the interval from surgery to the return of bowel function seems to be somewhat shorter for the RARC patients compared to the open surgery patients in the few studies to evaluate this endpoint. The return of bowel function is an important determinant of length of stay (and, by extension, cost) and may also have implications for quality of life and return to baseline nutritional status and functional status. Therefore, these early findings should be confirmed in larger, prospective randomized studies, and the downstream effects of early return of bowel function should be explored in greater depth.

Use of Pain Medication

One potential benefit of minimally invasive surgical approaches is the reduction in postoperative pain and, with that, a lower use of narcotic usage [39]. Narcotic use has a significant impact on bowel function and contributes to postoperative ileus, one of the most common complications of radical cystectomy [31]. Therefore, various strategies are employed to reduce postoperative pain and narcotic use among cystectomy patients, including use of NSAIDs and novel opioid antagonists that reduce these side effects [40]. If the difference in postoperative pain and narcotic use were markedly different between the open and robotic operations, the minimally invasive approach may represent an alternative strategy for reducing postoperative pain and ameliorating its downstream consequences.

In a randomized trial comparing open to robot-assisted radical cystectomy, Nix et al. showed significantly lower use of narcotic medication in the robotic group compared to the open surgery patients (89 vs. 147 morphine equivalents, $p=0.0044$) [25]. With this reduction in postoperative narcotic usage, there was a statistically significant reduction in the interval to return of bowel function, and a significant reduction in length of stay, suggesting that reduced postoperative pain may drive these downstream outcomes. In addition to the potential benefits for bowel function and length of stay, one would expect that a 40 % reduction in the use of narcotic pain medications would have a clinically meaningful impact on the patient's postoperative quality of life.

In a subsequent nonrandomized study from the same group, intracorporeal urinary diversion was associated with lower use of narcotic medications postoperatively (57.6 vs. 93.2 morphine equivalents, $p=0.042$), providing another potential mechanism for decreasing postoperative pain and narcotic usage [27].

In summary, the data on postoperative narcotic utilization after RARC, while intriguing, are very limited and preclude making any broad conclusions. This important outcome deserves further study to determine whether, in fact, RARC patients have reduced postoperative pain compared to open cystectomy patients, and, if so, whether that difference manifests in clinically meaningful differences in quality of life, return of bowel function, and length of stay.

Length of Stay and Use of Intensive Care Units

Length of stay (LOS) is second only to OR time in driving the cost of robotic vs. open cystectomy [5]. A shorter LOS for RARC could mitigate the higher costs associated with longer operative time, higher use of disposable items in the OR, and amortization of the robot itself. On the other hand, lower LOS is associated with higher rates of readmission in many situations, which would tend to drive up overall cost. Therefore, studies reporting LOS should also report readmission rates, though few do.

With length of stay (LOS), there is quite a bit of variability from one institution to the next and even more variability across countries, presumably due to differences in culture and healthcare systems. Looking at studies within the USA, the mean LOS ranged between 4.9 and 8.1 days among studies that included 50 or more patients [3, 10, 11]. Among these studies, Pruthi et al. report a mean LOS of 4.9 days, with a 30-day readmission rate of only 11 %, which compares favorably with other series reporting readmissions after cystectomy Pruthi et al. [10]. Factors associated with longer LOS included perioperative complication [11, 13] and surgeon/institution experience [3].

A German study with 84 patients had a mean LOS of 17.7 days (range 10–33), and a British series of 50 patients had a mean LOS of 10 days (range 5–24), demonstrating that there are large differences in discharge practices across countries, with European hospitals tending to have longer LOS than US hospitals [2, 7].

In studies comparing the open and robotic approaches, LOS was consistently lower in the robotic cohorts [5, 20, 21, 23–25], most often by 1–2 days, and the difference was statistically significant in three of the five studies. As indicated above, decreased use of narcotics and earlier return of bowel function in the robotic series may contribute to an earlier discharge from the hospital. Decreased blood loss and use of transfusion may also play a role. Theoretically, there may also be less fluid shift and metabolic demand after RARC compared to open cystectomy, which could influence discharge, but the data are not available to support or refute this hypothesis. Overall, though a shorter length of stay has a tangible impact on overall cost of the procedure and may predict a shorter convalescence.

Complications

The morbidity associated with radical cystectomy has been reported to range from 30 to 60 % even at high-volume tertiary referral centers [31, 42]. The scope of complications associated with robot-assisted radical cystectomy is very similar to open cystectomy, yet there are reported differences in the frequency of overall and specific types of complications between the two surgical techniques. While contemporary reporting of complications associated with radical cystectomy has improved with the use of standardized classification systems (i.e., Clavien grading), the exact reasons as to why differences in complication rates exist between the two techniques is not well understood. Recent studies have provided further insight into the frequency, distribution, and severity of complications associated with RARC.

Overall Complication Rates Associated with Robot-Assisted Cystectomy

The majority of studies investigating complication rates associated with RARC originate from single institution cohorts that are limited by relatively modest sample sizes. When standardized reporting of complications has been performed, minor/low grade complications were associated with Clavien grades 1 and 2 and major or high grade complications were associated with Clavien grades ≥3. In one study of 50 patients undergoing RARC, the overall perioperative complication rate was reported to be 34 % [7]. The majority of these complications (71 %) were classified as minor events. Another study of 79 consecutive patients undergoing RARC with extracorporeal urinary diversion reported one or more complications within 90 days of surgery in 49 % of patients. Approximately 79 % of complications were classified as low grade and zero mortalities were reported for this cohort of patients [11]. A summary of common complications associated with RARC and the frequency range of events is shown in Table 15.3.

Table 15.3 Types and frequencies of complications associated with robot-assisted radical cystectomy

System	Frequency	Reference
Gastrointestinal	7–31 %	[7, 10, 11, 13, 23]
Infectious	2–41 %	[7, 10, 11, 13, 23]
Genitourinary	3–13 %	[7, 11, 13, 23]
Wound	4–7 %	[7, 23]
Pulmonary	1–4 %	[7, 13, 23]
Cardiac	2–11 %	[10, 11, 13, 23]
Bleeding	1–4 %	[7, 23]
Thromboembolic	3–7 %	[10, 11, 13, 23]
Neurologic	0–2 %	[7, 13, 23]

In a single institution study with a larger cohort size, an overall complication rate of 36 % was reported with only 8 % of patients experiencing high grade complications [10]. Gastrointestinal events (7 %) were the most frequent type of complications followed by infectious (6 %), and cardiac-related problems (4 %) [10]. In another report of 156 consecutive patients who underwent RARC, 52 % of patients experienced a complication within 90 days of surgery [43]. At a median follow-up of 9 months, 65 % of patients experienced some type of postoperative complication. Approximately 41 % complications were classified as minor. The most frequent types of complications were classified as gastrointestinal (31 %), infectious (25 %), and genitourinary (13 %). The 90-day mortality rate was 5.8 % [43].

The distribution of complications associated with RARC appears to be similar to open cystectomy. Among the various studies which have reported outcomes related to RARC, the majority of complications have been classified as minor. One of the most frequent types of complications associated with RARC is gastrointestinal (postoperative ileus) which is not surprising given the requirement for a bowel anastomosis as part of the urinary diversion. The overall mortality rate associated with RARC has been reported to be 0–6 % which is comparable to open cystectomy [10, 43].

Comparing Complications: Robot-Assisted Versus Open Cystectomy

A number of studies have attempted to compare robot-assisted and open cystectomy using a variety of methods. Propensity-matched analysis of robotic versus open cystectomy has demonstrated that fewer deaths and overall complications were associated with RARC compared to open cystectomy (0 % vs. 2.5 % and 49.1 % vs. 63.8 %, respectively) [44]. Use of parenteral nutrition was lower for RARC compared to open cystectomy (6.4 % vs. 13.3 %), but median lengths of stay were similar. While the overall inpatient complication rate was found to be lower for RARC compared to open cystectomy, no complication subtype (i.e., cardiac, respiratory, genitourinary, wound, vascular) was found to be significantly different between the two surgical techniques. These data suggest that no single complication was responsible for the overall difference between the two cohorts [44]. In this population-based comparative study, RARC was associated with less parenteral nutrition use and fewer inpatient complications and deaths compared to open cystectomy.

Another single institution, matched analysis of robotic versus open cystectomy also demonstrated similar perioperative outcomes between the two techniques [45]. No differences in minor or major complications were observed. Length of stay was also similar for the two groups. The most frequent complication was postoperative ileus which occurred in 22 % and 25 % of robotic and open cystectomy cases, respectively. The 30-day readmission rate, return to operating room, and need for interventional procedures were similar for both groups. There were no mortalities observed in the RARC cohort at 30 and 90 days. The 30- and 90-day mortality rate for open cystectomy in this cohort was 1 % and 3 %, respectively. A multi-institutional study of 227 patients undergoing RARC demonstrated that 30 % of patients experienced a complication with 7 % of patients having Clavien grade 3 or higher severity [46]. Decreased age and increased ASA score were predictors of higher Clavien complication score.

In another series of 187 open and robotic cystectomies performed by a single surgeon, the overall complication rate at 30 days was significantly lower in the robotic group (41 %) compared to the open group (59 %) [23]. The rate of high-grade (Clavien grades 3–5) complications was also found to be lower for RARC compared to open cystectomy (17 % vs. 31 %) [23]. Infection was the most common complication followed by gastrointestinal and cardiac-related problems. The types of complications were similar in both surgical groups. A prospective randomized trial comparing open versus RARC demonstrated reduced ileus in patients who underwent RARC [25]. No significant difference was observed between the two surgical groups with regard complications reported as mean Clavien units, however, multivariable analysis showed a trend towards fewer complications in the robotic group when controlling for other known variables [25]. A summary of complication rates reported among studies that have compared robotic and open cystectomy is shown in Table 15.4.

Learning Curve and Complication Rates

Assessing proficiency in performing robot-assisted radical cystectomy remains challenging and there is no standardized definition for the learning curve associated with a surgeon's initial experience with this technique. The number of cases required to achieve proficiency with RARC has been reported to be as few as 20, however, the learning curve can be quite variable and is dependent upon a number of factors including individual surgeon experience, patient selection, and case volume. Several studies have examined the relationship between the learning curve and complication rates. A single institution analysis of 60 RARC cases showed that complications decreased as a function of learning curve progression from 70 % in the first tertile to 30 % in each of the second and third tertiles [3]. In a cohort of 45 patients who underwent RARC and

Table 15.4 Complication rates: robotic versus open cystectomy

Complication	Robotic (%)	Open (%)	*R* vs. *O*	Significance	References
Major complications	*31*	*17*	*R*>*O*	*p* = 0.03	[23]
Overall complications at 30 days	*41*	*59*	*R*<*O*	*p* = 0.04	
Overall complications at 90 days	62	48	*R*=*O*	*p*=0.07	
Clavien units (median)	2.3	2.6	*R*=*O*	*p*=0.5622	[25]
Clavien units (adjusted mean)	1.7	2.8	*R*=*O*	*p*=0.0503	
Death	*0*	*3*	*R*<*O*	*p* < 0.001	[44]
Use of TPN	*6*	*13*	*R*<*O*	*p* = 0.046	
Cardiac	6	10	*R*=*O*	*p*=0.110	
Respiratory	15	18	*R*=*O*	*p*=0.421	
Genitourinary	7	11	*R*=*O*	*p*=0.112	
Wound	5	8	*R*=*O*	*p*=0.185	
Vascular	2	4	*R*=*O*	*p*=0.316	
Overall complications	*49*	*64*	*R*<*O*	*p* = 0.035	
Readmission <30 days	28	20	*R*=*O*	*p*=0.25	[45]
Reoperation <30 days	10	4	*R*=*O*	*p*=0.15	
Overall complications <30 days	66	62	*R*=*O*	*p*=0.65	
Overall complications >30 days	26	29	*R*=*O*	*p*=0.69	

Statistically significant differences between the open and robot-assisted approaches are shown in italics

intracorporeal urinary diversion, there was a significant decrease in late (>30 days) complications over time [47].

No significant differences in complication rates were attributable to sequential case number in 164 consecutive patients from the initial series reported from another institution [48]. Approximately 64 % of patients experienced an intraoperative or postoperative complication with the majority of these (76 %) being classified as minor. Grades of complications were similar between sequential case number groups with the exception of Clavien grade 5 complications of which 75 % occurred in the first 50 cases [48]. A 4 % mortality rate was reported and there was no significant difference between patients who died in the initial 50 cases compared to those who died in subsequent cases. The overall hospital readmission rate was 36 % and was not significantly different between sequential case groups. While sequential case number was not significantly associated with increased incidence of complications, it was associated with shorter operative times in this series [48].

Perioperative neurologic complications related to prolonged surgery in steep Trendelenburg have been described in at least two patients undergoing RARC [49]. In these patients, neurological deterioration occurred following extubation and was attributed to cerebral edema. Prevention of these types of complications is especially relevant during the learning curve phase when longer operative times are more likely to occur.

Complications of Robot-Assisted Cystectomy with Intracorporeal Urinary Diversion

Extracorporeal urinary diversion is performed in the vast majority of robot-assisted cystectomy series. There are limited reports on complications associated with RARC and intracorporeal urinary diversion. Early studies that have explored intracorporeal ileal conduit reconstruction have primarily described technical feasibility of the procedure, however, certain types of complications may be unique to this surgical approach. Iatrogenic necrosis of the ileal conduit has been described as a result of vascular pedicle injury from retraction of the specimen bag [4]. In another study of 45 patients who underwent RARC with intracorporeal urinary diversion, the early (≤30 days) complication rate was 40 % and the late (>30 days) complication rate was 30 % [47]. The frequency of minor (Clavien grades 1 and 2) complications during early and late perioperative time periods was 17 % and 13 %, respectively.

Predictors of Complications Associated with Robot-Assisted Cystectomy

Patients with bladder cancer are typically older and have medical comorbidities that may be associated with the development of complications related to radical cystectomy. Preoperative risk factors including age, prior abdominal surgery, COPD, BMI, cardiac risk, and ASA score did not significantly influence complications in 66 patients undergoing RARC [28]. In this study, advanced age was associated with higher cardiac risk and an increased likelihood of admission to the intensive care unit. Higher ASA score was associated with an increased risk of overall hospital stay. A history of prior abdominal surgery correlated with more frequent unscheduled postoperative clinic visits. The frequency of minor and major complications was equivalent (24 %) at 3 months following surgery and the overall mortality rate was 1.6 % [28].

Significant risk factors for postoperative complications on univariate analysis of a single-institution experience of 79 patients included preoperative renal insufficiency, EBL≥500 mL, and intraoperative intravenous fluids of >5,000 mL. Preoperative renal insufficiency and intravenous fluids of >5,000 mL were significantly associated with overall complications on multivariate analyses [11]. Risk factors that were significantly associated with high-grade (Clavien grades 3–5) complications on multivariable analyses included: age≥65 years, EBL≥500 mL, and intravenous fluids >5,000 mL [11].

In another study of 156 patients undergoing RARC, multiple risk factors (i.e., gender, age, BMI, chemotherapy, smoking history, case #, ASA, EBL, diversion type) were analyzed to determine the association with perioperative complications [43]. No risk factor was significant in predicting a complication on uni- or multivariable analyses. On univariable analysis, BMI was a significant negative predictor of a high-grade complication, but on multivariable analysis no single risk factor was significant in predicting a complication [43]. In a series of 187 open and robotic cystectomies, the overall complication rate was lower in the robotic group (41 %) compared to the open group (59 %). Logistic regression analysis showed that surgical technique (RARC) was an independent predictor of fewer overall and major complications [23].

Conclusions

The majority of studies published to date have demonstrated comparable outcomes for RARC compared to open cystectomy. In the small number of studies comparing perioperative outcomes between open and RARC (including the only randomized trial to date), most studies show longer operative time for robotic surgery, but lower blood loss, shorter time to recovery of bowel function and shorter length of stay. Complications associated with RARC are generally minor (Clavien grades 1 and 2), and multiple studies that have directly compared robotic to open cystectomy have demonstrated fewer overall complications in patients undergoing RARC. As physicians, patients, and payers strive to determine the optimal surgical approach for the treatment of bladder cancer, perioperative outcomes and complications will be among the most important outcomes on which to focus because of their impact on patient quality of life, recovery, and cost. Ongoing randomized clinical trials comparing robotic to open cystectomy will further define the role of this minimally invasive surgical technique for the treatment of bladder cancer.

Since the main impetus for the development of minimally invasive surgery is to reduce surgical morbidity, such an evidence-based analysis of perioperative outcomes and complications is essential reading for all who perform this procedure.

Editors' Commentary

Erik P. Castle and Raj S. Pruthi

In the small number of studies comparing perioperative outcomes between open and robot-assisted radical cystectomy (RARC), most have shown longer operative times for robotic surgery, but lower blood loss, shorter time to recovery of bowel function, and shorter length of stay. In addition, our experience has also noted reduced pain and narcotic requirement and a more rapid physical convalescence for these patients. The authors also show that the complications associated with RARC are generally minor, and multiple studies that have directly compared robotic to open cystectomy have demonstrated fewer overall complications in patients undergoing RARC.

The authors are correct in their comments that perioperative outcomes and complications will be among the most important outcomes measured as physicians, patients, and payers analyze the evidence to determine the optimal surgical approach for the treatment of bladder cancer. Such outcomes are highly relevant based on their significant impact on patient quality of life, recovery, and cost. To date, the robotic approach to cystectomy appears to provide acceptable operative, pathological, and short-term clinical outcomes—seemingly duplicating the principles and practices of the time-tested open surgical technique.

References

1. Torrey RR, Chan KG, Yip W, et al. Functional outcomes and complications in patients with bladder cancer undergoing robotic-assisted radical cystectomy with extracorporeal indiana pouch continent cutaneous urinary diversion. Urology. 2012;79:1073–8.
2. Treiyer A, Saar M, Kopper B, Kamradt J, Siemer S, Stockle M. [Robotic-assisted laparoscopic radical cystectomy: evaluation of functional and oncological results]. Actas Urol Esp. 2011;35(3):152–7.
3. Richards KA, Kader K, Pettus JA, Smith JJ, Hemal AK. Does initial learning curve compromise outcomes for robot-assisted radical cystectomy? A critical evaluation of the first 60 cases while establishing a robotics program. J Endourol. 2011;25(9):1553–8.
4. Rehman J, Sangalli MN, Guru K, et al. Total intracorporeal robot-assisted laparoscopic ileal conduit (Bricker) urinary diversion: technique and outcomes. Can J Urol. 2011;18(1):5548–56.
5. Martin AD, Nunez RN, Castle EP. Robot-assisted radical cystectomy versus open radical cystectomy: a complete cost analysis. Urology. 2011;77(3):621–5.
6. Lavery HJ, Martinez-Suarez HJ, Abaza R. Robotic extended pelvic lymphadenectomy for bladder cancer with increased nodal yield. BJU Int. 2011;107(11):1802–5.
7. Khan MS, Elhage O, Challacombe B, Rimington P, Murphy D, Dasgupta P. Analysis of early complications of robotic-assisted radical cystectomy using a standardized reporting system. Urology. 2011;77(2):357–62.
8. Jonsson MN, Adding LC, Hosseini A, et al. Robot-assisted radical cystectomy with intracorporeal urinary diversion in patients with transitional cell carcinoma of the bladder. Eur Urol. 2011;60(5):1066–73.
9. Akbulut Z, Canda AE, Ozcan MF, Atmaca AF, Ozdemir AT, Balbay MD. Robot-assisted laparoscopic nerve-sparing radical cystoprostatectomy with bilateral extended lymph node dissection and intracorporeal studer pouch construction: outcomes of first 12 cases. J Endourol. Sep 2011;25(9):1469–79.
10. Pruthi RS, Nielsen ME, Nix J, Smith A, Schultz H, Wallen EM. Robotic radical cystectomy for bladder cancer: surgical and pathological outcomes in 100 consecutive cases. J Urol. 2010;183(2):510–4.
11. Kauffman EC, Ng CK, Lee MM, et al. Critical analysis of complications after robotic-assisted radical cystectomy with identification of preoperative and operative risk factors. BJU Int. 2010;105(4):520–7.
12. Kang SG, Kang SH, Lee YG, et al. Robot-assisted radical cystectomy and pelvic lymph node dissection: a multi-institutional study from Korea. J Endourol. 2010;24(9):1435–40.
13. Hayn MH, Hussain A, Mansour AM, et al. The learning curve of robot-assisted radical cystectomy: results from the International Robotic Cystectomy Consortium. Eur Urol. Aug 2010;58(2):197–202.
14. Yuh B, Butt Z, Fazili A, et al. Short-term quality-of-life assessed after robot-assisted radical cystectomy: a prospective analysis. BJU Int. 2009;103(6):800–4.
15. Woods M, Thomas R, Davis R, et al. Robot-assisted extended pelvic lymphadenectomy. J Endourol. 2008;22(6):1297–302.
16. Park SY, Jeong W, Choi YD, Chung BH, Hong SJ, Rha KH. Yonsei experience in robotic urologic surgery-application in various urological procedures. Yonsei Med J. 2008;49(6):897–900.
17. Murphy DG, Challacombe BJ, Elhage O, et al. Robotic-assisted laparoscopic radical cystectomy with extracorporeal urinary diversion: initial experience. Eur Urol. 2008;54(3):570–80.
18. Mottrie A, Schatteman P, Fonteyne E, Rotering J, Stockle M, Siemer S. [Robot-assisted laparoscopic

radical cystectomy]. Urologe A. 2008;47(4):414. 416–9.
19. Abraham JB, Young JL, Box GN, Lee HJ, Deane LA, Ornstein DK. Comparative analysis of laparoscopic and robot-assisted radical cystectomy with ileal conduit urinary diversion. J Endourol. 2007;21(12): 1473–80.
20. Rhee JJ, Lebeau S, Smolkin M, Theodorescu D. Radical cystectomy with ileal conduit diversion: early prospective evaluation of the impact of robotic assistance. BJU Int. 2006;98(5):1059–63.
21. Galich A, Sterrett S, Nazemi T, Pohlman G, Smith L, Balaji KC. Comparative analysis of early perioperative outcomes following radical cystectomy by either the robotic or open method. JSLS. 2006;10(2): 145–50.
22. Hemal AK, Abol-Enein H, Tewari A, et al. Robotic radical cystectomy and urinary diversion in the management of bladder cancer. Urol Clin North Am. 2004;31(4):719–29. viii.
23. Ng CK, Kauffman EC, Lee MM, et al. A comparison of postoperative complications in open versus robotic cystectomy. Eur Urol. 2010;57(2):274–81.
24. Pruthi RS, Wallen EM. Robotic assisted laparoscopic radical cystoprostatectomy: operative and pathological outcomes. J Urol. 2007;178(3 Pt 1):814–8.
25. Nix J, Smith A, Kurpad R, Nielsen ME, Wallen EM, Pruthi RS. Prospective randomized controlled trial of robotic versus open radical cystectomy for bladder cancer: perioperative and pathologic results. Eur Urol. 2010;57(2):196–201.
26. Coward RM, Smith A, Raynor M, Nielsen M, Wallen EM, Pruthi RS. Feasibility and outcomes of robotic-assisted laparoscopic radical cystectomy for bladder cancer in older patients. Urology. 2011;77(5): 1111–4.
27. Pruthi RS, Nix J, McRackan D, et al. Robotic-assisted laparoscopic intracorporeal urinary diversion. Eur Urol. 2010;57(6):1013–21.
28. Butt ZM, Fazili A, Tan W, et al. Does the presence of significant risk factors affect perioperative outcomes after robot-assisted radical cystectomy? BJU Int. 2009;104(7):986–90.
29. Yuh B, Padalino J, Butt ZM, et al. Impact of tumour volume on surgical and pathological outcomes after robot-assisted radical cystectomy. BJU Int. 2008;102(7):840–3.
30. Scheer A, Martel G, Moloo H, et al. Laparoscopic colon surgery: does operative time matter? Dis Colon Rectum. 2009;52(10):1746–52.
31. Shabsigh A, Korets R, Vora KC, et al. Defining early morbidity of radical cystectomy for patients with bladder cancer using a standardized reporting methodology. Eur Urol. 2009;55(1):164–74.
32. Wang GJ, Barocas DA, Raman JD, Scherr DS. Robotic vs open radical cystectomy: prospective comparison of perioperative outcomes and pathological measures of early oncological efficacy. BJU Int. 2008;101(1):89–93.
33. Chang SS, Cookson MS, Baumgartner RG, Wells N, Smith Jr JA. Analysis of early complications after radical cystectomy: results of a collaborative care pathway. J Urol. 2002;167(5):2012–6.
34. Bostrom PJ, Kossi J, Laato M, Nurmi M. Risk factors for mortality and morbidity related to radical cystectomy. BJU Int. 2009;103(2):191–6.
35. Amato A, Pescatori M. Perioperative blood transfusions for the recurrence of colorectal cancer. Cochrane Database Syst Rev. 2006;1:CD005033.
36. Morgan TM, Barocas DA, Chang SS, Phillips S, Salem S, Clark PE, Penson DF, Smith JA Jr, Cookson MS. The relationship between perioperative blood transfusion and overall mortality in patients undergoing radical cystectomy for bladder cancer. Urol Oncol, Epub ahead of print September 7, 2011. PMID: 21906965.
37. Stokes ME, Ye X, Shah M, et al. Impact of bleeding-related complications and/or blood product transfusions on hospital costs in inpatient surgical patients. BMC Health Serv Res. 2011;11:135.
38. Gregg JR, Cookson MS, Phillips S, et al. Effect of preoperative nutritional deficiency on mortality after radical cystectomy for bladder cancer. J Urol. 2011;185(1):90–6.
39. Wilson CH, Sanni A, Rix DA, Soomro NA. Laparoscopic versus open nephrectomy for live kidney donors. Cochrane Database Syst Rev. 2011;11: CD006124.
40. Buchler MW, Seiler CM, Monson JR, et al. Clinical trial: alvimopan for the management of post-operative ileus after abdominal surgery: results of an international randomized, double-blind, multicentre, placebo-controlled clinical study. Aliment Pharmacol Ther. 2008;28(3):312–25.
41. Stimson CJ, Chang SS, Barocas DA, et al. Early and late perioperative outcomes following radical cystectomy: 90-day readmissions, morbidity and mortality in a contemporary series. J Urol. 2010;184(4): 1296–300.
42. Stein JP, Lieskovsky G, Cote R, et al. Radical cystectomy in the treatment of invasive bladder cancer: long-term results in 1,054 patients. J Clin Oncol. 2001;19(3):666–75.
43. Hayn MH, Hellenthal NJ, Hussain A, Stegemann AP, Guru KA. Defining morbidity of robot-assisted radical cystectomy using a standardized reporting methodology. Eur Urol. 2011;59(2):213–8.
44. Yu HY, Hevelone ND, Lipsitz SR, et al. Comparative analysis of outcomes and costs following open radical cystectomy versus robot-assisted laparoscopic radical cystectomy: results from the US Nationwide Inpatient Sample. Eur Urol. 2012;61(6):1239–44.
45. Styn NR, Montgomery JS, Wood DP, et al. Matched comparison of robotic-assisted and open radical cystectomy. Urology. 2012;79(6):1303–9.
46. Smith AB, Raynor M, Amling CL, et al. Multi-institutional analysis of robotic radical cystectomy for bladder cancer: perioperative outcomes and

complications in 227 patients. J Laparoendosc Adv Surg Tech A. 2012;22(1):17–21.
47. Schumacher MC, Jonsson MN, Hosseini A, et al. Surgery-related complications of robot-assisted radical cystectomy with intracorporeal urinary diversion. Urology. 2011;77(4):871–6.
48. Hayn MH, Hellenthal NJ, Seixas-Mikelus SA, et al. Is patient outcome compromised during the initial experience with robot-assisted radical cystectomy? Results of 164 consecutive cases. BJU Int. 2011;108(6):882–7.
49. Pandey R, Garg R, Darlong V, Punj J, Chandralekha, Kumar A. Unpredicted neurological complications after robotic laparoscopic radical cystectomy and ileal conduit formation in steep trendelenburg position: two case reports. Acta Anaesthesiol Belg. 2010;61(3): 163–6.

Surgical Avoidance and Management of Operative Complications

16

Angela Smith and Michael Woods

Introduction

As already emphasized throughout this book, the development of robotic surgery has helped refine the more challenging technique of laparoscopic cystectomy, paving the way for robot-assisted radical cystectomy as a feasible alternative to the open method. Since the first reported series in 2003, there has been a marked increase in the number of manuscripts focusing on perioperative and postoperative outcomes following robot-assisted radical cystectomy (RARC).

While open radical cystectomy is associated with overall complication rates approaching 70 % when utilizing strict reporting criteria [1], complication rates following RARC vary widely. This disparity likely results from differences in reporting methodology and duration of postoperative follow-up, thus representing a major limitation when comparing techniques and institutions. In this chapter, we will briefly review these perioperative and postoperative outcomes while also discussing avoidance and management of complications during robot-assisted radical cystectomy (RARC).

A. Smith, M.D. • M. Woods, M.D. (✉)
Department of Urology, The University of North Carolina at Chapel Hill, Chapel Hill, NC, USA
e-mail: Michael_woods@med.unc.edu

Review of Perioperative and Postoperative Complications

The existing literature on perioperative and postoperative complications is primarily compromised of single center series reporting complication rates for RARC. These rates vary widely in the literature presumably due to difficulty in event capture, as many RARC complications occur at local, non-tertiary hospitals, and are therefore not systematically collected or reported. Additionally, a number of prior studies did not adhere to standard reporting guidelines, such as the MSKCC (Memorial Sloan Kettering Cancer Center) grading system or the modified Clavien–Dindo classification system [1, 2]. However, recent studies routinely report complication categorizations following these criteria.

Several single center series now exist, many reporting complication rates for RARC. Kauffman et al. published their complication data on a series of 79 consecutive patients after RARC [3]. While 49 % of patients experienced complications within 90 days when using a standardized reporting system, most were minor, with infectious complications (41 %) occurring most commonly, followed by gastrointestinal (27 %) and thromboembolic events (10 %). Another series by Treiyer et al. evaluate 84 consecutive RARC patients with overall and major 30-day Clavien complication rates of 53 % and 12 %, respectively [4]. In another European series, Khan et al. reported outcomes of

E.P. Castle and R.S. Pruthi (eds.), *Robotic Surgery of the Bladder*, DOI 10.1007/978-1-4614-4906-5_16,

their first 50 robotic cystectomies [5]. The Clavien 90-day complication rate was 34 %, with major complications occurring in 10 % of this cohort. Despite use of a standardized complication reporting system, a major limitation of this study revolves around its selection bias, with the selected population representing only half of patients undergoing cystectomy at their institution.

Addressing this limitation seen in many single case reports, Hayn et al. studied 156 consecutive patients undergoing the procedure and calculated an overall complication rate of 52 % within 90 days, including a 33 % major complication and a 21 % readmission rate [6]. The authors classified all complications using the MSKCC system. The most common complications reported in Hayn's series were gastrointestinal (31 %), infectious (25 %), and genitourinary (13 %). As suggested above, the study is noteworthy in that all cystectomies at this institution were performed robotically. However, limitations of single institution studies are well known and have led to the construction of multi-institutional analyses, which provide more robust and generalizable data.

Kang et al. describes a multi-institutional evaluation of complications during and after RARC in seven participating Korean institutions [7]. Retrospectively analyzing data from 104 patients, the authors reported an overall complication rate of 27 % using the modified Clavien system, with 7.7 % considered major complications and 19 % minor complications. Intraoperative complications represented 3.8 % of the total number of complications, with three conversions to open surgery. Two were secondary to adhesions with one due to an external iliac vein injury. Our own multi-institutional study expands on this data through inclusion of a larger sample size of 227 patients spread between four institutions [8]. The overall complication rate was 30 % with 7 % having a major complication as defined by the Clavien classification system, with no perioperative deaths. Interestingly, younger patients in this series were more likely to experience complications.

Comparisons Between Robot-Assisted and Open Radical Cystectomy

While understanding robotic complication rates is an important tool in quality assurance, another important comparison is contrasting robotic procedures with the standard, open technique. A number of studies have offered comparisons between the robotic and open procedures, but the vast majority remain nonrandomized studies, which are inherently limited by patient selection and other selection biases.

Ng et al. performed a prospective cohort study of 187 consecutive patients (104 ORC and 83 RARC) who underwent radical cystectomy [9]. Thirty- and ninety-day Clavien complications revealed a higher overall rate in the open group at 30 days (59 % vs. 41 %, $p=0.04$), as well as a significant increase in major complications (30 % vs. 10 %; $p=0.007$). At 90 days, the overall complication rate, while greater in the open cohort, was not statistically significantly different. However, there did appear to be more major complications in the open cohort at 90 days (31 % vs. 17 %; $p=0.03$). In a multivariate analysis controlling for a variety of comorbidities, RARC remained an independent predictor of fewer overall and major complications at both 30 and 90 days. The types of complications observed were similar to those in contemporary open series, including gastrointestinal, infectious, thromboembolic, and stomal events. Although this study was strengthened by prospective data collection, a large sample size, and procedures performed by a single surgeon, it remains limited by its observational methodology.

Only one randomized trial comparing ORC and RARC has been published to date [10]. Nix et al. reported results of our prospective, randomized study, including 20 patients undergoing ORC and 21 in the RARC cohort. Although designed as a non-inferiority study comparing lymph node yield, several secondary endpoints were evaluated, including complication rate. Comparing those undergoing open and robotic procedures, no difference in complication rates were noted

(50 % vs. 33 %, respectively; $p=0.28$). In a multivariate analysis controlling for age, body mass index, and pathologic stage there was a trend toward a lower complication rate in the robotic group, but it did not reach statistical significance ($p=0.0503$). A multi-institutional, randomized study is currently in the recruitment phase, the results of which will clarify this question.

Factors Associated with Perioperative Complications

While comparisons between open and RARC remain important, a more clinically relevant question involves examining preoperative predictors of postoperative RARC complications. Butt et al. evaluated 3-month complication rates among 62 consecutive patients undergoing RARC at a single institution. Stratifying patients into low- and high-risk groups based on age, prior surgery, comorbidities, body mass index (BMI), revised cardiac risk index (RCRI) and ASA score, they examined whether any of these preoperative factors were predictive of increased risk of complications. Although they found no association between any of these factors and complications rates during this time interval, advanced age was independently associated with a higher RCRI score ($p=0.014$) and increased likelihood of admission to the ICU ($p=0.007$) [11]. Evaluating 90-day outcomes, minor complications occurred in 24 % of patients, while 24 % had a major complication, with 11 % requiring reoperation. The same author published a study evaluating the effect of BMI on outcomes of RARC. Assessing a cohort of 51 patients categorized by three BMI subgroups, no significant differences were noted in postoperative complication rates between the cohorts [12]. Expanding on this group of patients, a subsequent study of 156 patients revealed a negative association between increased BMI and high grade complications in univariate analysis [6]. However, no significant predictors for complications following RARC were noted in multivariate analysis.

In the same study described earlier in this chapter, Kauffman et al. used two reporting methods for complications (MSKCC grading system and modified Clavien systems) to identify predisposing risk factors of 79 consecutive patients with bladder cancer undergoing RARC by a single surgeon at a single institution [3]. Forty-nine percent of patients experienced one or more complications within 90 days of surgery with 16 % experiencing major complications. Multivariate analysis identified pre and intraoperative factors which predicted complications, including preoperative renal insufficiency and intraoperative intravenous fluids >5,000 mL where were independent predictors across grades. Greater age ≥65 years, blood loss ≥500 mL, and intraoperative intravenous fluids of >5,000 mL were predictive of high-grade complications.

As described above, we recently participated in a multi-institutional study examining perioperative outcomes of 227 patients from four institutions undergoing RARC [8]. ASA score was a significant predictor of complication rate with higher scores associated with higher complication grades ($p=0.0258$). Age (stratified by age 65) was found to be a significant predictor of worse complications ($p=0.0230$) with those <65 years being twice as likely to experience a higher Clavien complication rate when controlling for other variables. While this finding is certainly different from prior studies, this may be explained by selection bias. Older patients with more comorbidities may be selected for the open procedure, thereby limiting our sample to healthier older surgical candidates in the robotic cohort. Conversely, the majority of younger patients may have been offered the procedure, therefore skewing the results. Certainly, this is a recognized limitation of retrospective case series which will hopefully be resolved through anticipated findings of the ongoing multi-institutional randomized trial comparing ORC and RARC.

Learning Curve and Complication Correlation

While preoperative patient factors may serve as important predictors of subsequent complications, surgeon experience and the effect of the learning curve on the RARC procedure must also be acknowledged. Hayn et al. performed an analysis on their first 164 consecutive patients [13]. Dividing patients into three groups according to sequential case number (<50, 50–100, >100 cases), no significant differences were observed with both estimated blood loss as well as complication rates. Pruthi et al. similarly evaluated the learning curve for their initial 50 patients [14]. When evaluating estimated blood loss, a significant decline was observed after the 20th patient, but no further improvements were noted thereafter. Comparing complication rates between the first and second cohort of 25 patients, no differences were observed. Schumacher et al. published a report evaluating complications in 45 patients [15]. This series is unique since all diversions were created intracorporeally with 80 % of patients choosing an orthotopic neobladder. Dividing patients into three groups of 15 patients, no differences were noted in estimated blood loss between cohorts. However, a significant decrease was observed in late complications after the initial group of 15 patients. An important consideration includes the fact that 70 % of patients in this study underwent RARC in the last 3 years of the 7-year study period.

These studies offer conflicting data regarding the role of the learning curve for RARC, thereby making it difficult to draw definitive conclusions and provide recommendations of when a surgeon can expect to overcome these hurdles. Understandably, this is based on numerous factors, including the surgeon's prior experience, institutional support, patient selection, and many other variables. However, through our use of recommendations in this chapter, we hope to lessen the burden of the learning curve.

Avoidance of Perioperative Complications

Patient Selection

As we outline above, the incidence of complications following radical cystectomy remains significant regardless of approach. However, we believe that there are specific keys to avoiding operative complications when performing RARC. Here we offer several preventative strategies which may help reduce complications.

First, appropriate patient selection cannot be overemphasized during the primary stages of transition to RARC. As an initial case, we would recommend beginning with a thin male patient and non-bulky tumor. Because of several parallels drawn from the maneuvers used during robotic prostatectomy, a male patient will provide familiarity and comfort during the initial, most challenging steps involved in mastering the procedure. This will additionally lessen operative times early in the learning curve. Furthermore, patient size is often an important factor in the level of difficulty, with some of the most challenging RARC cases occurring in morbidly obese patients. Technical issues are often more challenging in obese patients, due to the need for appropriate retraction, which an especially difficult during left ureteral identification due to the large amount of epiploic, mesenteric, and retroperitoneal fat.

As a final recommendation, avoidance of locally advanced and large tumors is imperative. Bulky tumors can produce significant challenges with anterior retraction of the bladder during the posterior dissection. This particular problem will place the surgeon at risk for inadvertent entry into the bladder or rectal injury secondary to the lack of a posterior working space. We feel it is advisable to wait until surgeons have reached a more advanced stage in their learning curve before taking on these challenging cases.

Perioperative Pathways

While many complications during one's early operative experience may be avoided through patient selection, an emphasis should also be placed on standardized preoperative and postoperative pathways. From our experience, we have developed a "fast track" method to maximize outcomes and minimize morbidity. While many series in the literature continue the use of bowel preparation prior to cystectomy and urinary diversion, we have eliminated this based on recent colorectal literature suggesting no significant benefit [16]. To study this in our patient population, we evaluated two sequential case series of 70 patients undergoing radical cystectomy and urinary diversion. While the first patient group was given a regular diet with no mechanical preparation (other than an enema prior to surgery to reduce rectal distension), the second patient group underwent a preoperative mechanical bowel preparation with clear liquid diet, magnesium citrate, and an enema [17]. This study revealed no differences in overall complication rates (or gastrointestinal complications), length of stay, or return of bowel function between the two cohorts. Based on this evidence, we exclude a mechanical bowel preparation.

Postoperative pathways for radical cystectomy are equally important and also can benefit from standardization. Our recommended "fast track" program has been studied using 362 consecutive patients undergoing open or robot-assisted radical cystectomy and urinary diversion, each undergoing this perioperative care plan [18]. The plan includes extensive preoperative counseling with regard to expectations as well as an intraoperative surgical plan which includes DVT prophylaxis with sequential compression devices and TED hose, removal of the orogastric tube at the end of the procedure, and perioperative antibiotics in accordance with the American Urological Association guidelines, continued for 24 h postprocedure. Postoperatively, DVT prophylaxis is begun with early ambulation (on postoperative day 0–1), TED hose, and subcutaneous low molecular weight heparin (or unfractionated heparin if poor renal function) begun on postoperative day 1. Additionally, patients are given a pro-kinetic agent (metacloproamide 10 mg daily × 48 h), non-narcotic analgesics (e.g., ketorolac 30 mg IV q6h × 48 h, converted to celecoxib 200 mg po BID), and supplemental pain management with narcotics. The fast-track program emphasizes a strict dietary regimen, beginning with NPO status and chewing gum (ad lib) on postoperative day 1, 8 oz of noncarbonated clear liquids every 8 h on postoperative day 2, followed by unrestricted noncarbonated clear liquids on postoperative day 3, and finally a regular diet on postoperative day 4. Diet advancement is performed regardless of bowel function and is only held or decreased in the setting of vomiting or intractable nausea. With this pathway, we have found a lower rate of overall and gastrointestinal complications with a favorable complication profile [18]. This particular pathway represents the authors experience in the postoperative management of radical cystectomy patients. Other clinical care pathways have been published and ultimately postoperative care will depend on surgeon preference [19].

Equipment and Materials

Prior to embarking on a RARC, the use of proper equipment and materials is crucial to avoidance of complications. First, the robotic instruments most commonly used include a Fenestrated Bipolar instrument in the left robotic arm and Monopolar Scissors in the right. A Prograsp is most commonly used in the fourth robotic arm, but use of robotic bowel grasper is an alternative. The latter instrument is larger in length and can provide more depth with troublesome bowel retraction. However, if this instrument is used, it is imperative to visualize the instrument when changing its position due to the potential for damage of adjacent structures due to its size.

With regard to bedside assistant ports, the use of a 12-mm and 15-mm port is essential regardless if the assistant is placed on the right or left. The 15-mm port can be placed in the lateral position, and this larger port will allow easier extraction of lymph node packets as well as placement of a 15-mm extraction bag for the final specimen. The 12-mm assistant port is placed in the medial position, cephalad, and just medial to the left robotic arm (for a left-sided bedside assistant). This allows direct placement of an endovascular stapler to the pedicles of the bladder. If this port is placed lateral to the ipsilateral working arm, the approach to the bladder pedicle can be difficult as the stapler cannot articulate enough to overcome the acuity of the angle.

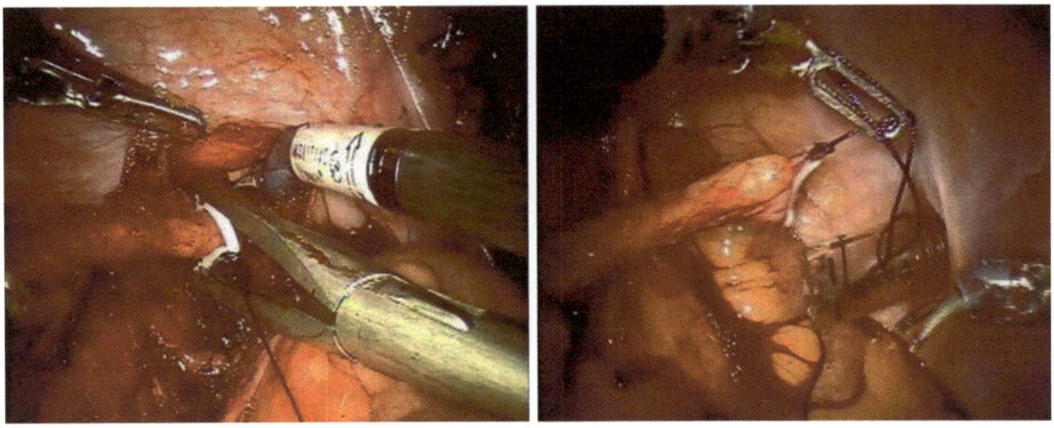

Fig. 16.1 Technique of ureteral clipping and division with pre-tied hem-o-lok clip

We use a bariatric/long stapler (Covidien EndoGIA Ultra XL, Mansfield, MA) which will easily reach the pelvis despite the fairly cephalad port location. As these are vascular pedicles, we often use tan Covidien 60 mm loads (for vascular/medium tissues). However, if one finds the pedicle too thick, a purple load can suffice in this situation, compressing tissue up to 2.25 mm in thickness, compared to tan reloads which compress up to 1.5 mm. Hem-o-lok (Weck, Research Triangle Park, NC) clips are also commonly used for portions of the cystectomy, with 15 mm (gold) clips recommended to allow control of larger tissue pedicles.

Intraoperative Techniques to Minimize Morbidity

We will now touch on several intraoperative techniques that can be employed to avoid postoperative complications. To start with, ureteral dissection is an important part of RARC. Ureteral strictures represent an extremely troubling late complication of urinary diversions, and the majority of these can be attributed to ischemia of the distal ureter, in some cases resulting from poor surgical technique during ureteral mobilization. Care must be taken to avoid tension during dissection. After dissection, a robotic arm is often employed to elevate the ureter, and due to the lack of tactile feedback, excessive tension may be unintentionally placed on the ureter. It is therefore essential to use visual cues to constantly assess this degree of tension. Additionally, it is imperative to leave periureteral tissue surrounding the ureter to allow for a non-ischemic anastomosis. A technique which we have found effective and efficient to minimize ureteral trauma involves the use of a pre-tied Hem-o-lok clip. We place a 15-mm clip with a 20-cm silk tie proximal to the site of ureteral transection. Once divided, the tie/clip functions as a secure stay for all future manipulation without direct handling of the ureter (Fig. 16.1).

An additional technique we utilize to minimize ureteral ischemia, limitation of proximal mobilization to just above the common iliac vessels allows for mobilization of the ureter away from the working field during extended pelvic lymphadenectomy while maintaining perforating vessels to the ureter above the aortic bifurcation. Although tempting, additional proximal dissection is rarely needed to complete the urinary diversion, even if done through a limited incision during extracorporeal reconstruction.

While a small incision is possible, it is still important to make a large enough incision to accommodate construction of the urinary diversion. This allows for creation of the ureteroenteric anastomosis without additional ureteral tension aggravated by a small incision. We believe that the benefits of a robotic approach will not be undone through limited extension of this incision.

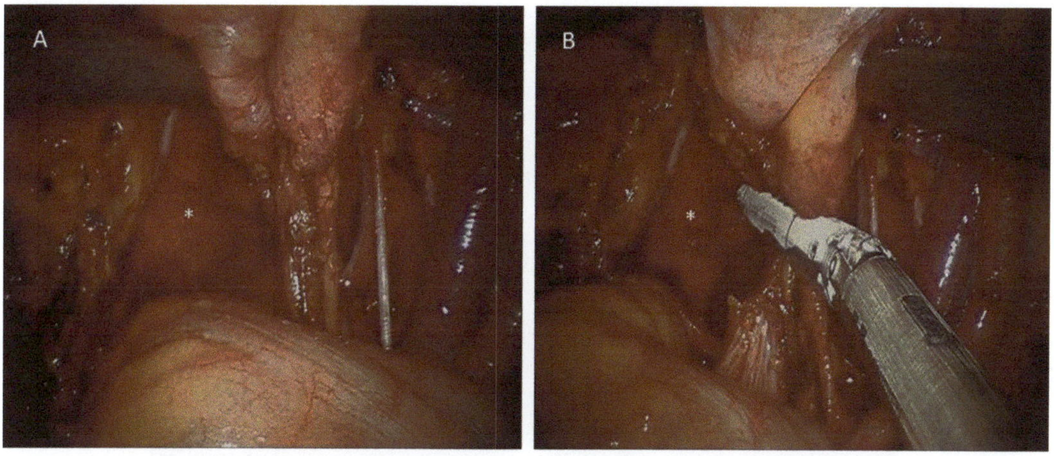

Fig. 16.2 (a) Isolation of right bladder pedicle after complete mobilization of the rectum. (b) Safe application of laparoscopic stapler above rectum (* = rectum)

Ultimately, performance of an incorporeal urinary diversion may help avoid tension-related insults to the ureteral blood supply.

While ureteral complications are certainly troublesome, a rectal injury can be a disastrous complication which could result in a colostomy, rectal fistula, and even death if unrecognized. When performing the posterior dissection in male patients, particular attention should be paid to careful and thorough mobilization of the rectum to avoid injury during division of the vascular pedicles. Our preference for division of these pedicles is with use of a vascular stapler. The posterior dissection usually becomes more difficult as one progresses distally, and it should be kept in mind that the rectum lies in a more anterior location when approaching the prostatic apex. We recommend allotting adequate time to fully mobilize the distal aspect of the rectum away from the prostate in much the same fashion as one prepares for neurovascular bundle preservation during a robot assisted radical prostatectomy. Once this is accomplished, the surgeon will be left with a narrow column of vascular tissue from the superior vesical artery to the prostatic apex. This will allow safe application of the vascular stapler above all rectal tissue as shown in (Fig. 16.2). When employing the stapler, we recommend the larger, more blunt blade be positioned medially to avoid inadvertent placement of the sharper, thinner blade into the rectum; also helpful is upward (anterior) articulation of the stapler away from the rectum.

If the separation of the bladder/prostate and rectum is difficult, we would then recommend proceeding cautiously through isolation of individual pedicles as one progresses distally, using Hem-o-lok (weck) clips for vascular control (Fig. 16.3). Blunt and sharp dissection should be employed avoiding the use of excessive cautery to thereby avert any thermal injury. If at any point a bulky tumor impedes visualization of the posterior plane, use of a 30° upward-facing lens may be warranted, which may improve visualization of the underside of the bladder.

Although the extirpative portion of RARC is undeniably the focus of the procedure, the prognostic and therapeutic benefits of an extended pelvic lymphadenectomy (PLND) at the time of radical cystectomy are also important and have been well established [20]. The ability to perform an adequate pelvic lymph node dissection during RARC has been a popular target for opponents of the robotic approach. However, this has been refuted by several authors [10, 21, 22], and we uphold that a meticulous dissection of any template can be performed robotically if the surgeon is committed to this goal. One of the most challenging aspects of the PLND is performing an adequate and safe dissection of the lymphatic

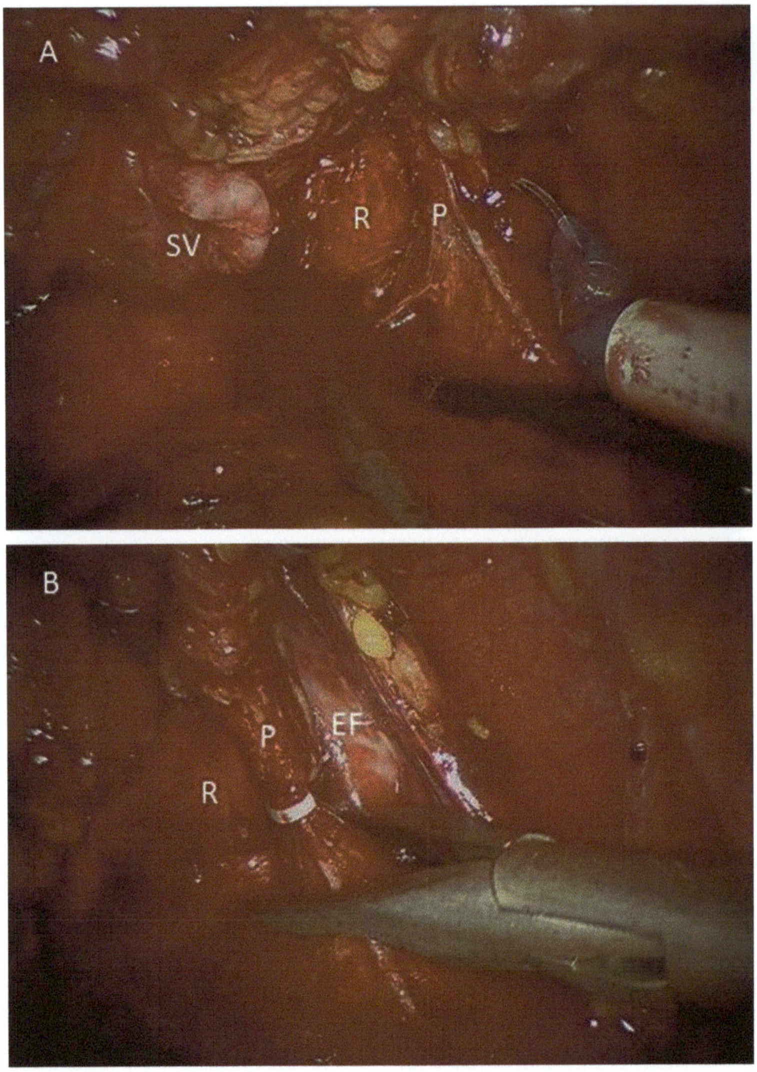

Fig. 16.3 (**a**) Distal right prostatic pedicle seen during a RARC where the application of a laparoscopic stapler would be potentially hazardous due to the proximity of the rectum. (**b**) Application of Hem-o-lok clip allowing precise division of pedicle anterior to rectum (R = rectum, P = pedicle, SV = seminal vesicle, EF = endopelvic fascia)

tissue in the bifurcation of the common iliac vessels. The difficulty of dissection can be decreased by medial mobilization of the external iliac vessels and all associated lymphatic tissue. This will expose the medial aspect of the psoas muscle and the most proximal aspect of the obturator nerve while releasing all lateral attachments of this nodal packet as shown in (Fig. 16.4a). It will further allow the surgeon to return to the medial side of the vessels and easily withdraw the entire lymph node packet from the bifurcation of the vessels (Fig. 16.4b). Overall, this will not only help decrease the risk of a vascular injury to the hypogastric vessels and alleviate the anxiety associated with dissection in this challenging area but also allow excellent access for the hypogastric vein dissection (Fig. 16.4c).

With the use of the above-mentioned advice for patient and instrument selection, perioperative care pathways, and intraoperative technique, we believe that many complications can be avoided.

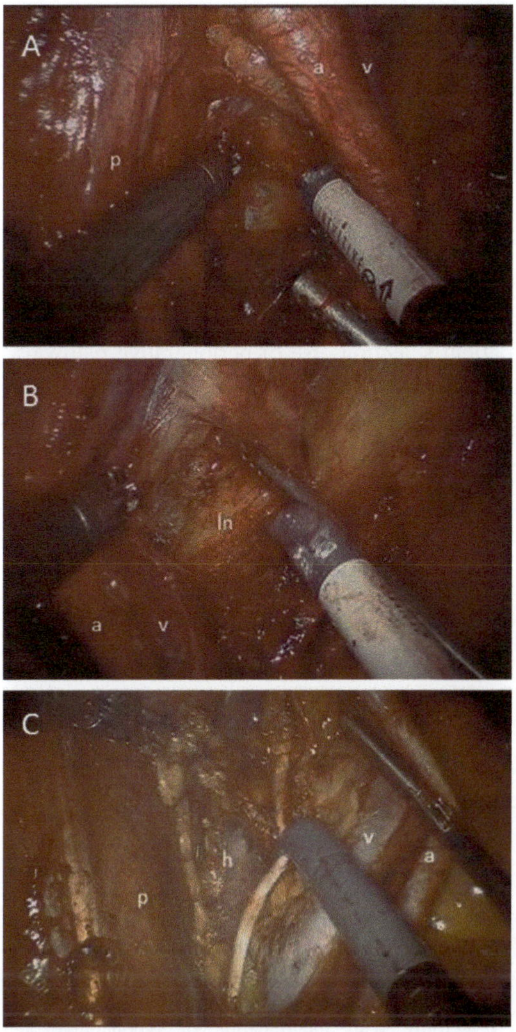

Fig. 16.4 (**a**) Medial mobilization of left external iliac vessels with the obturator/hypogastric lymph node packet. (**b**) Separation of lymph node packet from external iliac vessels. (**c**) Exposure of left hypogastric vein and obturator nerve (a = external iliac artery, v = external iliac vein, p = psoas muscle, ln = left hypogastric/obturator lymph node packet, h = hypogastric vein)

Management of Operative Complications

As described in the subsection above, avoidance of complications may be equally important to the ability of managing these same complications, most of which can be controlled robotically. Perhaps one of the most common intraoperative issues involves shortened ureteral length. Whether one has decreased length due to patient habitus or the necessity of decreasing length to attain negative margins, this can create difficulty in ureteroileal anastomoses. Furthermore, one can find additional length through elongation of the created ileal conduit (or neobladder limb). To enable adequate visualization of the anastomosis, one may need to lengthen the incision used for extracorporeal diversion, and the surgeon should not hesitate to do so, since this may decrease the possibility of ureteral tension and improve the quality of the anastomosis, reducing the chance of postoperative stricture.

While ureteral length may be a common intraoperative issue, a less common but more dangerous complication is intraoperative vascular injury, often experienced during lymph node dissection. Should this occur, vascular injuries can often be managed robotically. Additionally, a suture should be ready at all times to enable quick ligation of a bleeding vessel. In the setting of a venous injury the pneumoperitoneum should be increased to 20 mmHg to help tamponade the bleeding. In the case of a small to medium vessel with a visible stump or partial division, a clip may be employed. However, if a large en-face injury occurs (for example, in the external iliac vein), it may be necessary to grasp the opening (or apply pressure) with the left hand instrument (Fenestrated Bipolar) while placing a figure-of-eight suture around the defect with the contralateral hand. In this situation, the scissors in the right hand will need to be exchanged to a needle driver while the left hand maintains hemostasis. A shorter suture ($\leq$6 in.) will suffice and ensure ease of tying. In the event of a larger injury, proximal and distal control of the vessel may be required to adequately visualize and repair the defect. To accomplish this maneuver, the bedside assistant will likely be required to hold pressure on the injury while the console surgeon gains vascular control. Once the dissection is complete, either a tourniquet or laparoscopic bulldog clamps may be used. While controlling bleeding vessels, it is imperative to be cognizant of adjacent structures, particularly the obturator nerve, which can inadvertently be injured if one is not careful.

Equally disturbing but perhaps less emergent is the complication of a rectal injury. If an injury is encountered, consideration can be made for primary repair and closure, both of which may be accomplished robotically [23, 24]. If the patient has had radiation and appears to be a poor candidate for primary repair, one should consider colostomy with judicious use of general surgery consultation. It is important to stress preoperative counseling to these patients, so that they are made aware of this possibility before the day of surgery. However, if primary closure appears feasible, the edges of the defect should be freshened (and perhaps even resected further if cautery was the etiologic factor), and closure should proceed with at least two layers of absorbable suture (at the discretion of the surgeon) with some authors recommending a third imbricating layer of nonabsorbable suture [23]. An omental interposition may be performed, and we recommend the use of an intraperitoneal drain.

Conclusions

An increasing number of case series of robot-assisted radical cystectomy describe complication rates comparable to open series. Conflicting reports describe various preoperative factors as predictors of postoperative complications. Furthermore, learning curves complicate these predictors and should also be taken into account. Despite these variables, there are a number of considerations, including patient selection, equipment choice, perioperative pathways, and intraoperative technique that we have found to decrease postoperative complications and improve patient outcomes. We hope that this chapter provides a primer to best avoid and manage these complications, enabling the surgeon to achieve a smooth transition to performing robotic cystectomies.

Editors' Commentary

Erik P. Castle and Raj S. Pruthi

A successful outcome with radical cystectomy is not only related to surgical technique and safe extirpation of the bladder but also to factors such as patient selection and coordinated perioperative care. Indeed, minimally invasive surgery seeks to reduce surgical morbidity in all of its forms—including complications.

Indeed, perioperative outcomes and complications will be among the most important outcomes measured as physicians, patients, and payers. Such factors have a major impact on quality of care as well as cost of care. As such, it is highly relevant that surgeons strive to reduce complications and improve outcomes through appropriate patient selection, use of perioperative pathways, and proper intraoperative techniques. These highly experienced authors provide an insightful description of these important considerations to reduce complications and improve outcomes. Hopefully, the reader will be able to shorten their own learning curve by adopting the lessons and techniques put forth in this chapter.

References

1. Shabsigh A, Korets R, Vora KC, et al. Defining early morbidity of radical cystectomy for patients with bladder cancer using a standardized reporting methodology. Eur Urol. 2009;55(1):164–74.
2. Dindo D, Demartines N, Clavien PA. Classification of surgical complications: a new proposal with evaluation in a cohort of 6336 patients and results of a survey. Ann Surg. 2004;240(2):205–13.
3. Kauffman EC, Ng CK, Lee MM, et al. Critical analysis of complications after robotic-assisted radical cystectomy with identification of preoperative and operative risk factors. BJU Int. 2010;105(4):520–7.
4. Treiyer A, Saar M, Kopper B, Kamradt J, Siemer S, Stockle M. [Robotic-assisted laparoscopic radical cystectomy: evaluation of functional and oncological results]. Actas Urol Esp. 2011;35(3):152–7.
5. Khan MS, Elhage O, Challacombe B, Rimington P, Murphy D, Dasgupta P. Analysis of early complications of robotic-assisted radical cystectomy using a standardized reporting system. Urology. 2011;77(2):357–62.
6. Hayn MH, Hellenthal NJ, Hussain A, Stegemann AP, Guru KA. Defining morbidity of robot-assisted radical cystectomy using a standardized reporting methodology. Eur Urol. 2011;59(2):213–8.
7. Kang SG, Kang SH, Lee YG, et al. Robot-assisted radical cystectomy and pelvic lymph node dissection: a multi-institutional study from Korea. J Endourol. 2010;24(9):1435–40.
8. Smith AB, Raynor M, Amling CL, et al. Multi-institutional analysis of robotic radical cystectomy for bladder cancer: perioperative outcomes and

complications in 227 patients. J Laparoendosc Adv Surg Tech A. 2012;22(1):17–21.
9. Ng CK, Kauffman EC, Lee MM, et al. A comparison of postoperative complications in open versus robotic cystectomy. Eur Urol. 2010;57(2):274–81.
10. Nix J, Smith A, Kurpad R, Nielsen ME, Wallen EM, Pruthi RS. Prospective randomized controlled trial of robotic versus open radical cystectomy for bladder cancer: perioperative and pathologic results. Eur Urol. 2010;57(2):196–201.
11. Butt ZM, Fazili A, Tan W, et al. Does the presence of significant risk factors affect perioperative outcomes after robot-assisted radical cystectomy? BJU Int. 2009;104(7):986–90.
12. Butt ZM, Perlmutter AE, Piacente PM, et al. Impact of body mass index on robot-assisted radical cystectomy. JSLS. 2008;12(3):241–5.
13. Hayn MH, Hellenthal NJ, Seixas-Mikelus SA, et al. Is patient outcome compromised during the initial experience with robot-assisted radical cystectomy? Results of 164 consecutive cases. BJU Int. 2011;108:882–7.
14. Pruthi RS, Smith A, Wallen EM. Evaluating the learning curve for robot-assisted laparoscopic radical cystectomy. J Endourol. 2008;22(11):2469–74.
15. Schumacher MC, Jonsson MN, Hosseini A, et al. Surgery-related complications of robot-assisted radical cystectomy with intracorporeal urinary diversion. Urology. 2011;77(4):871–6.
16. Bucher P, Gervaz P, Soravia C, Mermillod B, Erne M, Morel P. Randomized clinical trial of mechanical bowel preparation versus no preparation before elective left-sided colorectal surgery. Br J Surg. 2005;92(4):409–14.
17. Raynor MC, Lavien G, Nielsen M, Wallen EM, Pruthi RS. Elimination of preoperative mechanical bowel preparation in patients undergoing cystectomy and urinary diversion. Urol Oncol. 2013;31:32–5.
18. Pruthi RS, Nielsen M, Smith A, Nix J, Schultz H, Wallen EM. Fast track program in patients undergoing radical cystectomy: results in 362 consecutive patients. J Am Coll Surg. 2010;210:93–9.
19. Chang SS, Cookson MS, Baumgartner RG, Wells N, Smith Jr JA. Analysis of early complications after radical cystectomy: results of a collaborative care pathway. J Urol. 2002;167(5):2012–6.
20. Poulsen AL, Horn T, Steven K. Radical cystectomy: extending the limits of pelvic lymph node dissection improves survival for patients with bladder cancer confined to the bladder wall. J Urol. 1998;160(6 Pt 1):2015–9. discussion 20.
21. Davis JW, Gaston K, Anderson R, et al. Robot assisted extended pelvic lymphadenectomy at radical cystectomy: lymph node yield compared with second look open dissection. J Urol. 2011;185(1):79–83.
22. Lavery HJ, Martinez-Suarez HJ, Abaza R. Robotic extended pelvic lymphadenectomy for bladder cancer with increased nodal yield. BJU Int. 2011;107(11):1802–5.
23. Yee DS, Ornstein DK. Repair of rectal injury during robotic-assisted laparoscopic prostatectomy. Urology. 2008;72(2):428–31.
24. Kheterpal E, Bhandari A, Siddiqui S, Pokala N, Peabody J, Menon M. Management of rectal injury during robotic radical prostatectomy. Urology. 2011;77(4):976–9.

Cost of Robot-Assisted Radical Cystectomy

17

David A. Green and Douglas S. Scherr

An estimated 70,530 new cases of urothelial carcinoma of the bladder (UCB) were diagnosed in the USA in 2010, resulting in 14,680 deaths [1] representing one of the costliest malignancies to treat in the USA [2]. The cost of treatment burden encompasses both the office-based procedures used to monitor patients as well as the surgical therapies employed to treat muscle-invasive, progressive, or high-risk disease as well as the costs inherent to treatment-related complications. Radical cystectomy (RC) with bilateral pelvic lymph node dissection (PLND) with or without neoadjuvant chemotherapy is the gold-standard treatment for non-metastatic high-risk non-muscle-invasive and muscle-invasive UCB, resulting in excellent local control, providing a cure for most patients with organ-confined UCB [3].

However, this potentially curative operation has a relatively high complication rate [4], upon which minimally invasive surgical techniques may be able to improve. Robot-assisted prostatectomy has achieved unprecedented market penetration in the treatment of clinically localized prostate cancer, now accounting for the majority of radical prostatectomy performed in the USA [5]. With the widespread acceptance of robotic assistance for prostate cancer surgery, the expansion into other urologic cancers such as bladder cancer, is inevitable, and in certain centers of excellence robot-assisted radical cystectomy (RARC) is now offered to essentially all patients who present with the oncologic indication for extirpative bladder surgery [6]. However, long-term comparative oncologic data remain sparse, although short-term RARC data are encouraging [7]. Given this, it is important to keep in mind economic predictions stating that healthcare costs will represent up to 20 % of the US' gross domestic product 10 years from now [8]. Indeed, the cost of purchase and yearly maintenance of the robotic surgical platform is approximately $1.65M and $150K, respectively (Intuitive Surgical, Sunnyvale, CA). As long-term data evolve on oncologic and functional outcomes after RARC, we most continuously reexamine the cost of our treatment choices, and ideally, the cost effectiveness of those choices.

Several cost analyses comparing ORC and RARC have been recently performed all at centers of excellence with broad experience in both the open and robotic technique. Those studies from Smith et al. [9], Martin et al. [10], and Lee et al. [11] comprise the majority of the data upon which this chapter is based. An additional study was performed by the latter group, further comparing the three cost analyses [12]. Of course, these well-designed analyses suffer from the same limitations as do all retrospectively conducted studies, but one limitation specific to cost analyses deserves particular mention. Cost-effectiveness analyses are the optimal methods to study economic considerations as they

D.A. Green • D.S. Scherr, M.D. (✉)
Department of Urology, Weill Medical College of Cornell University, 525 East 68th Street, New York, NY 10021, USA
e-mail: dss2001@med.cornell.edu

E.P. Castle and R.S. Pruthi (eds.), *Robotic Surgery of the Bladder*, DOI 10.1007/978-1-4614-4906-5_17,

pertain to health outcomes, where the unit of measure is typically $/quality adjusted life year (QALY). Such an analysis requires laboriously collected utility data which prescribes evidenced based "weights" to various health states. Unfortunately, in the bladder cancer literature, primary utility data is lacking, and prior studies have relied upon extrapolation from other similar health states [13]. To impute extrapolated utility data to model RARC vs. ORC cost effectiveness, a comparison which lacks strong oncologic data, would require too many assumptions and significantly dilute the conclusions that one could draw from such a study. Thus, the authors of the studies that we focus on here performed cost-identification analyses, which quantify economic resources involved, but not the benefits derived from their expenditure [12].

Smith et al. [9] captured data from 20 consecutive RARC and 20 ORC performed at their institution just prior to the time of their study. These authors stratified expenditures into fixed and variable costs, which were then further categorized as operating room (OR) or hospital costs. Fixed OR costs included base costs in addition to disposables, including endovascular stapling devices. Robotic cases added the per case cost of the robot itself which was calculated by dividing the sum of the 5-year amortized purchase price and yearly maintenance contract by the number of robotic cases performed institutionally per year, 288 in this case. Variable OR costs depended on the length of the procedure and were comprised of OR personnel and anesthesia time. These authors assumed that RARC and ORC fixed hospital costs were the same because the patients were placed on an identical clinical pathway regardless of surgical technique. Variable hospital costs derived from transfusion-related expenses and length of stay calculations. Costs associated with complications were not modeled because this group previously found no difference in their own complication rates between surgical techniques [14].

The mean fixed OR costs for RARC vs. ORC were greater by $1,634 ($4,032 vs. $2,398) OR variable costs were also greater by $570 ($7,798 vs. $7,228) because of increased OR time, with each hour of OR time costing $1,902. Variable hospital costs were higher in the ORC group by $564 ($4,982 vs. $4,418) by $564 because of a higher incidence of transfusions, and a longer hospital stay, which added $658 per day. Overall, the authors concluded that purchase and maintenance is the main driver of cost with the overall cost difference between RARC and ORC at $1,640, accounting for the greatest difference between modalities. An editorial written in response to this article suggested using multi-institutional costing data in future models as well as regression models to account for confounders specific to a given institution such as case mix and other local characteristics [15].

Martin et al. [10] drew upon the Mayo clinic RARC experience to compare associated costs with ORC using two different methods. Per case robot costs were calculated based on 300 cases per year. First, they performed Monte Carlo analysis to determine which factors (LOS, OR time, case volume, OR supply cost, and robot cost) had the greatest influence upon cost. Then, they analyzed direct and indirect costs computed from their institutional experience, including costs related to complications occurring within 30 days postoperatively. Actual cost values were not reported in this study, for proprietary reasons, in favor of percentage differences in cost.

The results of their first model showed that OR time and LOS were the primary determinants of cost. Not surprisingly, the cost of the robot figures materially into the cost difference from ORC. If one assumes that the robot is donated to the institution, leaving only the costs of the maintenance contract, 42 robotic cases annually are required to achieve cost equivalence with ORC. If the institution purchases the robot as well as the maintenance contract, 113 robotic cases annually are required to achieve cost equivalence with ORC. The second portion of their analysis averaged direct and indirect costs of 19 and 14 consecutive RARC and ORC patients at the authors' institution. Confirming what Smith et al. [9] found, when only direct costs were considered, ORC was 16 % less costly than RARC. However, when secondary costs were considered, including but not limited to LOS, transfusions, and

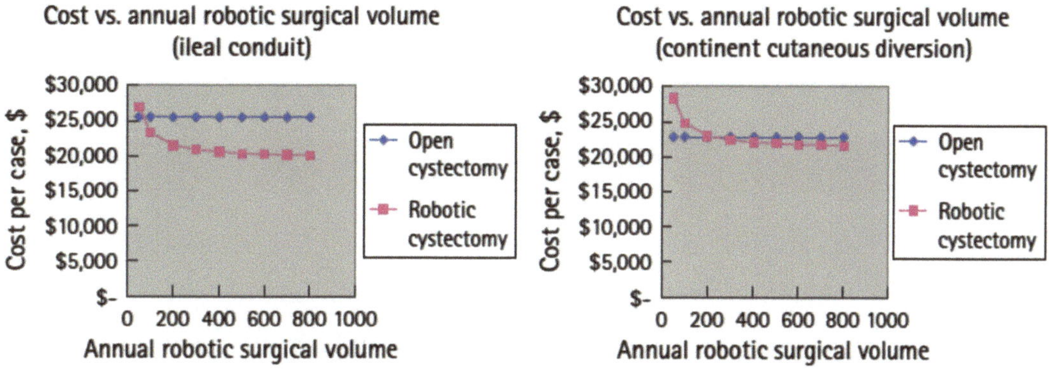

Fig. 17.1 One-way sensitivity analysis of annual robotic surgical volume across ileal conduit (IC) and continent cutaneous diversion (CCD). Reprinted with the permission of the authors

complications, RARC showed a 38 % cost advantage over ORC.

Lee et al. [11] built upon these two prior studies by considering the effect of different urinary diversions on cost as well as the cost of complications occurring within the 90-day postoperative period. Data from 83 RARC and 103 ORC were considered. Direct costs were derived from the Medicare resource-based relative value scale (MRBRVS), a standard fee schedule in the USA [16] and per case robot costs were based upon an annual volume of 361 robotic cases. Complication costs were calculated by multiplying the rate of a complication by the cost of treating the complication (i.e., MRBRVS procedural related costs) or institutional data for hospitalization costs.

Again, confirming the findings of Smith et al. [9] and Martin et al. [10], ORC outperformed RARC for all diversion types by ($13–$1,085) if only direct costs were considered. However, as Martin et al. [10] showed, the cost of complications for RARC vs. ORC did make a substantial difference, and in fact for patients undergoing either an ileal conduit (IC) ($1,624 vs. $7,202; $p<0.001$) or a continent cutaneous diversion (CCD) ($1,911 vs. $2,520; $p<0.001$), RARC conferred a cost advantage over ORC. This is consistent with the same groups' work that showed fewer major complications in their RARC series vs. the comparative ORC group (17 % vs. 31 %) [6]. Presumably, the lower incidence of major complications conferred a lower cost of treating complications overall. However, the cost–benefit diminished as the complexity of the urinary diversion increased and for patients undergoing orthotopic neobladder, the cost advantage of RARC over ORC disappeared.

Several sensitivity analyses in this study explored the effect of varying the different factors (annual surgical volume, LOS, daily hospitalization cost) that influence overall cost. Annual robotic surgery volume could decline to 62 and 225 institutionally, while maintaining cost equivalence between RARC and ORC, for patients undergoing IC and CCD, respectively (Fig. 17.1). ORC LOS could decrease to 4.5 and 7.5 days, while maintaining cost equivalence between RARC and ORC, for patients undergoing IC and CCD, respectively. ORC LOS could be as long as 9.6 days before RARC and ORC were cost equivalent in patients undergoing orthotopic neobladder (Fig. 17.2). RARC daily hospitalization costs could decrease to $468 and $827, while maintaining cost equivalence between RARC and ORC, for patients undergoing IC and CCD. Daily hospitalization costs could increase to $1,825 before RARC and ORC were cost equivalent in patients undergoing orthotopic neobladder (Fig. 17.3).

In sum, the studies described confirmed that RARC is more expensive than ORC in a direct cost analysis, but the additional cost impact can be abrogated by cost savings associated with lower complication rates in RARC patients as compared to those undergoing ORC. Additionally, hospital and surgical factors such as institutional robotic volume, LOS, hospitalization cost, and

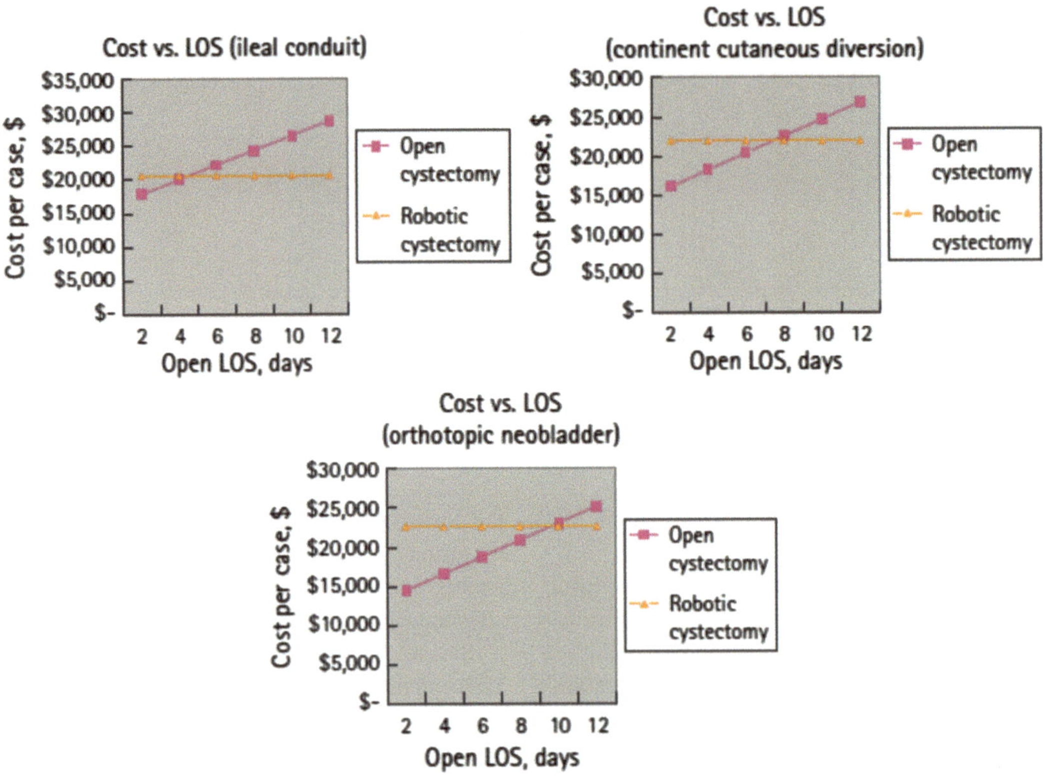

Fig. 17.2 One-way sensitivity analysis of open radical cystectomy (ORC) length of stay (LOS) across all types of urinary diversions. Reprinted with the permission of the authors

choice of urinary diversion can materially affect cost calculations.

There are many limitations to the cost analysis performed to date comparing RARC and ORC. Most importantly, each study draws from a single institution cohort making comparisons between studies problematic as health systems vary greatly, including measurement of costs and complications [17,18]. For example, in the study of Smith et al. [9] and Martin et al. [10], OR duration was the same or shorter for RARC vs. ORC, while in the study of Lee et al. [12], OR times were longer for patients undergoing RARC. It is difficult to fully understand all factors contributing to institutional differences in OR duration when all surgeons involved are highly experienced surgeons. Another major source of potential bias is the nonrandomized fashion in which ORC and RARC cohorts are assembled. For example, there are doubtless, immeasurable factors that contribute to a surgeon's decision to elect one urinary diversion over another, and these decisions can be a source of potential bias.

An important institutional factor implicit in all three of these previously mentioned cost studies is the relatively large institutional yearly robotic surgical volume. Cost calculations overall, were based on robotic volumes of approximately 300 annual cases. Even with the robotic startup and maintenance costs defrayed by large case volumes, the per case direct robotic costs still dominated all analyses. Thus, most small, community hospitals are unlikely to achieve anything near cost equivalence in a RARC vs. ORC comparison. In fact, the cost-effective incorporation of a RARC program requires the presence of a robust overall robotics program. As the prevalence of bladder cancer requiring radical surgery will never equal the prevalence of prostate cancer patients undergoing radical surgery, radical prostatectomy volume must facilitate cost-effective RARC. Furthermore, the trend towards centralization of complicated medi-

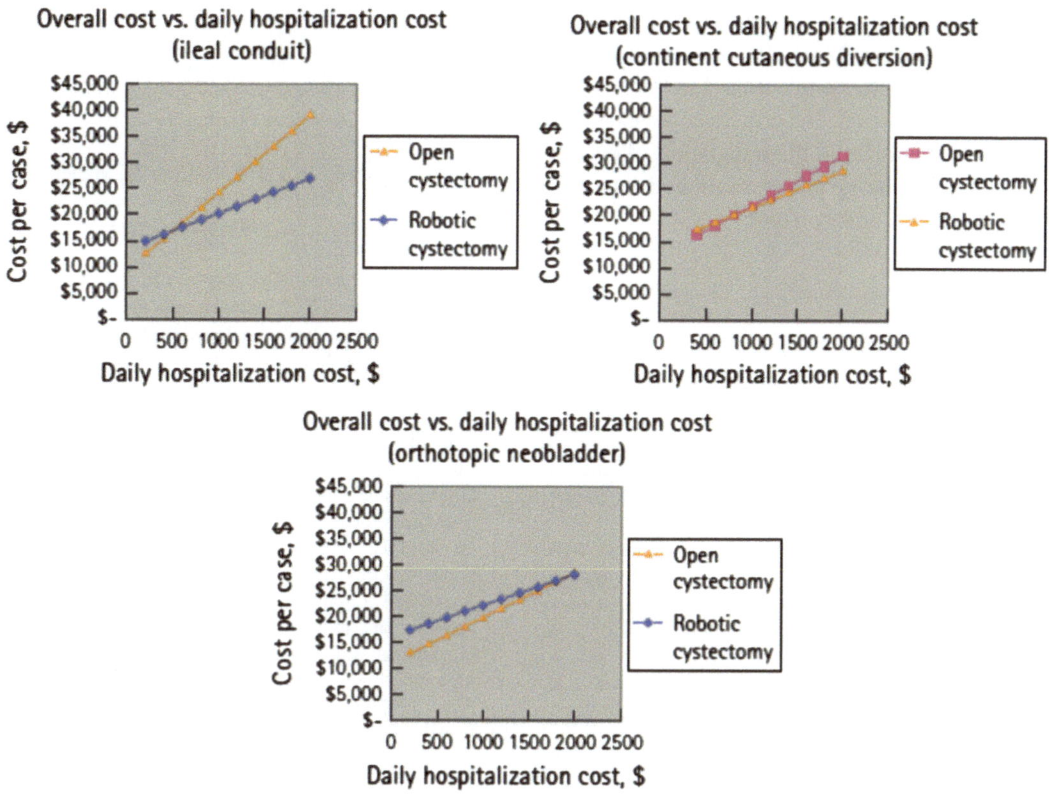

Fig. 17.3 One-way sensitivity analysis of daily hospitalization costs across all types of urinary diversion. Reprinted with the permission of the authors

cal care to tertiary care centers, may facilitate not only improve oncologic and functional outcomes but also keep per patient costs from soaring. Last, to optimally study economic considerations in bladder cancer, costing data along with utility data should be collected in a prospective fashion as a part of randomized controlled trials comparing ORC to RARC. Only through these types of studies can we truly begin to understand not just the cost of RARC, but the cost effectiveness of this evolving therapy.

Editors' Commentary

Erik P. Castle and Raj S. Pruthi

When new technology is introduced into health care, cost considerations become a large concern and must be critically analyzed in order to determine whether the added costs are offset by the benefits provided to patients and health care as a whole. In this chapter, the authors review the few analyses that have been performed for RARC. The problem with any cost analysis is that it is very difficult to assess true "cost" as there are many definitions of this term. When we talk about cost are we referring to "cost to the hospital," "cost to the patient," "cost to the third party payers," or "cost to health care"? Furthermore, cost to a hospital depends on contracts that are negotiated with industry and how their own internal accounting is performed for capital costs in the operating room. Depreciation and bottom line calculations further complicate the issue. What is certain is that new technology is rarely inexpensive and health care continues to become more expensive every day. We hope that increased utilization will drive cost down but until that happens, robotic technology will continue to be an expensive tool for surgeons. It may be that procedures such as RARC may be limited to high volume centers to compensate for the start-up and day-to-day costs. Nevertheless, we expect to see a continued rise in the integration of robotic technology in the operating room and look forward to future studies on cost.

References

1. Jemal A, Siegel R, Xu J, Ward E. Cancer statistics, 2010. CA Cancer J Clin. 2010;60:277–300.
2. Botteman MF, Pashos CL, Redaelli A, Laskin B, Hauser R. The health economics of bladder cancer: a comprehensive review of the published literature. Pharmacoeconomics. 2003;21:1315–30.
3. Stenzl A, Cowan NC, De Santis M, Kuczyk MA, Merseburger AS, Ribal MJ, et al. Treatment of muscle-invasive and metastatic bladder cancer: update of the EAU guidelines. Actas Urol Esp. 2012;36(8):449–60.
4. Skinner DG, Crawford ED, Kaufman JJ. Complications of radical cystectomy for carcinoma of the bladder. J Urol. 1980;123:640–3.
5. Lowrance WT, Eastham JA, Savage C, Maschino AC, Laudone VP, Dechet CB, et al. Contemporary open and robotic radical prostatectomy practice patterns among urologists in the United States. J Urol. 2012;187:2087–92.
6. Ng CK, Kauffman EC, Lee MM, Otto BJ, Portnoff A, Ehrlich JR, et al. A comparison of postoperative complications in open versus robotic cystectomy. Eur Urol. 2010;57:274–81.
7. Challacombe BJ, Bochner BH, Dasgupta P, Gill I, Guru K, Herr H, et al. The role of laparoscopic and robotic cystectomy in the management of muscle-invasive bladder cancer with special emphasis on cancer control and complications. Eur Urol. 2011;60:767–75.
8. Wayne A. Health-care spending to reach 20% of U.S. economy by 2021. Bloomberg business week. June 13, 2012. http://www.businessweek.com/news/2012-06-13/health-care-spending-to-reach-20-percent-of-u-dot-s-dot-economy-by-2021. Accessed 6 Aug 2012.
9. Smith A, Kurpad R, Lal A, Nielsen M, Wallen EM, Pruthi RS. Cost analysis of robotic versus open radical cystectomy for bladder cancer. J Urol. 2010;183:505–9.
10. Martin AD, Nunez RN, Castle EP. Robot-assisted radical cystectomy versus open radical cystectomy: a complete cost analysis. Urology. 2011;77:621–5.
11. Lee R, Ng CK, Shariat SF, Borkina A, Guimento R, Brumit KF, et al. The economics of robotic cystectomy: cost comparison of open versus robotic cystectomy. BJU Int. 2011;108:1886–92.
12. Lee R, Chughtai B, Herman M, Shariat SF, Scherr DS. Cost-analysis comparison of robot-assisted laparoscopic radical cystectomy (RC) vs open RC. BJU Int. 2011;108:976–83.
13. Kulkarni GS, Alibhai SM, Finelli A, Fleshner NE, Jewett MA, Lopushinsky SR, et al. Cost-effectiveness analysis of immediate radical cystectomy versus intravesical Bacillus Calmette-Guerin therapy for high-risk, high-grade (T1G3) bladder cancer. Cancer. 2009;115:5450–9.
14. Pruthi RS, Wallen EM. Robotic-assisted laparoscopic radical cystoprostatectomy. Eur Urol. 2008;53:310–22.
15. Makarov DV. Editorial comment. J Urol. 2010;183:509.
16. Wasserman Y. Physician's fee reference 2006. 23rd ed. Milwaukee, WI: Medical Publishing, Ltd; 2006.
17. Zehnder P, Gill IS. Cost-effectiveness of open versus laparoscopic versus robotic-assisted laparoscopic cystectomy and urinary diversion. Curr Opin Urol. 2011;21:415–9.
18. Scales CD, Jones PJ, Eisenstein EL, Preminger GM, Albala DM. Local cost structures and the economics of robot assisted radical prostatectomy. J Urol. 2005;174:2323–9.

Questions and Concerns of Robotic Approaches to Bladder Cancer Surgery

18

Katherine Theisen, Ken Haberman, and Badrinath R. Konety

Introduction

It is projected that 56,000 men and 18,000 women will be newly diagnosed with bladder cancer in 2012, and approximately 15,000 individuals with bladder cancer will die from their disease [1]. Bladder cancer is the eighth leading cause of death in men and the fourth most common cancer, with transitional cell carcinoma comprising 90 % of these cases. While the incidence of new cases in males has been stable since 2004, the incidence of bladder cancer in women has been steadily increasing (0.3 % per year) [1].

Most new cases of bladder cancer arise in patients >70 years of age, and though approximately 80 % of newly diagnosed cases are non-muscle invasive, as many as 70 % may recur after treatment and up to 25 % will progress to muscle invasive disease [2]. Open radical cystectomy with lymphadenectomy is the gold standard therapy for any patient with muscle-invasive bladder cancer and non-muscle invasive cancer that is high risk or refractory to intra-vesicular therapy. And while open radical cystectomy has witnessed a decrease in associated morbidity and mortality over the years, there remains a high rate of complications, exceeding 60 % in some large series [3, 4]. The mortality rate has been reported to be approximately 3 % [5, 6]. With hopes of decreasing cystectomy-related morbidity and recovery time, there is growing interest in the use of minimally invasive approaches to radical cystectomy, specifically with employment of the surgical robot.

Robot Gaining Ground

The introduction of the Intuitive Surgical da Vinci robot in laparoscopic pelvic surgery has changed the way many surgeons think about operations in this area. First used in radical prostatectomy, the three-dimensional visualization with endo-wrist tools providing six degrees of movement and tremor dampening has allowed the rapid adoption of a minimally invasive technique that had otherwise been limited to expert laparoscopists. It has gained such widespread acceptance in radical prostatectomy, that it is now the most used surgical technique for removal of the prostate. Though still somewhat controversial, several studies have shown equivalent if not better outcomes with use of the robot compared to open surgery when evaluating intra and perioperative parameters for radical prostatectomy, as well as continence, potency,

K. Theisen, B.S. • K. Haberman, M.D.
Department of Urology and Institute for Prostate and Urologic Cancers, University of Minnesota, Minneapolis, MN, USA

B.R. Konety, M.D., M.B.A. (✉)
Department of Urology and Institute for Prostate and Urologic Cancers, University of Minnesota, Minneapolis, MN, USA

Department of Urology and Institute for Prostate and Urologic Cancers, University of Minnesota, 420 Delaware Street SE, MMC 394, Room B536, Minneapolis, MN, USA
e-mail: brkonety@umn.edu

E.P. Castle and R.S. Pruthi (eds.), *Robotic Surgery of the Bladder*, DOI 10.1007/978-1-4614-4906-5_18,

quality of life, and most importantly long-term oncologic outcomes [7].

Given the positive experience with prostatectomy, the robot has been employed to perform a number of other urologic procedures including nephrectomy, partial nephrectomy, and even microsurgical procedures with equivalent success [8, 9]. With the higher degree of maneuverability provided by the newer da Vinci models, the robot has solidified its utility in the surgical armamentarium of urologists. However, with the added complexity, larger anatomic scope, and more commonly aggressive disease seen in muscle-invasive bladder cancer, the use of the robot in radical cystectomy has been approached more cautiously.

The first report of robot assistance in radical cystectomy came from Beecken et al. [10] who performed the operation including an intracorporeal urinary diversion in 8.5 h. This was shortly followed by Menon et al. [11] who reported on a series of 17 patients. These and more recent studies confirmed feasibility of the procedure and suggest possible advantages to robot-assisted radical cystectomy (RARC) including decreases in pain, blood loss, hospital stay, and time to recovery. However, there remain concerns that implementation of this minimally invasive, technically challenging approach will lead to unnecessarily long operating times, increased positive surgical margins due to decreased tactile feedback, and decreased lymph node yields due to operation in an enclosed space. This would undoubtedly result in sub-par oncologic outcomes compared to open surgery. In this chapter, we seek to analyze the current literature to address a few of the issues and controversies surrounding the acceptability of robotic assistance for the performance of radical cystectomy.

Pelvic Lymph Node Dissection: Does Robot-Assisted Pelvic Lymphadenectomy Allow for Adequate Diagnostic and Therapeutic Efficacy?

The most common sites for metastasis in patients with bladder cancer are to the pelvic lymph nodes, with approximately 25 % of patients having lymph node metastases at diagnosis [5, 12]. It has been well established that removal of these nodes improves survival with a decreased rate of local recurrence. A "standard" LND (obturator fossa posteriorly, genitofemoral nerves laterally, hypogastric vessels distally, to bifurcation of common iliac proximally and including node of Cloquet and tissue around deep circumflex vein) has been traditionally accepted as adequate in the treatment with cystectomy [13, 14]. However, more recent studies have reported that as many as 31 % of patients with lymph node positive disease will have metastases outside the range of a "standard" LND; metastasizing to levels above the bifurcation of the aorta and to presacral nodes [12, 15, 16]. Skinner [17] showed that an "extended" LND (standard dissection plus nodes extending to aortic bifurcation and pre-sacral region) resulted in improved long-term survival in patients with lymph node positive disease. Since that time there has been an increasing body of evidence to support a survival benefit in patients undergoing more extensive LND [13, 18–21]. Given the apparent survival benefits of an "extended" LND, and the evidence that it can be performed without increasing the morbidity of the procedure, several authors have recommended that "extended" LND be a necessary component of the management for muscle-invasive bladder cancer [16, 22–24].

Without time consuming additional port placement and redocking procedures, robot-assisted laparoscopy is limited by a fixed camera port position, with subsequent constraints on the direction and field of view not encountered with open surgery. Similarly the robotic arms, despite their high level of dexterity, have limited travel (25 cm) which may prevent access throughout the pelvis. Some have argued that this theoretical mobility and vision restriction would compromise lymphadenectomy such that an "extended" LND is not feasible. This alone could likely result in poorer oncologic outcomes compared to standard open techniques and present an argument against the use of a robotic approach to bladder cancer.

Menon et al. [11] published the first series of RARC with lymphadenectomy on 17 patients revealing feasibility and safety. The initial reports from robot-assisted cystectomy with LND series

Table 18.1 Lymph node yield from "extended" pelvic lymph node dissection

References	Number of patients (RC vs. OC)	Mean nodes RC (range)	Mean nodes OC (range)	Complications from ePLND
Abraham et al. [81]	10	22.3 (13–42)		NR
Wang et al. [43]	33	17 (6–32)		0
Woods et al. [26]	27	12.3 (7–20)		0
Guru et al. [34]	100	21		0
Gamboa et al. [58]	41	25 (4–68)		3
Guru et al. [49]	26	25.5 (13–56)		1
Lavery et al. [82]	15	41.8 (18–67)		0
Pruthi et al. [41]	100	19 (8–40)		NR
Nix et al. [32]	41 (21 vs. 20)	19 (12–30)	18 (8–30)	NR
Richards et al. [33]	70 (35 vs. 35)	16 (11–24)	15 (11–22)	NR
Kauffman et al. [83]	85	19 (0–56)		NR
Khan et al. [59]	50	17 (9–28)		1
Schumacher et al. [36]	14	32 (19–52)		5
Davis et al. [30]	11	43 (19–63)	4 (0–8)[a]	NR

Results from various trials reporting lymph node yields from extended pelvic lymph node dissection from robot-assisted radical cystectomy alone or comparison to open cystectomy There were no statistically significant differences for lymph node yields in the studies that directly compared OC versus RC

[a]Nodes removed during second-look open LND following robotic extended LND

RC robot-assisted radical cystectomy, *OC* open cystectomy

mostly performed dissections within the boundaries of "limited" (obturator region) and "standard" LND templates [25]. However, more recently studies have explored the acceptability and feasibility of robotic "extended" LND. Table 18.1 shows a list of studies that have performed robot-assisted "extended" LND. When evaluated, the robot-assisted LND only added an additional 30–45 min of operation time and was not associated with increased morbidity/mortality [26–28]. In general, the lymph node count has been the only measure by which to compare the adequacy of the node dissection. However, it is an imperfect measure since the number of lymph nodes counted is dependent on both the manner in which the specimens are submitted to pathology and the technique used by the pathologist [29, 30]. Despite its drawbacks, lymph node yields in a range of 10–20 have been shown to confer a survival benefit in several open series [13, 18–21, 31]. By comparison, all robotic series noted in Table 18.1 were able to obtain mean lymph node counts of greater than 16 with only a few studies having counts less than 10 nodes. Notably, in two separate prospective randomized trials comparing open and RARC, lymph node yields were not statistically different while employing identical anatomic lymphadenectomy templates [32, 33].

An additional small, but provocative study by Davis et al. [30] looked directly at the number of lymph nodes leftover by robot-assisted "extended" LND through the use of a second look open LND. A total of 11 patients underwent robot-assisted LND by a single surgeon, and each robotic LND was immediately followed by a second-look open LND by a different team of surgeons to extract any leftover nodal tissue. The mean lymph node yield was 43 (range 19–63) with a median of 93 % of all lymph nodes retrieved removed by the robotic technique. Interestingly, the newer da Vinci S system allowed for even higher retrieval rates with a range of 83–100 % of all lymph nodes removed robotically compared to 70 and 75 % in each of the two procedures using the older da Vinci machine.

Surgeon learning and experience with the robotic platform may also be an important factor affecting lymph node yield. Of concern, Guru et al. [34] found a significant increase in lymph node yield over time which plateaued at the 30th case. Similarly, Hayn et al. [35] found that lymph node yield increased 73 % when surgeons had performed >50 RARC's compared to those who had performed <30 cases. On the other hand, several other studies found no change in lymph node yields with increasing experience/volume [27, 36, 37]. Therefore, available data on the effects of early experiences with RARC on lymph node yield remains controversial.

Given the abundance of reports including two small randomized trials, it appears that robot-assisted extended lymphadenectomy up to the aortic bifurcation is technically feasible and safe, yielding lymph node counts on par with open surgery. With the varied initial results, further evaluation of the surgical learning curve is needed to determine whether early experience with RARC sacrifices acceptable lymph node yields. However, it appears that, when using lymph node counts as a surrogate for the extent of lymph node dissection (LND), robot-assisted lymphadenectomy does not represent an inferior surgical intervention compared to open lymphadenectomy, and, all other factors being equal, we would expect similar long-term oncologic outcomes.

Positive Margin Rate: Can the Robot-Assisted Approach Match or Improve on the Open Approach?

Whereas there exists some controversy on lymph node yield as a surrogate for adequate surgical resection, it is well established that the completeness of the primary resection plays a critical role in oncologic outcomes following treatment for bladder cancer. A positive surgical margin at time of radical cystectomy has been shown to be an independent predictor of disease recurrence, metastatic progression, and cancer-specific mortality [19, 38–40]. The overall positive margin rates in large series of open radical cystectomy have ranged from 4 to 9 %, with slightly higher rates in advanced disease [19, 38–40]. As a result of such studies and the importance of surgical margins in patient survival, Herr et al. [19] recommended a surgical benchmark of less than 10 % positive surgical margin rate for all cystectomies and less than 15 % positive margin rate for advanced (≥pT3) disease.

Though the use of the surgical robot can improve visualization with the 3D, 10× magnifications available with the stereoscopic laparoscope, questions arise as to whether visual cues alone are sufficient for determining the extent of surgical resection. Some argue that the lack of tactile sensation may compromise the ability to assess the level of tumor extension, particularly with pT3/pT4 disease, thus leading to a higher rate of positive margins. Are surgical margin rates similar between robotic versus open cystectomies? Does the stage of the tumor have an effect?

Table 18.2 shows a list of the robot-assisted cystectomy studies and their rates of positive surgical margins. The overall incidence of positive surgical margins at the time of robot-assisted radical cystectomy has ranged from 0 to 7.2 %, with most of the studies showing an overall positive surgical margin rate <10 %, which meets the standard set by series of open radical cystectomy. However, the data raises concern for the rates of positive surgical margins in more advanced disease. There also exists the potential for significant unaccounted for selection bias in many of these retrospective and/or nonrandomized reports. Early studies that reported 0 % positive margins often did not report the breakdown of organ confined versus more advanced disease and, these being early experiences, may have bias toward selecting patients with less aggressive disease for RARC. More recently, however, there have been reports which include significant numbers of patients with pT3/pT4 disease. In one of the larger multi-institutional trials, Hellenthal et al. [40] used the IRCC database to show an overall positive margin rate of 6.8 % in 513 patients undergoing robot-assisted radical cystectomy. However, the positive margin rate increased to 16.6 % when considering pathologic stage ≥pT3; a rate slightly above the standard suggested by Herr et al. [19]. Patients in this study with pT4 disease were found to have a positive margin rate of 39 %. Another larger retrospective study by Guru et al. [34] showed an overall

Table 18.2 Rates of positive surgical margins from trials of robotic and open cystectomy

References	Number of patients (RC vs. OC)	Total PSM RC: *n* (%)	Total PSM OC: *n* (%)	PSM in pT3/T4 RC: *n* (%)	PSM in pT3/pT4 OC: *n* (%)
Beecken et al. [10]	1	0			
Menon et al. [11]	17	0			
Hemal et al. [78]	24	0			
Rhee et al. [70]	30 (7 vs. 23)	0	0	0	0
Galich et al. [42]	37 (13 vs. 24)	0	3 (12.5)	0	3 (20)
Wang et al. [43]	54 (33 vs. 21)	2 (6)	3 (14)	2 (22)	3 (25)
Guru et al. [34]	100	7 (7)		7 (13)	
Richards et al. [33]	70 (35 vs. 35)	1 (3)	3 (9)	1 (7)	2 (13.3)
Ng et al. [44]	187 (83 vs. 104)	6 (7.2)	9 (8.7)	6 (19)	9 (20.5)
Nix et al. [32]	41 (21 vs. 20)	0	0	0	0
Hellenthal et al. [40]	513	35 (6.8)		31 (17)	
Pruthi et al. [41]	100	0		0	
Khan et al. [59]	50	1 (2)		1 (7)	
Schumacher et al. [36]	45	1 (2.2)		1 (10)	
Nepple et al. [45]	65 (36 vs. 29)	2 (6)	2 (7)	2 (12)	2 (17)
Davis et al. [30]	11	0		0	

The total number of positive margins is shown followed by the rate of positive surgical margins in patients with non-organ-confined disease (pT3/pT4)
n number of patients, *PSM* positive surgical margins, *RC* radical cystectomy, *OC* open cystectomy

positive surgical margin rate of 7 % for 100 patients undergoing RARC, with the positive margin rate increasing to 13 % in the patients with advanced disease. Pruthi et al. [41] found no positive margins in a cohort of 100 patients undergoing RARC. However, when looking at the patient population included in the trial, most of the patients (87 %) had pathologic stage ≤pT2.

Several nonrandomized comparisons have been performed comparing open and RARC but these are generally single-institution case series with surgeon preference governing which patients received an open vs. robot-assisted approach [33, 42–45]. As seen from the data in Table 18.2, overall positive margin rates were actually slightly higher in the open group, though in most studies this did not reach statistical significance [33, 42–45]. This trend persists when only pT3/pT4 patients were analyzed. However, these differences again did not reach statistical significance and the studies were not powered to detect these differences [33, 42, 44, 45]. Though some series had similar stage breakdown between cohorts [42, 44, 45], they may have suffered from other unaccounted selection bias. Others clearly were early robot experiences with a significant bias toward more difficult cases being performed open [43]. The only published prospective randomized trial comparing open and robotic was reported by Nix et al. [32]. The patient populations did not differ with respect to pathologic stage, and there were no patients in either cohort that had positive surgical margins. Though the absolute number of patients was relatively low and there were a disproportionate number of patients with ≤pT2, this last study would suggest non-inferiority of robot-assisted radical cystectomy compared to open surgery in pT2 or lower disease when possible bias is controlled for by randomization. However this study was not powered to detect difference in positive margin rates between groups and hence additional studies with that specific endpoint in mind are required to truly answer that question.

While a direct comparison of positive margins to open cystectomy is important, there is also the need to assess changes in positive margin rates over time as surgeons are progressing on their learning curves. Similar to lymph node yields, if there were a significant increase in positive

Table 18.3 Medium-length follow-up reports of oncologic outcomes following robot-assisted radical cystectomy

References	Number of patients	Mean follow-up	Overall survival (%)	Recurrence-free survival (%)	Disease-specific survival (%)
Dasgupta et al. [57]	20	23 mo	95	90	95
Pruthi et al. [41]	100	21 mo	91	85	94
Kauffman et al. [83]	85	18 mo	79	71	85
Nepple et al. [45]	36	12 mo	68	72	75
Martin et al. [84]	59	36 mo	69	71	72

margins during early robotic experiences, it may be irresponsible to implement use of the robot since positive margins result in substantial consequences to oncologic outcomes [19, 38–40]. While Guru et al. [34] found a significant decrease in positive margin rate from their first to fourth cohort, other studies found no change in positive margin rate with increasing surgeon experience/volume [27, 36, 37]. Therefore, the available data on the effect of RARC on positive margins (both compared to open and along surgeons' learning curves) is controversial. All training surgeons must remember the oncologic principles of radical cystectomy and prioritize their operation to maximize patient outcomes.

It is important to remember that measures of positive margins, in addition to lymph node yields, are only surrogates for oncologic outcomes. The true measure of oncologic efficacy of a procedure is the effect on overall and disease-free survival. Unfortunately, there is limited long-term follow-up among patients undergoing RARC so discussion is therefore limited to short and medium-term follow-up. Table 18.3 shows results from a few studies reporting oncologic outcomes following RARC. However, the follow-up time across studies ranged from 1 to 3 years. While the overall survival, disease-specific survival, recurrence-free survival rates are promising and deemed comparable to results from an open series by Stein et al. [5], they do not allow for adequate comparison due to limited follow-up periods and bias toward performing RARC on patients with less aggressive disease.

Currently, we are left with comparisons to historical controls, case series, one small randomized trial, and studies with limited follow up to assess (1) the ability to obtain an adequate resection with the surgical robot and (2) the long-term oncologic efficacy of this approach. From the data available for stage T2 or lower disease, it appears that a number of groups have shown the ability to match or even improve on historically acceptable positive margin and lymph node yield rates. For more advanced disease, the data are not as clear since many of the cohorts had positive margin rates greater than 15 %. There is currently an ongoing large multicenter randomized trial which should be able to more definitively assess this concern. Until then, and until more studies report on the long-term follow-up after RARC, patient selection for robot-assisted radical cystectomy should be made carefully, and one should abide by the surgical benchmarks from studies of ORC [19] that serve as surrogates for optimizing long term oncologic outcomes.

Should Urinary Diversions Be Performed Intracorporeally for Robot-Assisted Cystectomy?

Surgeons employing a pure laparoscopic approach to radical cystectomy have demonstrated the feasibility of intracorporeal (IC) urinary diversion, but this was never widely adopted due to the technical challenges. In fact, purely laparoscopic intracorporeal urinary diversion was associated with significantly more complications along with higher blood loss, longer operative times, and increased time to ambulation and oral intake when compared to extracorporeal (EC) urinary diversion [46]. Despite these short comings, the smaller incisions, decreased bowel exposure, and reduced tissue manipulation creates the potential for decreased pain, decreased fluid imbalances with perhaps subsequent advantages in time to bowel function return and overall recovery. Does the use of the surgical robot improve results of intracorporeal diversion compared to a pure laparoscopic approach? Have the theoretical advantages been demonstrated?

The first robot-assisted radical cystectomy (RARC) involved an intracorporeal urinary diversion [10]. The total operating time was 8.5 h, but the blood loss was only 200 ml and the reservoir was considered functionally and oncologically excellent at 5 months follow-up. Another early attempt at RARC with IC diversion by Balaji et al. [47] included three patients all of whom had operative times greater than 10 h, but similarly had nominal mean blood loss of 250 ml and good postoperative functional outcomes at 2 months.

Since these early attempts, there has been continued interest with reports of additional small series showing promising results. Pruthi et al. [48] compared the perioperative outcomes among 12 patients undergoing RARC and IC to 20 patients receiving RARC and EC diversion during the same period. The overall operative time was significantly longer in patients who underwent the IC diversion; 5.3 h versus 4.2 h in the EC cohort, but not as substantial as that seen in the earliest reports. There was, however, no difference in mean blood loss, time to return of bowel function, time to discharge, or the number of complications. A benefit of the IC method was evidenced by a significantly decreased narcotic requirement in the group receiving an IC diversion.

Recently, Guru and colleagues [49] published data on their initial experience with IC conduit diversion in which they found no difference in operative times compared to EC diversion. A total of 26 patients underwent RARC; the first 13 patients received an EC diversion and the last 13 an IC conduit diversion. There was no difference in overall operative time. The difference in diversion times alone trended toward but did not reach significance (159 min for IC versus 120 min EC, $P=0.058$). The groups did not differ in number of complications or other perioperative parameters (mean blood loss, lymph node yield, time to oral feeds, and length of hospital stay), and the mean time for IC diversion decreased over sequential case number which suggests a rapid learning curve. Lastly, Smith et al. [50] reported on a multi-institution, multi-surgeon experience with RARC with regard to operative outcomes. There were 227 patients in the study with a mixture of EC and IC diversions performed. The 30-day complication rate was 30 % with 7 % major complications. Multivariate analysis showed that the type of diversion was not associated with postoperative complications.

Unfortunately, there is a lack of evidence comparing IC versus EC while subdividing for type of urinary diversion. This is an important consideration because different types of urinary diversion represent different levels of difficulty and pose a risk for different associated complication rates and operative times when performed intracorporeally. Lee et al. [51] compared RARC with EC versus ORC and found significantly longer operative times in RARC with EC for ileal conduit and orthotopic neobladders, but not for continent cutaneous diversions. This study supports the variability in operative time as a function of diversion type during RARC. Additional studies are needed to determine which (if any) diversion types confer an unsuitable risk to patient outcome if performed intracorporeally.

Current assessment suggests that in experienced hands there is a place for intracorporeal urinary diversion in the armamentarium of urologists, with some evidence for improvement in pain and non-inferiority across other measures. However, inferences should be made with caution as these studies were not randomized trials and therefore were subject to selection bias that accompanies early attempts with new procedures; patients tended to be younger with fewer comorbidities or a lower stage disease in order to optimize tolerability to a potentially prolonged procedure. We currently believe that the potential advantages of the intracorporeal method have not been fully demonstrated and thus, except in the most expert hands, do not outweigh the associated disadvantages or potential complications.

Furthermore, longer studies and follow-up are required to confirm that other complications such as stricture rate are not adversely affected.

Does Restriction of Movement in an Enclosed Pelvis During Robot-Assisted Radical Cystectomy Result in Increased Ureteral Skeletonization and Stricture Formation?

Proponents of minimally invasive surgery cite that one of the advantages over open surgery is that there are fewer surgical-related complications [52]. However, a theoretical concern exists that robot-assisted radical cystectomy (RARC), with its lack of tactile feedback and limited workspace, may lead to excessive tissue skeletonization and devascularization resulting in an increased frequency of delayed complications, specifically ureteral–intestinal anastomic strictures. Anastomotic strictures are a well-known occurrence in open radical cystectomy with urinary diversion with an overall incidence ranging from 2 to 4 % [53–56], but have been reported as high as 10 % [4, 53]. While it is not fully known why ureteral anastomotic strictures develop, there are number of factors thought to play a role: tissue ischemia, tissue tension, inflammation from urinary leak, and/or suturing errors. While studies have sought to determine risk factors for stricture formation [53, 55, 56], the results remain inconclusive and/or controversial over the extent any of these play in stricture formation.

With RARC in addition to the potential issues related to ureteral skeletalization, there exists particular concern on the ability to fully mobilize the left ureter allowing for a tension free anastomosis. The rate of ureteral anastomotic stricture formation reported among the various RARC series has ranged from 1.5 to 10 % [44, 57–59]. This is similar to the reports from large series of open radical cystectomy. Thus, early data may suggest that RARC has similar stricture rates as ORC.

However, the emerging use of intracorporal urinary diversion (a diversion limited to minimally invasive surgery) could theoretically play a role in decreasing the relative risk of stricture formation in RARC compared to ORC. It has been proposed [36] that urinary diversion performed extracorporally may be a risk factor in stricture formation due to increased mobilization required for the appropriate tissue exposure required for suturing. With this in mind, perhaps employment of more intracorporeal diversions will decrease tissue mobilization and subsequently the incidence of ureteral strictures associated with urinary diversion. Evidence to support this theory comes from studies performing RARC with extracorporeal diversions that reported stricture rates from 8 to 10 % [49, 57, 59] which are at the high end of the range for ORC. Further, Guru et al. [49] compared the two types of diversion in their series and found a 7.9 % stricture rate in the extracorporeal group and 0 % in their intracorporeal group. However, a stricture rate of 7.3 % was reported in a group of patients undergoing intracorporeal diversion which may argue against this theory [58]. However, this study did not perform a comparison to patients undergoing open surgery, so it is hard to assess the relative difference in stricture rates between open and robotic approaches. Overall, definitive conclusions are limited because of the small sample sizes, few direct comparisons, and highly variable stricture rates regardless of the diversion type reported in different studies.

Perhaps the greatest hindrance to full realization of the risk of stricture formation in RARC is the lack of long-term follow-up. To date, many of the studies of RARC have either been (1) feasibility studies or (2) reports on the perioperative and short-term outcomes following the procedure. Thus, many of the current studies likely did not follow patients long enough to report on stricture formation since studies of ORC have shown stricture formation can occur at a time point ranging from 8.8 months [54] to 1 year [4]. This is an area that will need close monitoring and more studies employing long-term follow-up to determine whether this technology confers increased or unique complications or whether perhaps provides an opportunity to reduce the complication risks associated with ORC. As of this time it does not appear that there is a significant increase risk of stricture formation with RARC compared to open cystectomy, though availability of additional data in the future may shed more light on this issue.

Does Robot-Assisted Radical Cystectomy Confer Increased Risk of Direct Tumor Spread from Tumor Spillage or Port Site Recurrence?

In addressing oncologic outcomes between robot and open radical cystectomy, in addition to issues related to positive margins and extent of lymph node dissection, one must also address concerns about aspects of the robotic technique that may generate risks for cancer recurrence not realized in open surgery; specifically, the possibility for port site metastases or increased local recurrence secondary to local spread from tumor spillage in a closed abdomen.

One concern that directly arises from the issue of minimally invasive surgery is the risk of port site metastasis, especially with highly aggressive tumors. The exact etiology of port site metastases is unknown and so any effort to confidently prevent occurrence in RARC is difficult. Some authors have proposed different methods to prevent port site metastases in patients with bladder cancer including the use of meticulous dissection, the use endobags for specimen extraction [60], avoiding specimen morcellation, and ensuring adequate seal of laparoscopy trocars to prevent chimney effect of a pneumoperitoneum [61]. Regardless of the method employed, this concern has failed to become reality as only one case of port site metastasis has been reported in the literature [61], occurring at 10 months. Similarly, studies employing minimally invasive surgery for colorectal, uterine, and other urologic malignancies have shown no or minimal incidence of port site metastases [62–64].

Another concern, given the closed peritoneal space and additional access sites from laparoscopic ports, is that a robotic approach may be more susceptible to spillage-related cancer recurrence. Urothelial cell carcinoma is known to be aggressive with numerous descriptions from open surgery reporting local spread from spillage or access tracts including suprapubic and percutaneous nephrostomy tubes. Thus, meticulous effort to avoid urine spillage has become a requirement in open surgery. Proposed techniques to avoid spillage of urine during robot-assisted radical cystectomy (RARC) include meticulously avoiding puncture of the bladder, carefully clipping the ureters before dissection, and ensuring adequate stapling, clipping, or suturing of the urethral stump [65]. Similarly, most studies publishing their RARC technique have also reported their efforts toward preventing urine leak/tumor spillage. To date, no studies have reported local disease recurrence secondary to documented seeding from tumor spillage. Pruthi et al. [41] reported an inadvertent bladder puncture intraoperatively but noted no urine spillage at the time and did not report any local recurrence from suspected seeding from tumor spillage in any of their patients at a mean follow-up of 21 months. However, with accrual of additional data, the true risk of tumor spillage and local recurrence will become clear.

With lack of good data surrounding documented spillage or use of laparoscopic ports causing local recurrence in RARC overall local recurrence rates may serve as a surrogate. Looking at the studies with longest follow-up, there does not appear to be a change in local recurrence rates over 1–2 year observed follow-up [66–68] suggesting that techniques and caution employed during surgery are preventing this concern from rising to clinical significance.

Is There a Learning Curve Associated with RARC, and If So, Are Patient Outcomes Sacrificed During Early Surgeon Experiences?

Like any new technology, the surgical robot will only gain universal acceptance as a treatment modality for cystectomy if it can be incorporated safely and efficiently into the practice of established surgeons. It is of utmost importance that the oncologic standards of this operation be upheld regardless of technical approach, because such an oversight would unquestionably sacrifice patient outcome and survival [19]. As we've noted in the preceding sections, in many instances, based upon various criteria, RARC appears to be as good as and in some cases superior to ORC. However, much of this work comes from high volume centers experienced with the use of the robot. Are these results replicable by less experienced surgeons? Is there a learning curve associated with RARC? If so, will the initial use of RARC by surgeons lower on their learning curves sacrifice patient outcomes?

One might make the assumption that more experience and familiarity with any procedure results in better patient outcomes. Unfortunately, quantitation of how much experience is required to effectively perform a RARC is difficult because the heterogeneity of the patients as well as the surgeons' prior experience can play a significant role. There is also no definitive variable that can be used to judge the effectiveness of the procedure. We have previously noted the mixed results seen in evaluating the learning curve by looking at lymph node yields and positive margin rates. Factors that have been evaluated in relation to experience/volume that we will discuss here include the operating time and complication rates.

Operative Time

The ability to withstand anesthesia and the overall physical stresses of an operation are serious considerations when deciding if a patient is a candidate for surgery. This is particularly true for patients with bladder cancer who tend to have serious illnesses with multiple comorbidities. Therefore, it is imperative to limit the length of surgery for all patients in order to reduce possible risks associated with an operation. The use of minimally invasive surgery generates its own risk-conferring variables; specifically, the use of steep Trendelenburg positioning and carbon dioxide to induce pneumoperitoneum, which is itself a time-dependent stressor. These factors can cause serious strain on patients, especially those with poor lung function. Radical cystectomy regardless of surgical approach should have the goal of minimizing operative times to minimize the risk of surgical-related complications.

The initial studies of robot-assisted radical cystectomy (RARC) with intracorporeal urinary diversions reported operative times as long as 10 h [10, 47], far surpassing the average 4.3 h open cystectomy at that time [69]. This was very disconcerting and caused question of the appropriateness of robotic surgery.

Several studies have since published on operative times between open and robot-assisted radical cystectomy at their institutions. While initial trials reported a significantly longer operative time in patients undergoing RARC compared to ORC (even with extracorporeal diversion) [42, 43, 70], more recent published studies demonstrate a trend toward decreasing operative times comparable to that of ORC [30, 35, 58].

Several studies seeking to specifically address the learning curve in RARC have reported improvement in operative times with increased experience. Schumacher et al. [36] divided 45 patients into 3 cohorts to assess their learning curve with RARC and found a significant decrease in mean operative times over the 3 cohorts. Similarly, Hayn et al. [35] used the IRCC to assess the outcomes of 496 patients undergoing RARC by 21 different surgeons at 14 different institutions and found a significant decrease in operative time when surgeons had performed >50 RARCs compared to those who performed <30. Guru et al. [34] analyzed the learning curve from 100 consecutive patients, while Richards et al. [37] used data from their first 60 patients undergoing RARC; both studies showed a trend toward decreased operative times (just missing statistical significance). Guru et al. [34] also showed a plateau for operative time occurring at the 16th case but all the surgeons were fellowship trained in robotic surgery, likely shifting the learning curve. Unfortunately, these studies employed multiple surgeons so the learning curve is more of a facility-based learning curve with respect to procedure volume rather than an individual learning curve generalizable to all Urologists. There is a report of a single-surgeon experience from Pruthi et al. [27] who used data from their initial 50 patients divided into 5 cohorts. They found a decrease in operating time that plateaued after the 20th case. Again, however, this surgeon was seasoned in robot-assisted prostatectomy, so familiarity with the robot likely lowered his plateau. Despite the drawbacks to this work, one might expect continued improvement in operative times during the first 15–20 cases for a well-experienced robotic surgeon, but perhaps as many as 50 cases may be required to approach more optimum efficiency for a more robot-naïve surgeon.

Lastly, while there may be an increase in operative time during early surgeon experience with RARC, it may be comforting to note that perioperative complication rates following RARC have not been significantly greater than ORC and actually have shown a trend toward fewer complications in some studies (discussed in detail below). This suggests that differences in operative time to date have not been responsible for increasing complications in patients undergoing RARC. Further, studies of complications following RARC have found no association between operative time and complication rate [50, 71]. However, interpretation of these data should be made with caution and full awareness that early studies with robotic surgery have tended to select for patients with fewer comorbidities to ensure optimal ability to handle any increased stress from the procedure. As surgeons gain more experience with RARC (and with decreasing operative times), one could expect to see a more widely distributed patient population undergoing the procedure from which more generalizable conclusions can be drawn.

Complications

An important concern when addressing the learning curve with RARC is the effect of initial experiences on postoperative complications. Theoretically, one might speculate that robot-naïve surgeons may be more likely to have surgical complications simply from lack of comfort/knowledge of the subtleties of the procedure. While Richards et al. [37] found a significant decrease in their complication rates over 60 patients, other studies failed to show a change in complication rates over time [27, 34]. Interestingly, Schumacher et al. [36] reported a trend toward fewer complications over time and actually found a significant decrease in the number of late complications (>30 days). Therefore, again, there is controversy regarding the presence of a significant learning curve when the presence of complications is used as a surrogate for effectiveness.

Another factor affecting the learning curve for a RARC is the surgeon's prior experience with any robotic surgery, including prostatectomy and/or nephrectomy. One might think that familiarity with the technology would allow more rapid advancement through the learning curve with RARC. Hayn et al. [72] used the IRCC database to assess the outcomes of 496 patients undergoing RARC by 21 different surgeons at 14 different institutions. The surgeons were divided into four groups based on previous robot-assisted radical prostatectomy (RARP) experience (<50, 51–100, 101–150, >150). There was a significant association between more robotic experience and (1) decreased operative time, (2) decreased EBL, (3) increased lymph node yield, and (4) increased pathologic stage. In fact, there was a 20 % decrease in operative time and a 31 % increase in lymph node yield when surgeons had performed 51–100 RARPs compared to <50 RARPs. Interestingly, this trend toward better outcomes was witnessed only between the first two groups of surgeons. There was actually a detrimental effect on these operative parameters when surgeons had performed 101–150 and >150 RARPs. Further, this worsening trend did not disappear when the authors controlled for pathologic stage of disease. The authors hypothesized that surgeons with very large RARP experience may not have had the time for or interest in open radical cystectomy, while surgeons with less RARP experience may have more open cystectomy experience due to different subspecialization. Thus, the possibility that surgeons with less RARP experience have more experience with open radical cystectomy would likely have granted them the advantage in early experience with RARC.

When assessing the feasibility and practicality of incorporating a new technique/procedure into surgical practice, one must consider the benefits versus potential harm to the patient. In RARC, it is important to assess whether a patient's perioperative and oncologic outcomes are sacrificed when physicians are early in their learning curve. Unfortunately, the evidence from the studies noted above is not conclusive. While there appears to be a consistent decrease in operative time, other critical parameters in predicting patient outcomes following RARC have varied. Of most concern is the association some studies have shown between initial surgeon experiences and a higher rate of positive surgical margins, higher complication rates, and fewer lymph nodes removed. These variables are significant predictors of morbidity and mortality and must not be ignored. Thus, further investigation with well-controlled trials is needed to better characterize the learning curve associated with RARC. Characterization of this learning curve is important because it would determine the acceptability of this technology's universal implementation and help set realistic expectations for surgeons attempting to master this technique.

Are the Costs Associated with the Use of Robotic Technology Greater than Open? If So, Is It Too Substantial to Warrant Its Use?

Bladder cancer has the highest lifetime treatment costs per patient [73]. With rising healthcare costs and widespread pressure to reduce expenditures, a discussion of robot versus open radical cystectomy would not be complete without considering the differences in cost associated with the two techniques. For radical cystectomy there are costs associated with the operation, including anesthesia time, surgeon fee, instrument costs, and with the robot a significant acquisition and maintenance fee [74]. How this robotic equipment cost factors into the average procedural cost is highly dependent on hospital volume. There are also hospitalization related costs which can include medications, blood transfusions, and daily room cost which is directly related to length of stay. Follow-up, including imaging, laboratory tests, and physician time will also contribute. Finally, complication-related costs are something that have not always been addressed but are critical to take into account. Konety et al. [75] presented evidence that post-cystectomy complications can drastically impact hospital charges imparting a cumulative effect on charges mostly through extended length of hospital stay. They report that a single complication can increase the charges for treatment by $15,000 [75].

Several groups have attempted to analyze the cost difference, taking some or all of these factors into account. Smith et al. [76] analyzed the fixed and variable costs, further subcategorized by operating room and hospital costs, between 20 robotic and 20 open radical cystectomies. Overall, there was a higher financial cost of $1,640 associated with robotic versus open surgery. This higher cost of robotic surgery was largely due to differences in operating room costs ($1,634 more for RARC) driven primarily by the amortized acquisition cost of the robot itself as well as maintenance fees and the increased average operative time. However, comparison of hospital costs favored RARC because of a shorter average hospital stay and decreased transfusion requirements. They did not take into account differences in complications or analgesic needs postoperatively because in earlier work, they had noted similar values for these parameters [27]. This study also did not specific the type of urinary diversion used which can greatly impact length of surgery, thus influencing costs. Interestingly, each day of hospitalization represented a loss of $658, while each hour in the operating room represented $1,902. Thus, decreasing operative times as a result of increased surgeon experience and refinement of technique may make RARC a more cost-effective procedure. These data suggest that the cost differential ratio between hospital stay and operative time is approximately 1:3 meaning that hospital stay would have to come down by 3 days to compensate for each hour of increased operative time.

With the operative time, length of stay, and complication rates being such significant driving forces in cost related to radical cystectomy, any increased cost associated with using a robot in the operating room has the potential to be completely offset by improvements in these areas. Martin et al. [77] did consider procedure-associated complications in their analysis of costs when they compared 14 open to 19 robot-assisted cystectomies. All cases were assumed to use ileal conduit diversions. Costs were divided into direct (surgeon fees, purchase and maintenance of robot, anesthesia fees, operating room costs, length of stay, and blood transfusion costs) and indirect costs (complications and their associated treatments and readmissions up to 30 days postoperatively). There was a 16 % higher direct cost of RARC (driven by operating room costs) that was offset by the 60 % less expensive hospitalization costs. This resulted in a 38 % overall decreased cost of the robot approach [74, 77]. The authors reported that complications and readmission rates are major drivers of differences in cost.

Similarly, Lee et al. [51] performed cost analysis of RARC and ORC while including costs resulting from complications and readmissions for up to 90 days postoperatively. In contrast to the previous two studies, Lee et al. [51] stratified costs by type of urinary diversion. The investigators found higher direct costs for RARC (which included surgeon fee, per-case cost of robot, disposable instruments, utilization cost, and anesthesia cost) but this higher cost was offset by lower indirect costs (length of stay and complication-associated costs). The investigators found that length of hospital stay was the most significant driving factor in offsetting the costs of RARC. However, upon subcategory analysis, the higher direct cost of RARC was only offset for ileal conduit (IC) and continent cutaneous diversions (CCD), not for orthotopic neobladders (ON). As a result, the authors concluded that RARC would be most cost efficient in patients receiving IC, but less advantageous for CCD or ON (probably because they are more complex diversions resulting in longer operating times). Further, the complication rates were equivalent between ORC and RARC groups but trended toward fewer complications in RARC resulting in an indirect cost difference that favored RARC. These data suggest that the high costs associated with RARC may be offset if fewer complications and a shorter length of hospital stay are seen.

As with other suggestions and conclusions made in this chapter, it is again important to keep in mind the likelihood of patient selection bias that is present in early studies with RARC; specifically, that the difference in complications and operative times could be a result of different patient comorbidities or disease severity prior to the operation rather than a direct result of RARC versus ORC [59, 71]. Variations in hospital policy, insurance reimbursement rates, and geographic region will also affect calculated cost effectiveness. The studies discussed here would suggest that the high costs associated with acquisition and maintenance of a robot can be offset by shorter hospital stays and decreased complications as compared to ORC. However, until more studies are performed across a range of institutions and geographic regions, with better controlled patient populations, extrapolations from these studies should be made critically and cautiously and specific to every institution's financial structure, case volume, and surgeon experience. An ongoing multi-institutional randomized study comparing robotic and open radical cystectomy should provide answers to some of these questions.

Are There Benefits of Robot-Assisted Radical Cystectomy That Are Not Realized in Open Radical Cystectomy That Would Make RARC a Superior Option in the Treatment of Bladder Cancer?

In prior sections we have addressed different controversies surrounding robot-assisted radical cystectomy by providing evidence that suggests non-inferiority compared to open radical cystectomy—the gold standard treatment of bladder cancer. However, if RARC is to be widely implemented, we would hope to see specific advantages as well. Several potential benefits have been suggested including decreased blood loss, decreased length of hospital stay, decreased complications, and faster recovery.

Table 18.4 Comparison of perioperative parameters following robotic and open radical cystectomy

References	Number of patients (RC vs. OC)	EBL RC (range)	EBL OC (range)	mean LOS RC: *n* (range)	mean LOS OC: *n* (range)	Complications RC: *n* (%)	Complications OC: *n* (%)
Rhee et al. [70]	30 (7 vs. 23)	479[a]	1,109	11	13	NR	NR
Galich et al. [42]	37 (13 vs. 24)	500 (100–1,000)[a]	1,250 (300–10,200)	8 (4–23)[b]	10 (6–35)	2 (15.4)	4 (16.7)
Wang et al. [43]	54 (33 vs. 21)	400 (100–1,200)[a]	750 (250–2,500)	5 (4–18)[b]	8 (5–28)	7 (21)	5 (24)
Ng et al. [44]	187 (83 vs. 104)	460 (161–759)[a]	1,172 (256–2,088)	5.5 (3–28)[b]	8 (3–60)	37 (44.6)[c]	64 (61.5)
Nix et al. [32]	41 (21 vs. 20)	258[a]	576	5.1	6	7 (33)	10 (50)
Richards et al. [33]	70 (35 vs. 35)	360 (260–600)[a]	1,000 (500–2,000)	7 (6–9)[b]	8 (7–15)	21 (60)	23 (65.7)
Nepple et al. [45]	65 (36 vs. 29)	675[a]	1,497	7.9	9.6	NR	NR

EBL estimated blood loss in milliliters, *LOS* length of hospital stay in days
[a]Mean EBL of RC significantly less than OC
[b]Mean LOS RC significantly less than OC
[c]Number of complications following RC significantly less than OC

Perioperative Parameters

The first reports of robot-assisted radical cystectomy provided evidence that this technique offers decreased intraoperative blood loss compared to open cystectomy. Menon et al. [11] reported a mean blood loss of 150 ml, while Hemal et al. [78] reported a mean of 100 ml. This is very appealing when compared to a study during the same time period of open cystectomy [79] which sought to decrease the amount of blood loss associated with the procedure; despite all attempts the mean blood loss was still 600 ml with a third of patients requiring transfusion [79]. Other studies of ORC have shown mean blood loss from 1,000 to 1,300 ml [3, 80]. Similarly, Table 18.4 shows various studies comparing RARC to ORC, with significantly decreased blood loss associated with RARC across studies.

These studies also show a benefit in length of hospitalization with mean length of stay ranging from 5 to 11 days for RARC and 8 to 13 days for ORC (Table 18.4). Though the data are promising, it is important to realize that these trials were not randomized and likely were subject to selection bias in an attempt to minimize difficulty and complications while attempting a new surgical technique.

The first randomized trial comparing ORC to RARC was reported by Nix et al. [32] who compared the perioperative differences between the two techniques and reported significantly less blood loss, time to flatus, time to bowel movements, and less inpatient narcotic needs. They found no difference in hospital stay between groups. However the study was not adequately powered to answer all of these questions. Overall, these studies point toward improved perioperative outcomes with RARC compared to ORC.

Complications

Postoperative complications are a well-known consequence of radical cystectomy. And while we previously addressed complications following RARC during initial surgeon experience, we have yet to directly compare complications between open and robotic approaches. However, until recently, such comparisons have been limited because of a lack of standardized reporting system. With the more widespread reporting of complications using the Clavien system, comparison of complication rates between RARC and ORC has become more feasible. A large series of open radical cystectomy from Memorial Sloan-Kettering Cancer Center reported complication rates using the Clavien system [3]. They found that 64 % of patients experienced a complication within 90 days of ORC. The authors discussed that their complication rate was higher than previously reported with ORC but that this was likely due to the detailed nature of the Clavien system and extension of reporting out to 90 days.

Though the Clavien system can help standardized comparisons across studies, not all groups have reported using this method. One study that employed the Clavien classification was by Ng et al. [44], reporting that patients undergoing ORC had significantly higher rates of overall and major complications at 30 days. And, though the overall complications were not different at 90 days between these groups, there were still significantly more major complications in the ORC group. This study suggests that RARC could possibly result in fewer major complications; however, since this was a nonrandomized trial, it is unclear whether patient selection bias contributed to differences in complication rates. The only randomized trial comparing RARC and ORC from Nix et al. [32] also used the Clavien system and found no differences in the complication rates between RARC and ORC, but the study was not powered to detect differences in complication rates. Other comparison studies not using the Clavien system have reported variable complication rates ranging from 15 to 60 % (Table 18.4) [32, 33, 42–44], with several showing no differences in the overall complication rates between RARC and ORC [33, 42, 43]. With variations in reporting and the concern for selection bias, the true effect of RARC on postoperative complications is still undetermined and requires further study using standardized reporting systems.

Recovery

Lastly, with the less invasive nature of the robotic approach, some theorize a faster long-term recovery. This is a difficult parameter to assess, but two studies have looked at timing to initiation of chemotherapy to address this. Nix et al. [32] compared 21 patients undergoing RARC to 20 undergoing ORC and found a significant difference in the time to adjuvant chemotherapy initiation; 6.7 weeks in RARC versus 8.8 weeks in ORC which they attributed to quicker time to recovery after surgery. Pruthi et al. [41] studied 100 patients undergoing RARC, 18 of which required adjuvant chemotherapy with a mean time to initiation of 7.2 weeks. The authors compared their results to an age-matched cohort of 20 patients undergoing ORC at their institution and found a mean time to chemotherapy initiation of 10.2 weeks. With the need for good overall health and functional status before initiation of chemotherapy, the decreased time to initiation provides some preliminary evidence that RARC may confer a more rapid recovery. But again, the speedier recovery in some patients may be related to selection bias and baseline performance status. Since the choice of adjuvant chemotherapy is also not based on uniform criteria, time to such therapy may be influenced by a variety of factors. This further confounds the use of the variable of time to adjuvant chemotherapy as an outcome variable outside of a controlled study. However, these data do suggest that patients undergoing RARC may recover more quickly than those undergoing ORC. This will certainly benefit those needing to go onto adjuvant chemotherapy.

In conclusion, it appears that robotic approaches may hold significant promise in improving certain outcomes while ensuring adequate cancer control from a complex procedure such as radical cystectomy. Early data indicate that several concerns pertaining to the use of robotic surgery such as adequacy of resection, adequate node dissection, and complication rates are not of substantial merit. There appear to be some potential benefits to RARC in reduction of blood loss, reduced length of stay, and even decreased complication rates. Additional data that will become available from large cohort studies and ongoing randomized trials will further help clarify these issues and delineate the role of robotic surgery as applied to radical cystectomy.

Editors' Commentary

Erik P. Castle and Raj S. Pruthi

Robotic techniques in bladder cancer surgery must continue to duplicate the surgical principles of open radical cystectomy with regard to the extirpative portion of the procedure, the ability to perform adequate lymphadenectomy, and the urinary diversion. While the potential benefits of robotics for radical cystectomy are well defined, the universal acceptance of this technique has been met with some resistance because of concerns about unique issues and complications surrounding the application of robotic surgery. The authors provide a thoughtful and evidence-based examination of the potential areas of concerns ranging from oncologic efficacy to perioperative complications to the learning curve and costs. Those initiating a robot-assisted radical cystectomy program are strongly encouraged to understand these potential concerns and be sure to evaluate and address such issues when applying robotics to their own clinical practice.

References

1. American Cancer Society. Cancer facts and figures 2012. Atlanta: American Cancer Society; 2012.
2. Hall MC, Chang SS, Dalbagni G, Pruthi RS, Seigne JD, Skinner EC, et al. Guideline for the management of nonmuscle invasive bladder cancer (stages Ta, T1, and Tis): 2007 update. J Urol. 2007;178(6): 2314–30.
3. Shabsigh A, Korets R, Vora KC, Brooks CM, Cronin AM, Savage C, et al. Defining early morbidity of radical cystectomy for patients with bladder cancer using a standardized reporting methodology. Eur Urol. 2009;55:164–76.
4. Shimko MS, Tollefson MK, Umbreit EC, Farmer SA, Blute ML, Frank I. Long-term complications of conduit urinary diversion. J Urol. 2011;185:562–7.
5. Stein JP, Lieskovsky G, Cote R, Groshen S, Feng AC, Boyd S, et al. Radical cystectomy in the treatment of invasive bladder cancer: long-term results in 1054 patients. J Clin Oncol. 2001;19:666–75.
6. Konety BR, Dhawan V, Allareddy V, Joslyn SA. Impact of hospital and surgeon volume on in-hospital mortality from radical cystectomy: data from the health care utilization project. J Urol. 2005;173(5): 1695–700.
7. Wilson T, Torrey R. Open versus robotic-assisted radical prostatectomy: which is better? Curr Opin Urol. 2011;21(3):200–5.
8. Parekattil SJ, Cohen MS. Robotic microsurgery 2011: male infertility, chronic testicular pain, postvasectomy pain, sports hernia pain and phantom pain. Curr Opin Urol. 2011;21(2):121–6.
9. Benway BM, Bhayani SB. Surgical outcomes of robot-assisted partial nephrectomy. BJU Int. 2011; 108(6):955–61.
10. Beecken WD, Wolfram M, Engl T, Bentas W, Probst M, Blaheta R. Robotic-assisted laparoscopic radical cystectomy and intra-abdominal formation of an orthotopic ileal neobladder. Eur Urol. 2003;44(3): 337–9.
11. Menon M, Hemal AK, Tewari A, Shrivastava A, Shoma AM, El-Tabey NA, et al. Nerve-sparing robot-assisted radical cystoprostatectomy and urinary diversion. BJU Int. 2003;92(3):232–6.
12. Vazina A, Dugi D, Shariat SF, Evans J, Link R, Lerner SP. Stage specific lymph node metastasis mapping in radical cystectomy specimens. J Urol. 2004;171: 1830–4.
13. Leissner J, Hohenfellner R, Thuroff JW, Wolf HK. Lymphadenectomy in patients with transitional cell carcinoma of the urinary bladder; significance for staging and prognosis. BJU Int. 2000;85(7):817–23.
14. Colston J, Leadbetter W. Infiltrating carcinoma of the bladder. J Urol. 1936;36:669–89.
15. Leissner J, Ghoneim MA, Abol-Enein H, Thuroff JW, Franzaring L, Fisch M, et al. Extended radical lymphadenectomy in patients with urothelial bladder cancer: results of a prospective multicenter study. J Urol. 2004;171(1):139–44.
16. Stein JP, Quek ML, Skinner DG. Lymphadenectomy for invasive bladder cancer: I. Historical perspective and contemporary rationale. BJU Int. 2006;97(2): 227–31.
17. Skinner DG. Management of invasive bladder cancer: a meticulous pelvic node dissection can make a difference. J Urol. 1982;128(1):34–6.
18. Herr HW, Bochner B, Dalbagni G, Machele Donat S, Reuter VE, Bajorin DF. Impact of the number of lymph nodes retrieved on outcome in patients with muscle invasive bladder cancer. J Urol. 2002;167(3): 1295–8.
19. Herr HW, Faulkner JR, Grossman HB, Natale RB, deVere White R, Sarosdy MF, et al. Surgical factors influence bladder cancer outcomes: a cooperative group report. J Clin Oncol. 2004;22(14):2781–9.
20. Poulsen AL, Horn T, Steven K. Radical cystectomy; extending limits of pelvic lymph node dissection improves survival for patients with bladder cancer confined to the bladder wall. J Urol. 1998;160(6): 2015–9.
21. Konety BR, Joslyn SA, O'Donnell MA. Extent of pelvic lymphadenectomy and its impact on outcome in patients diagnosed with bladder cancer: analysis of data from the surveillance, epidemiology and end results program data base. J Urol. 2003;169(3): 946–50.

22. Huang GJSJ. Open radical cystectomy with lymphadenectomy remains the treatment of choice for invasive bladder cancer. Curr Opin Urol. 2007;17(5):369–75.
23. Dorin RP, Skinner EC. Extended lymphadenectomy in bladder cancer. Curr Opin Urol. 2010;20:414–20.
24. Singh I. Robot-assisted pelvic lymphadenectomy for bladder cancer - where have we reached by 2009. Urology. 2010;75(6):1269–74.
25. Schumacher MC, Jonsson MN, Wiklund NP. Does extended lymphadenectomy preclude laparoscopic or robot-assisted radical cystectomy in advanced bladder cancer? Curr Opin Urol. 2009;19:527–32.
26. Woods M, Thomas R, Davis R, Andres PE, Ferrigni RG, Cheng J, et al. Robot-assisted extended pelvic lymphadenectomy. J Endourol. 2008;22(6):1297–302.
27. Pruthi RS, Smith A, Wallen EM. Evaluating the learning curve for robot-assisted laparoscopic radical cystectomy. J Endourol. 2008;22(11):2469–74.
28. Guru KA, Sternberg K, Wilding GE, Tan W, Butt ZM, Mohler JL, et al. The lymph node yield during robot-assisted radical cystectomy. BJU Int. 2008;102(2): 231–4.
29. Bochner BH, Herr HW, Reuter VE. Impact of separate versus en bloc pelvic lymph node dissection on the number of lymph nodes retrieved in cystectomy specimens. J Urol. 2001;166(6):2295–6.
30. Davis JW, Gaston K, Anderson R, Dinney CPN, Grossman HB, Munsell MF, et al. Robot assisted extended pelvic lymphadenectomy at radical cystectomy: lymph node yield compared with second look open dissection. J Urol. 2011;185(1):79–84.
31. Fang AC, Ahmad AE, Whitson JM, Ferrell LD, Carroll PR, Konety BR. Effect of a minimum lymph node policy in radical cystectomy and pelvic lymphadenectomy on lymph node yields, lymph node positivity rates, lymph node density, and survivorship in patients with bladder cancer. Cancer. 2010;116(8): 1901–8.
32. Nix J, Smith A, Kurpad R, Nielsen ME, Wallen EM, Pruthi RS. Prospective randomized controlled trial of robotic versus open radical cystectomy for bladder cancer: perioperative and pathologic results. Eur Urol. 2010;57:196–201.
33. Richards KA, Hemal AK, Kader K, Pettus JA. Robot assisted laparoscopic pelvic lymphadenectomy at the time of radical cystectomy rivals that of open surgery: single institiution report. Urology. 2010;76(6):1400–4.
34. Guru KA, Perlmutter AE, Butt ZM, Piacente P, Wilding GE, Tan W, et al. The learning curve for robot-assisted radical cystectomy. JSLS. 2009;13:509–14.
35. Hayn MH, Hussain A, Mansour AM, Andrews PE, Carpentier P, Castle E, et al. The learning curve of robot-assisted radical cystectomy: results from the international robotic cystectomy consortium. Eur Urol. 2010;58:197–202.
36. Schumacher MC, Jonsson MN, Hosseini A, Nyberg T, Poulakis V, Pardalidis NP, et al. Surgery-related complications of robot-assisted radical cystectomy with intracorporeal urinary diversion. Urology. 2011;77:871–7.
37. Richards KA, Kader K, Pettus JA, Smith JJ, Hemal AK. Does the initial larning curve comparomise outcomes for robot-assisted radical cystectomy? A critical evaluation of the first 60 cases while establishing a robotics program. J Endourol. 2011;25(9):1553–8.
38. Dotan ZA, Kavanagh K, Yossepowitch O, Kaag M, Olgac S, Donat M, et al. Positive surgical margins in soft tissue following radical cystectomy for bladder cancer and cancer specific survival. J Urol. 2007;178: 2308–13.
39. Novara G, Svatek RS, Karakiewicz PI, Skinner E, Ficarra V, Fradet Y, et al. Soft tissue surgical margin status is a powerful predictor of outcomes after radical cystectomy: a multicenter study of more than 4,400 patients. J Urol. 2010;183:2165–70.
40. Hellenthal NJ, Hussain A, Andrews PE, Carpentier P, Castle E, Dasgupta P, et al. Surgical margin status after robot assisted radical cystectomy: results from the International Robotic Cystectomy Consortium. J Urol. 2010;184:87–91.
41. Pruthi RS, Nielsen ME, Nix J, Smith A, Schultz H, Wallen EM. Robotic radical cystectomy for bladder cancer: surgical and pathological outcomes in 100 consecutive cases. J Urol. 2010;183:510–5.
42. Galich A, Sterrett S, Nazemi T, Pohlman G, Smith L, Balaji KC. Comparative analysis of early perioperative outcomes following radical cystectomy by either the robotic or open method. JSLS. 2006;10:145–50.
43. Wang GJ, Barocas DA, Raman JD, Scherr DS. Robotic vs open radical cystectomy: prospective comparison of perioperative outcomes and pathological measures of early oncological efficacy. BJU Int. 2008;101(1):89–93.
44. Ng CK, Kauggman EC, Lee M, Otto BJ, Portnoff A, Ehrlich JR, et al. A comparison of postoperative complications in open versus robotic cystectomy. Eur Urol. 2010;57:274–82.
45. Nepple KG, Strope SA, Grubb RL, Kibel AS. Early oncologic outcomes of robotic vs. open radical cystectomy for urothelial cancer. Urol Oncol. 2011; epublish ahead of print.
46. Haber GP, Crouzet S, Gill IS. Laparoscopic and robotic assisted radical cystectomy for bladder cancer: a critical analysis. Eur Urol. 2008;54:54–64.
47. Balaji KC, Yohannes P, McBride CL, Oleynikov D, Hemstreet GP. Feasibility of robot-assisted totally intracorporeal laparoscopic ileal conduit urinary diversion: initial results of a single institutional pilot study. Urology. 2004;63(1):51–5.
48. Pruthi RS, Wallen EM. Robotic-assisted laproscopic pelvic lymphadenectomy for bladder cancer: a surgical atlas. J Laparoendosc Adv Surg Tech. 2009;19(1): 23–7.
49. Guru KA, Seixas-Mikelus A, Hussain A, Blumenfeld AJ, Nyquist J, Chandrasekhar R, et al. Robot-assisted intracorporeal ileal conduit: Marionette technique and initial experience at Roswell Park Cancer Institute. Urology. 2010;76:866–72.
50. Smith AB, Raynor M, Amling CL, Busby E, Castle E, Davis R, et al. Multi-institutional analysis of robotic

radical cystectomy for bladder cancer: perioperative outcomes and complications in 227 patients. J Laparoendosc Adv Surg Tech A. 2012;22(1):17–21.
51. Lee R, Chughtai B, Herman M, Shariat SF, Scherr DS. Cost-analysis comparison of robot-assisted laparoscopic radical cystectomy (RC) vs open RC. BJU Int. 2011;108:976–83.
52. Cha EK, Wiklund NP, Scherr DS. Recent advances in robot-assisted radical cystectomy. Curr Opin Urol. 2011;21:65–70.
53. Mattei A, Birkhaeuser FD, Baermann C, Warncke SH, Studer UE. To stent or not to stent perioperatively the ureteroileal anastomosis of ileal orthotopic bladder substitutes and ileal conduits? Results of a prospective randomized trial. J Urol. 2008;179:582–6.
54. Evangelidis A, Lee E, Karellas M, Thrasher JB, Holzbeierlein J. Evaluation of ureterointestinal anastomosis: Wallace vs Bricker. J Urol. 2006;175(5):1755–8.
55. Hautmann RE. The oncologic results of laparoscopic radical cystectomy are not (yet) equivalent to open cystectomy. Curr Opin Urol. 2009;19:522–6.
56. Regan JB, Barrett DM. Stented versus nonstented ureteroileal anastomoses: is there a difference with regard to leak and stricture? J Urol. 1985;134(6):1101–3.
57. Dasgupta P, Rimington P, Murphy D, Challacombe B, Hemal A, Elhage O, et al. Robotic assisted radical cystectomy: short to medium-term oncologic and functional outcomes. Int J Clin Pract. 2008;62(11):1709–14.
58. Gamboa AJ, Young JL, Dash A, Abraham JB, Box GN, Omstein DK. Pelvic lymph node dissection and outcome of robot-assisted radical cystectomy for bladder carcinoma. J Robot Surg. 2009;3:7–12.
59. Khan MS, Elhage O, Challacombe B, Rimington P, Murphy D, Dasgupta P. Analysis of early complications of robotic-assisted radical cystectomy using a standardized reporting system. Urology. 2011;77:357–62.
60. Ghavamian R, Hakimi AA. Lymph node dissection for bladder cancer: the issue of extent and feasibility in the minimally invasive era. Expert Rev Anticancer Ther. 2009;9(12):1783–92.
61. El-Tabey NA, Shoma AM. Port site metastases after robot-assisted laparoscopic radical cystectomy. Urology. 2005;66:1110-e1–3.
62. Martel G, Boushey RP. Laparoscopic colon surgery: past, present and future. Surg Clin North Am. 2006;86(4):867–97.
63. Seracchioli R, Ventruoli S, Ceccarini M, Cantarelli M, Ceccaroni M, Pignotti E, et al. Is total laparoscopic surgery for endometrial carcinoma at risk of local recurrence? A long-term survival. Anticancer Res. 2005;25(3c):2423–8.
64. Tanaka K, Hara I, Takenaka A, Kawabata G, Fujisawa M. Incidence of local and port site recurrence of urologic cancer after laparoscopic surgery. Urology. 2008;71(4):728–34.
65. Hubert J. Laparoscopic cystectomy and robotic-assisted cystectomy. In: Lokeshwar VB, Merseburger AS, Hautmann SH, editors. Bladder tumors: molecular aspects and clinical management New York. New York, NY: Humana; 2011. p. 365–76.
66. Chade DC, Laudone VP, Bochner BH, Parra RO. Oncological outcomes after radical cystectomy for bladder cancer: open versus minimally invasive approaches. J Urol. 2010;183:862–70.
67. Challacombe BJ, Bochner BH, Dasgupta P, Gill I, Guru K, Herr H, et al. The role of laparoscopic and robotic cystectomy in the management of muscle-invasive bladder cancer with special emphasis on cancer control and complications. Eur Urol. 2011;60:767–75.
68. Smith AB, Raynor MC, Pruthi RS. Peri- and postoperative outcomes of robot-assisted radical cystectomy (RARC). BJU Int. 2011;108:969–75.
69. Lowrance WT, Rumohr JA, Change SS, Clark PE, Smith JA, Cookson MS. Contemporary open radical cystectomy: analysis of perioperative outcomes. J Urol. 2008;179:1313–8.
70. Rhee JJ, Lebeau S, Smolkin M, Theodorescu D. Radical cystectomy with ileal conduit diversion: early prospective evaluation of the impact of robotic assistance. BJU Int. 2006;98:1059–63.
71. Butt ZM, Fazili A, Tan W, Wilding GE, Filadora V, Kim HL, et al. Does the presence of significant risk factors affect perioperative outcomes after robot-assisted radical cystectomy? BJU Int. 2009;104:986–90.
72. Hayn MH, Hellenthal NJ, Hussain A, Andrews PE, Carpentier P, Castle E, et al. Does previous robot-assisted radical prostatectomy experience affect outcomes at robot-assisted radical cystectomy? Results from the International Robotic Cystectomy Consortium. Urology. 2010;76:1111–6.
73. Riley GF, Potosky AL, Lubitz JD, Kessler LG. Medicare payments from diagnosis to death for elderly cancer patients by stage at diagnosis. Med Care. 1995;33(8):828–41.
74. Zehnder P, Gill IS. Cost-effectiveness of open versus laparoscopic versus robotic-assisted laparoscopic cystectomy and urinary diversion. Curr Opin Urol. 2011;21:415–9.
75. Konety BR, Allareddy V. Influence of post-cystectomy complications on cost and subsequent outcome. J Urol. 2007;177(1):280–7.
76. Smith A, Kurpad R, Lal A, Nielsen M, Wallen EM, Pruthi RS. Cost analysis of robotic versus open radical cystectomy for bladder cancer. J Urol. 2010;183:505–9.
77. Martin AD, Nunez RN, Castle EP. Robot-assisted radical cystectomy versus open radical cystectomy: a complete cost analysis. Urology. 2011;77(3):621–5.
78. Hemal AK, Abol-Enein H, Tewari A, Shrivastava A, Shoma AM, Ghoneim MA, et al. Robotic radical cystectomy and urinary diversion in the management of bladder cancer. Urol Clin North Am. 2004;31:719–29.
79. Chang SS, Smith Jr JA, Cookson MS. Decreasing blood loss in patients treated with radical cystectomy: a prospective randomized trial using a new stapling device. J Urol. 2003;169(3):951–4.

80. Elhage O, Keegan J, Challacombe B, Murphey D, Rimington P, Khan MS, et al. A comparative analysis of open laparoscopic and robotic radical cystectomy for bladder cancer. J Endourol. 2007;21(S1):142.
81. Abraham JB, Young JL, Box GN, Lee HJ, Deane LA, Ornstein DK. Comparative analysis of laparoscopic and robotic-assisted radical cystectomy with ileal conduit urinary diversion. J Endourol. 2007;21(12): 1473–80.
82. Lavery HJ, Martinez-Suarez HJ, Abaza R. Tobotic extended pelvic lymphadenectomy for bladder cancer with increased nodal yield. BJU Int. 2011;107: 1802–05.
83. Kauffman EC, Ng CK, Lee MM, Otto BJ, Wang GJ, Scherr DS. Early oncological outcomes for bladder urothelial carcinoma patients treated with robotic-assisted radical cystectomy. BJU Int. 2011;107: 628–35.
84. Martin AD, Nunez RN, Pacelli A, Woods ME, Davis R, Thomas R et al. Robot-assisted radical cystectomy: intermediate survival results at a mean follow-up of 25 months. BJU Int. 2010;105:1706–09.

Robot-Assisted Surgery for Benign Disease of the Bladder

19

Christopher E. Wolter, Rafael N. Nunez, and Erik P. Castle

Introduction

Surgery of the bladder for benign disease and reconstruction is a varied and somewhat broad field. Because there are so many categories of procedures and scenarios of when they may arise, this chapter will cover the major reported procedures for benign bladder disease. Much of what has already been learned from robot-assisted radical cystectomy can be applied here, and the nuances and outcomes of these techniques applied to benign disease situations will be described. The more commonly described procedures of ureteral reimplantation, bladder diverticulectomy, bladder augmentation, and vesicovaginal fistula repair will be covered. In addition, simple cystectomy will be discussed. While this procedure does not vary greatly from radical cystectomy, which is covered in previous chapters, we will cover special circumstances and the authors' experience with this procedure.

Simple Cystectomy

While robot-assisted radical cystectomy is well described in the literature, there is actually very little written about robotic simple cystectomy. This is likely due to the fact that there are a large number of diagnoses that are treated with this procedure, and for the simple fact that this is not necessarily a very commonly performed surgery when compared to radical cystectomy. Considering that the extirpative part of radical cystectomy is very similar to simple cystectomy, it is therefore not surprising that simple cystectomy is not well described. In addition, the technical demands and margins of the procedure are not as exacting as for radical cystectomy. Given that the underlying reason for simple cystectomy is not cancer, incomplete removal of the bladder or simply a supra-trigonal cystectomy may be all that is necessary in some cases.

In males, there is very little difference in the operation when compared to radical cystectomy other than the fact that the surgeon may elect to leave the prostate in situ and lymph nodes are not removed. This is well described in previous chapters. In females, there are a few techniques that could be incorporated to make the robotic dissection even easier, especially if urethrectomy and/or vaginal sparing are chosen. Urinary diversion techniques can be chosen as described in previous chapters as well. Port placement is the same as it would be for radical cystectomy with the option of placing the assistant on the left side if an intracorporeal diversion is planned (Fig. 19.1).

For the female simple cystectomy, a discussion with the patient regarding urinary diversion type is important. If an ileal conduit or non-orthotopic diversion is chosen, the patient and surgeon should decide if the patient wants to keep her urethra.

C.E. Wolter, M.D. (✉) • R.N. Nunez, M.D.
E.P. Castle, M.D., F.A.C.S.
Department of Urology, Mayo Clinic,
5779 E. Mayo Blvd., Phoenix, AZ 85054, USA
e-mail: wolter.christopher@mayo.edu

E.P. Castle and R.S. Pruthi (eds.), *Robotic Surgery of the Bladder*, DOI 10.1007/978-1-4614-4906-5_19,

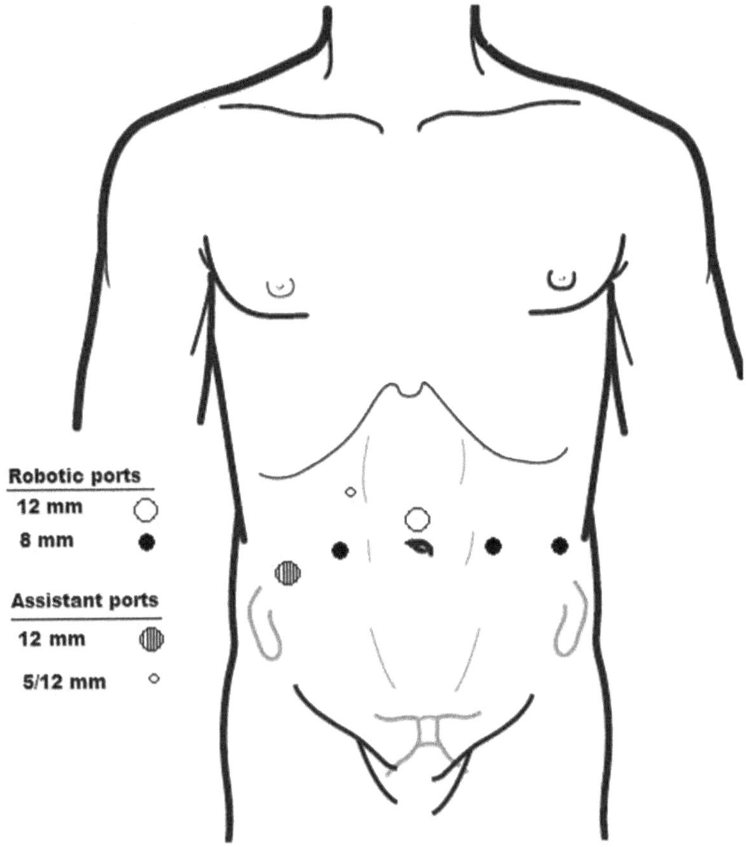

Fig. 19.1 Port placement for access to the bladder and ureter

Frequently the reasons for simple cystectomy often involve urethral pain and/or recurrent infections, so en-bloc removal of the entire urethra with the bladder is a good option. We approach this vaginally in our patients, and the periurethral and retropubic dissection is quite simple and straightforward from this direction. This approach also lends itself nicely if the patient has chosen a vaginal-sparing cystectomy as well. Simple vaginal wall advancement is all that is necessary to cover the defect left by removing the urethra. We liberally mobilize the vaginal wall and use a multilayered closure to prevent any possibility for later prolapse or herniation, using an interrupted absorbable suture on the deep and periostial structures, and a running absorbable suture on the vaginal mucosal edges.

Vaginal sparing is also easily initiated from a vaginal approach and can be done in conjunction with urethrectomy. In either case, we use a distal horizontal vaginal incision and then completely dissect the anterior vaginal wall from the bladder all the way to the vaginal cuff or cervix. If performing a urethrectomy as well, the urethra should be circumscribed, with the horizontal vaginal incision marking the inferior edge of the urethral incision. After carrying out the dissection and freeing the vagina from the bladder, the vagina is closed as described above in multiple layers. Later, when the bladder is approached robotically, it should already be completely free from the vagina. All that is necessary is to open the peritoneum over the vaginal cuff, and the space can easily be entered to take the bladder pedicles. The remainder of the operation is essentially the same as the previously described radical cystectomy.

It is important to recognize the potential for vaginal bleeding during vaginal sparing. Due to the fact that the vagina is extensively vascularized, the surgeon must pay attention to meticulous hemostasis following removal of the bladder. This will prevent delayed bleeds and pelvic hematomas which can complicate recovery. In addition, if the anterior vaginal wall dissection is approached vaginally, bleeding can occur within the vagina that may go unrecognized once the robot is docked and the robotic portion of the procedure is undertaken. Be sure to have all vaginal and pelvic bleeders controlled before proceeding with the robotic portion; otherwise one may find a pool of blood at the foot of the bed on the floor once the robot is undocked.

Whether performing sparing of the anterior vaginal wall or removing it, pelvic organ prolapse occurs at a high rate following simple or radical cystectomy. This is a product of disruption of the anterior and lateral support structures of the pelvic organs. One option is to perform a paravaginal repair using nonabsorbable suture to any available later support structures. The authors currently use zero polypropylene interrupted sutures at four points (two on each side) of the vagina. Unfortunately this only provides lateral support and anterior weakness can result in prolapse in some patients.

Another important consideration is the closure of the vaginotomy. The surgeon must remember that magnification can give the impression of large bites during closure and it is important to have a very strong closure of the vaginal wall. Herniation of intestinal contents as well as omentum through the vaginal closure has been anecdotally reported. In order to avoid this, the authors currently perform a "clam-shell" closure of the vagina in multilayer fashion with zero polyglactin suture. We also make sure to reinforce with interrupted sutures and manually check the integrity of the closure transvaginally at the completion of the procedure.

Important Technical Considerations

- The prostate may be left in situ in male patients allowing for minimal risk of post-op bleeding
- Vaginal approach to the anterior vaginal wall dissection and urethral dissection *prior* to robotic dissection
- Meticulous hemostasis of anterior vaginal wall following cystectomy to avoid delayed post-op bleeds
- Multilayer closure of vaginotomy if anterior vaginal wall not spared key to avoid post-op herniation

Ureteral Reimplantation

Stricture or fistula of the distal ureter is a rare outcome after pelvic surgery. Unfortunately, it is often discovered days to weeks after the inciting procedure has occurred, thus sometimes making management difficult. Regardless, even if it is recognized intraoperatively, it should be managed by ureteral reimplantation with or without a psoas hitch, or possibly even a Boari flap. This section will deal with techniques and pearls when performing reimplantation of the ureter for distal ureteral pathology.

Given the delicate nature of operating on the ureter, the procedure has not typically been performed in a pure laparoscopic approach, although it has been described [1]. Generally speaking, this is a pelvic operation, and the robotic approach suits this procedure very well. It has been described in multiple case series, with seemingly good efficacy [2]. Again, the main indications are distal ureteral stricture, distal ureteral TCC requiring reimplantation, and ureterovaginal fistula. All of these disease entities have been described being managed with robotic ureteral reimplantation [3, 4]. It should be noted that the authors would not recommend robot-assisted reimplantation of a ureter for upper tract urothelial cancer due to the risk of intraperitoneal spillage of cancer cells and limit this procedure for benign purposes.

The surgical approach for a robotic ureteral reimplant is similar to that of other pelvic operations, and standard robotic instrumentation is all that is typically necessary. One or two assistant ports are utilized as well, depending on the complexity of the procedure. Port placement is similar to that used for robot-assisted radical or simple cystectomy (Fig. 19.1). The third working robotic arm (fourth arm) should be placed to the opposite side of the ureter being reimplanted in order to be available for retracting the bladder. While this is technically a pelvic operation, on occasion, the laterality of the procedure can come into play, especially if the stricture is higher and a psoas hitch or Boari flap will be necessary. In these instances, it is better to rotate port placement towards the side of the reimplant slightly. Camera placement should also be sufficiently high as to not place the surgeon in a position where visualization becomes difficult.

The procedure typically begins with medial mobilization of the colon from either side in order to gain exposure of the ureter over the course of the psoas muscle before it courses over the iliac vessels. For the purposes of distal strictures, this is often a nonviolated plane, and dissection should be quite feasible here. The ureter should be circumferentially mobilized with care being taken not to skeletonize it. The ureter then should be traced into the pelvis to the level of the offending pathology and transected. Place a stay suture on the ureter to aid in delicate manipulation of the ureter as well as identification later.

Assessment of the type of reimplant needed should be made. The bladder should be prepared for this at this point in time. For a long ureter, simple mobilization of the bladder by releasing its anterior and superior attachments from the space of retzius and contralateral side may be all that is required. Once it is certain that the ureter can be reimplanted in a tension-free manor, a lateral trough through the peritoneum and detrusor should be made to the level of the mucosa. Generously spatulate the ureter and open the bladder mucosa the same distance. The ureteral mucosa should then be anastomosed to the bladder mucosa using a fine absorbable suture (4-0 polyglactin or similar). Following closure of one side of the anastomosis, a double-J stent should be passed into the ureter over a wire that is inserted through an assistant port and guided into the ureter by the robotic surgeon. The mucosal anastomosis can be completed and the overlying muscle and peritoneum may be reapproximated over the closure to provide additional security and to ensure a watertight closure.

More typically, the bladder will need to be mobilized more, and a psoas hitch or Boari flap will be necessary. The bladder should first be appropriately mobilized from the anterior and contralateral side, ligating and dividing the obliterated umbilical ligament and/or superior vesical pedicle if necessary. Filling the bladder will aid in this and will also give the surgeon an idea of how well mobilized the bladder is and whether it will reach adequately. After this, the psoas hitch should be done by suturing the bladder to the psoas muscle and tendon with a permanent suture, taking care to avoid the genitofemoral nerve.

If a Boari flap is necessary, the flap should be opened from about 3 cm cephalad from the bladder neck at this point. This should be done with the bladder full in order to estimate the size of the flap and location. It is very important to make a sufficiently wide flap in order to be able to roll into a tube following anastomosis of the ureter to the flap. A dreaded complication is a leak due to inability to close external layers of detrusor over the mucosal tube. The ureter should then be anastomosed in an end-to-side fashion laying the flap on the anteriorly spatulated ureter. A stent should be inserted as one would do open, and the Boari flap can be closed using a running absorbable 3-0 suture [5]. After completing the reimplant, the closure should be tested for leaks, and a catheter should be left in the bladder for 7–14 days, and a cystogram checked before removing the catheter. The stent should remain in place for 6 weeks, typically.

Important Technical Considerations

- Place the third working robotic arm (fourth arm) contralateral to the ureter to be repaired
- "Tension-free" anastomosis of the ureter to bladder mucosa
- Be sure to make the Boari flap wide enough for rolling into a tube and have adequate detrusor to roll over the mucosal closure

Bladder Diverticulectomy

Typically in adults, bladder diverticula are mainly acquired and in men with bladder outlet obstruction. This is typically secondary to BPH, but other obstructive processed can be to blame as well. Congenital diverticula can also be seen in children as well. For both of these groups of patients, a robotic approach for diverticulectomy is quite feasible and have been described in case series in the literature [6, 7]. While the overall concept of the procedure is straightforward, it can actually be a difficult surgical approach in certain instances, especially in men with bladder outlet obstruction. It should also be determined if diverticulectomy is even necessary in all cases. Diverticula with active urothelial cell carcinoma should be managed through an open retropubic/extraperitoneal approach to avoid intraperitoneal spillage of cancerous cells.

Preoperative imaging and cystoscopy should be performed to gain a detailed understanding of the location and size of the diverticulum and diverticular neck. Preoperative urodynamics are often misleading as to the presence of obstruction and the diverticulum can serve as a "pop-off" for the pressure. However, the underlying cause of the diverticulum should be addressed prior to or at the same time as the diverticulectomy.

Ureteral catheters or stents should first be placed in the OR if desired. The surgical approach is a standard positioning and port placement for a transperitoneal procedure. At the onset, the location of the diverticulum can be tricky to identify. It is often anterolateral to the ureteral orifice, but correlation with preoperative cystoscopy and imaging should always be confirmed. Often, a bulge in the peritoneum can be seen, and the peritoneum can safely be entered above the vas deferens in order to safely avoid the ureter [7]. Once the diverticulum is exposed, dissection should proceed to completely reveal the diverticulum down to its neck. At this point the diverticulum can be excised. If the neck of the diverticulum is difficult to identify, techniques to aid in this include endoscopic transillumination, catheter placement into the diverticulum, or intravesical dye instillation [8]. The authors have found bedside flexible cystoscopy with transillumination of the diverticulum to be most helpful. Occasionally, it is necessary or unavoidable that the diverticulum is entered. In this case, the edges can then be traced and the borders of the neck and bladder can be established, and the resection of the diverticulum can proceed accordingly. Closure of the defect in the bladder should be carried out in multiple layers with absorbable 3-0 and 2-0 polyglactin suture, a large foley catheter should remain in place and a cystogram should be checked in 10–14 days. An intraperitoneal drain should also be left as well. Ureteral stents should be removed 1–2 weeks after the foley catheter.

Important Technical Considerations

- Preoperative imaging and cystoscopy important for operative planning
- Consider bedside flexible cystoscopy into the diverticulum with transillumination to facilitate identification transabdominally

Augmentation Cystoplasty

Enterocystoplasty is a seldom used but useful procedure for small, contracted, high-pressure bladders in which conservative management has failed. Most frequently this is a consequence of neurogenic bladder. The robotic approach has been described numerous times in the pediatric literature, both with and without appendicovesicostomy [9], and it has also been reported in small series in adults.

Conceptually, this is a good application of robotic surgery, as an attempt to recreate the open procedure is very feasible. The procedure itself, however, is not without its challenges. The real trouble with this operation is the extensive amount of suturing required in preparing the bowel segment. While this can be somewhat alleviated by delivering the bowel through a small incision midprocedure to prepare the augment, it still needs to be sewn to the bladder itself in a watertight fashion. This is where the robot's dexterity and easy suturing really come into play. Completely intracorporeal augmentations have even been described with good results [10, 11].

The procedure proceeds with standard port placement and instrumentation for a pelvic procedure, with the camera port being placed at least 2 cm above the umbilicus in order to be able to

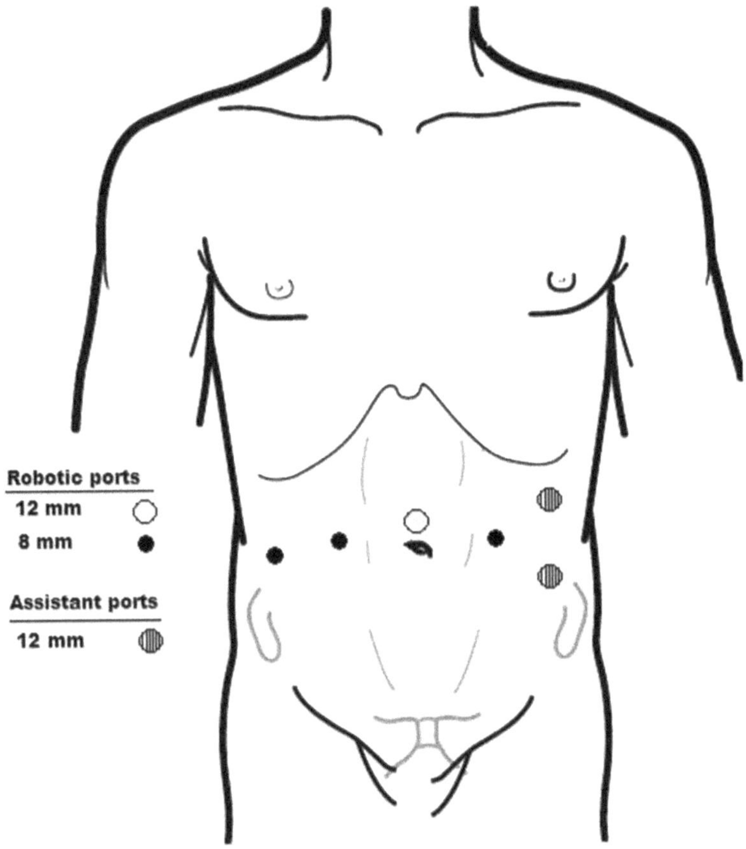

Fig. 19.2 Port placement in cases with intracorporeal bowel reconstruction—note assistant on left side of patient

visualize and identify the ileocecal junction. Quite frequently, the bladder dissection is fairly straightforward. A coronal or sagital opening can be made, and it should be large enough to allow for the final construct to be a spherical as possible. The choice of which direction is opened depends on the reach of the mesentery of the bowel and whether or not an appendicovesicostomy will be performed.

Twenty to thirty centimeter of bowel is typically utilized, although a larger augment can certainly be utilized if necessary. The segment of ileum should then be detubularized on the anti-mesenteric border and sewn into a "U"-configuration with running 2-0 suture. If a longer segment is used, as "S"-configuration may be needed. Try and keep the augment as symmetric a possible, avoiding an oblong or partially tabularized shape.

If an extracorporeal construct is chosen, then after identifying and tagging the desired bowel segment, the robot will need to be un-docked and the bowel can be delivered through a 4–6 cm incision. The augment can then be configured and then dropped back into the body. The bladder anastomosis should be completed with a running 2-0 polyglactin suture. Prior to completing the augment, a suprapubic cystostomy tube should be placed through the native bladder segment, and a drain should also be placed in the peritoneal cavity [9, 11].

If an intracorporeal construct is undertaken, it is best to put the bedside assistant on the left side of the bed with the third robotic arm on the patients left side (Fig. 19.2). Furthermore, the two assistant ports should be both 12 mm ports to allow for more option for angle of passage of laparoscopic staplers during harvest of the ileal segment to be used. The bowel anastomosis can be completed as described in previous chapters on intracorporeal diversion (Chaps. 11 and 12).

Important Technical Considerations

- If intracorporeal construct desired, place the bedside assistant on the left side for easier angle of approach for the laparoscopic staplers
- "U" or "S"-configuration of the detubularized ileum

Vesicovaginal Fistula Repair

Vesicovaginal fistula is a devastating complication of gynecologic surgery, penetrating trauma, or abdominopelvic radiation. The continuous incontinence is quite debilitating and extremely distressing. Traditionally, abdominal access to fistula repair involved an incision and a prolonged hospitalization, but the laparoscopic and subsequently robotic approaches have converted this to a minimally invasive procedure as well. While these fistulae can be repaired in a minimally invasive and well-tolerated vaginal approach with equal success, not all fistulae are amenable to this [12]. Again, this is another pelvic operation that is very well suited to robotic surgery, the visualization is excellent, and the procedure is mainly in a small region in the pelvis. All things being equal, the outcomes in robotic repair are equal to traditional open abdominal repair [13].

All patients with a suspected fistula should be carefully examined and cystoscopy should be performed. In the work up of the patient prior to repair, ureteral involvement should be determined, as this can be present in up to 10 % of patients. This can be either with imaging, dual dye tests, or retrograde pyelography in the OR. Once the extent and determination of location and size of the fistula is made, surgical correction can proceed. Distal vaginal fistulae or those at the vaginal cuff that are easily mobilized or accessible can be considered for vaginal repair. High fistulae, fixed or narrow vaginas, recurrent, and radiated fistulae should be considered for abdominal repair. The rationale for this is that a robust tissue interposition aids greatly in preventing recurrence, and the options for this are more readily available and feasible from a transperitoneal approach. Urine culture and antibiotics should be administered as indicated. Ureteral stents should be placed at the surgeon's discretion.

Once laparoscopic access is achieved, if an omental flap is planned, this should be secured prior to placing the patient in steep trendelenberg and docking the robot. The omentum can be assessed using basic laparoscopy, and if suitable, should be mobilized on its right gastroepiploic pedicle to reach into the pelvis. One or more long suture tags should be left on the omentum for easy identification once the patient is in trendelenberg during the robotic portion of the procedure. Robotic surgery can then proceed from this point. Given the nature of the cause of the fistula, bowel adhesions are frequently present, and need to be carefully dissected free from the vaginal cuff. A large, sturdy vaginal retractor should be utilized. If desired, a catheter, guide wire, or stent should be placed cystoscopically through the fistula tract to aid in identification. With maximal cephalad traction placed on the vaginal by the bedside assistant, the vesicovaginal space should be developed. This dissection should be carried right across the fistulous tract and beyond, allowing for good separation of the bladder and vagina. Development of this plane is often challenging, and use of electrocautery should be limited to preserve tissue integrity if possible. After coming across the fistula, if a stent or catheter was used for identification, this should be removed.

Standard principles of fistula management should be incorporated, including non-opposing closure lines, watertight closure, and interposition flaps. From the robotic approach, it is best to close the vaginal opening first in an orientation opposite the planned bladder closure. Following this, the interposition flap should be secured between the vagina and bladder. If using omentum that had already been harvested laparoscopically, the sutures that were left on it can be grasped and held in place with the third working arm of the robot. If omentum is not available, then using a flap of the overlying and readily available bladder peritoneum should be used. Regardless, make sure the flap is not under tension, and secure it in place with multiple interrupted

absorbable sutures. After this, the bladder can be closed. We prefer a multilayered closure. A foley catheter should be left in place, as well as a drain in the peritoneal cavity. A cystogram should be checked 10–14 days postoperatively. Reported robotic outcomes have been very favorable [13, 14].
Important Technical Considerations

- If an omental flap is planned, this should be created via a laparoscopic approach before placement of the patient in tendelenberg
- Placement of a wire in the fistula may be helpful during dissection
- Use nonopposing suture lines and interposition flaps

Conclusions

As one can see, the applications of robotic surgery are very effective. Again, as long as sound surgical principles are followed, the limits of what can be performed robotically go only as far as the surgeon's determination and imagination. As the field continues to advance, there is conceivably no procedure traditionally performed for benign urologic disease that cannot be performed robotically.

References

1. Reddy PK, Evans RM. Laparoscopic ureteroneocystostomy. J Urol. 1994;152:2057.
2. Baldie K, Angell J, Ogan K, et al. Robotic management of benign mid and distal ureteral strictures and comparison with laparoscopic approaches at a single institution. Urology. 2012;80:596.
3. Phillips EA, Wang DS. Current status of robot-assisted laparoscopic ureteral reimplantation and reconstruction. Curr Urol Rep. 2012;13:190.
4. Hemal AK, Nayyar R, Gupta NP, et al. Experience with robot assisted laparoscopic surgery for upper and lower benign and malignant ureteral pathologies. Urology. 2010;76:1387.
5. Kozinn SI, Canes D, Sorcini A, et al. Robotic versus open distal ureteral reconstruction and reimplantation for benign stricture disease. J Endourol. 2012;26:147.
6. Christman MS, Casale P. Robot-assisted bladder diverticulectomy in the pediatric population. J Endourol. 2012;26:1296.
7. Thiel DD, Young PR, Wehle MJ, et al. Robotic-assisted bladder diverticulectomy: tips and tricks. Urology. 2011;77:1238.
8. Moore CR, Shirodkar SP, Avallone MA, et al. Intravesical methylene blue facilitates precise identification of the diverticular neck during robot-assisted laparoscopic bladder diverticulectomy. J Laparoendosc Adv Surg Tech A. 2012;22:492.
9. Wille MA, Zagaja GP, Shalhav AL, et al. Continence outcomes in patients undergoing robotic assisted laparoscopic mitrofanoff appendicovesicostomy. J Urol. 2011;185:1438.
10. Passerotti CC, Nguyen HT, Lais A, et al. Robot-assisted laparoscopic ileal bladder augmentation: defining techniques and potential pitfalls. J Endourol. 2008;22:355.
11. Gundeti MS, Eng MK, Reynolds WS, et al. Pediatric robotic-assisted laparoscopic augmentation ileocystoplasty and Mitrofanoff appendicovesicostomy: complete intracorporeal–initial case report. Urology. 2008; 72:1144.
12. Chigbu CO, Nwogu-Ikojo EE, Onah HE, et al. Juxtacervical vesicovaginal fistulae: outcome by route of repair. J Obstet Gynaecol. 2006;26:795.
13. Gupta NP, Mishra S, Hemal AK, et al. Comparative analysis of outcome between open and robotic surgical repair of recurrent supra-trigonal vesico-vaginal fistula. J Endourol. 2010;24:1779.
14. Hemal AK, Kolla SB, Wadhwa P. Robotic reconstruction for recurrent supratrigonal vesicovaginal fistulas. J Urol. 2008;180:981.

Future Directions in Robotic Surgery for Bladder Cancer

20

Michele Billia, Muhammad Shamim Khan, and Prokar Dasgupta

Introduction

Radical cystectomy is currently accepted as the gold standard for treatment of MIBC and high risk NMIBC. This procedure can be performed using open, laparoscopic or robotic approach.

In 1991 R. Clayman performed the first laparoscopic radical nephrectomy and became the pioneer of the new era of minimally invasive surgery in urology. During the last 20 years, indications for laparoscopic surgery have expanded to include both ablative and reconstructive procedures for various indications. Its place in the armamentarium of urological and other surgical specialties is well established.

Laparoscopic surgery, however, generally has longer operative times than open surgery and requires a steeper learning curve due to the need for the surgeon to develop high skills for intracorporeal suturing and knotting; abilities which are required in the majority of urological procedures. These characteristics have been identified as the main limiting factors for widespread adaptation of laparoscopic surgery in urology. While many urology centres could not progress in technical expertise to venture starting technically challenging procedures like partial nephrectomy and radical prostatectomy, others suspended these programmes in favour of a standard open surgical approach [1].

In 2001, the era of robotic surgery (RS) began with the introduction of the Da Vinci surgical system® (Intuitive Surgical, Inc., Sunnyvale, California, USA, http://www.intuitivesurgical.com).

RS represents a further evolution of laparoscopy with better ergonomics, improved, higher magnification 3D vision and providing the surgeon the independence of controlling the camera and multiple instruments, which can reproduce the whole spectrum of movements of a human hand. This has made the most difficult steps of intra-corporeal knotting and suturing easier and quicker than laparoscopy. RS has become increasingly popular and, at many centres around the world, robotic radical prostatectomy has essentially become the standard of care for a localised prostate cancer.

As regards radical cystectomy, there is evidence that robot-assisted radical cystectomy (RARC) provides outcomes similar or even superior to laparoscopic and open radical cystectomy. However, long-term follow-up data are still lacking. There is a significant heterogeneity in the data reported in the literature in relation to approaches to urinary diversion.

In this chapter we analyse the possible future directions of robotic surgery for urinary bladder cancer with focus on our analysis of surgical access and instrumentation, techniques of urinary

M. Billia, M.D. (✉) • M.S. Khan
Department of Urology, Kings College London, Kings Health Partners, Guy's Hospital, Great Maze Pond, London, UK

P. Dasgupta
Kings College London, Kings Health Partners, Guy's Hospital, MRC Centre for Transplantation NIHR Biomedical Research Centre, London, UK

E.P. Castle and R.S. Pruthi (eds.), *Robotic Surgery of the Bladder*, DOI 10.1007/978-1-4614-4906-5_20,

diversions, simulation and training and future employment of chemical agents which could improve the detection rate of a early nodal metastasis.

Single-Site Surgery and Instrumentation

Laparoendoscopic single-site surgery (LESS) and natural orifice transluminal endoscopic surgery (NOTES) are relatively novel techniques in urology and have gained prominence in academic centres which have a strong interest for laparoscopic surgery.

NOTES can be defined as the penetration of hollow viscera with an endoscope in order to access the abdominal cavity and perform an intra-abdominal operation [2]. On the contrary, a LESS access can be obtained either by performing a single incision on the skin, through which a single multi-channel access platform is placed (*single port*) or by placing several low-profile ports through separate fascial incisions (*single site*) [3–5]. Single-port access is used most commonly, and there are several commercially available ports, including Triport and Quadport, Advanced Surgical Concepts, Ireland (see Figs. 20.1 and 20.2). The umbilicus is the most frequently chosen access site.

The lack of port placement triangulation and collision of instruments make LESS a challenging technique and requires an experienced laparoscopic surgeon. These tasks become even more demanding during reconstructive procedures when suturing is needed, and as a result instruments have been especially conceived to facilitate LESS. Application of robotic technology for single-port surgery has enhanced intracorporeal dissection and suturing, albeit the platform can be cumbersome. Therefore further refinements will need to occur before full utilisation of LESS.

LESS radical cystectomy (RC) has been attempted in highly selected patients, with or without robotic assistance and so far appears safe and feasible. Kaouk et al. were the first to report LESS robot-assisted radical cystectomy and bilateral pelvic lymph node dissection (PLND) in three patients (two men and one woman). All procedures were completed successfully and all patients underwent extracorporeal urinary diversion by extending the umbilical port site. The operative time was 315 ± 40 min, with minimal blood loss (217 ± 29 mL). The pathologic evaluation revealed negative margins and negative lymph node involvement (mean number of nodes 16 ± 3). At a minimum of 2 years of follow-up (range 24–26 months), no evidence of local recurrence or metastatic disease was detected.

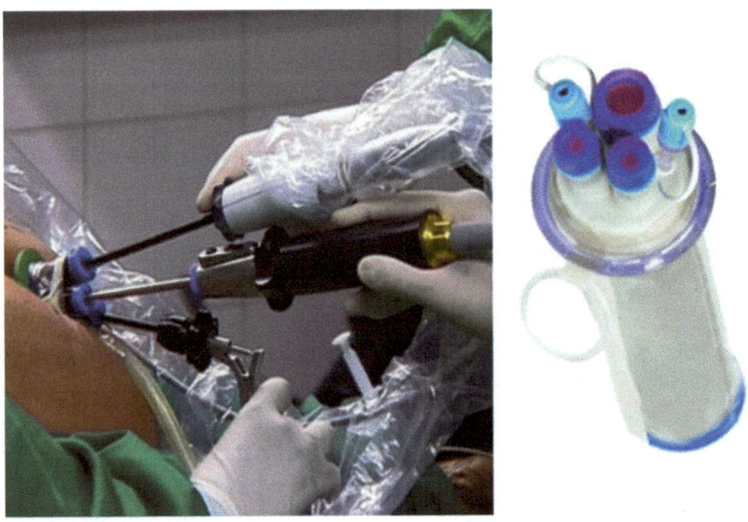

Fig. 20.1 Triport (R-Port), Advanced Surgical Concepts, Ireland. http://www.advancedsurgical.ie/TriPort/Default.166.html

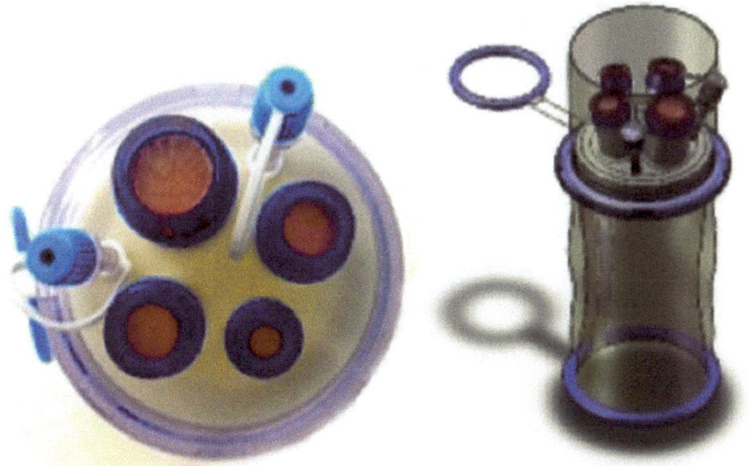

Fig. 20.2 Quadport, Advanced Surgical Concepts, Ireland. http://www.advancedsurgical.ie/QuadPort/Default.544.html

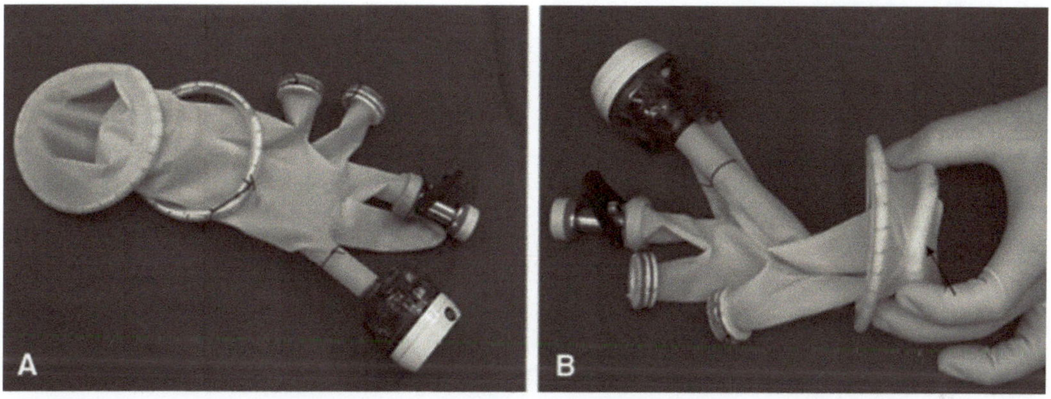

Fig. 20.3 (**a**) A homemade multichannel port was constructed of two stretchable rubber rings and a surgical glove. (**b**) The *outer* and *inner rings* of the multichannel port (*arrow* indicates the inner ring). Lin T et al. J Endourol. 2011 Jan;25(1):57–63

The same group has subsequently performed three robot-assisted LESS (R-LESS) radical cystectomy with intra-corporeal ileal conduit [6]. The Authors inserted an additional trocar that served as the stoma site. None of these were converted to open, although one rectal perforation in a patient who had previous brachytherapy was identified and repaired by R-LESS. Within a mean follow-up of 12.6 months (8–18), one patient developed deep vein thrombosis (DVT) and was managed medically. No patients had positive surgical margins on final histology.

Lin et al. described "hybrid-LESS" radical cystectomy with orthotopic neo-bladder reconstruction in a cohort of 12 patients [7]. A homemade multi-channel port, consisting of two stretchable rings and a surgical glove with trocars and valves attached to its fingers, was placed into a 4–5-cm midline incision in the lower abdomen and was used for laparoscopic instruments (see Figs. 20.3 and 20.4). Another sub-umbilical port was placed for the laparoscope. Extended pelvic lymph node dissection and radical cystectomy were completed laparoscopically; construction of the ileal neo-bladder was performed extra-corporeally and the neo-bladder was anastomosed to the urethral stump laparoscopically, with a slipknot running suture technique. No conversion

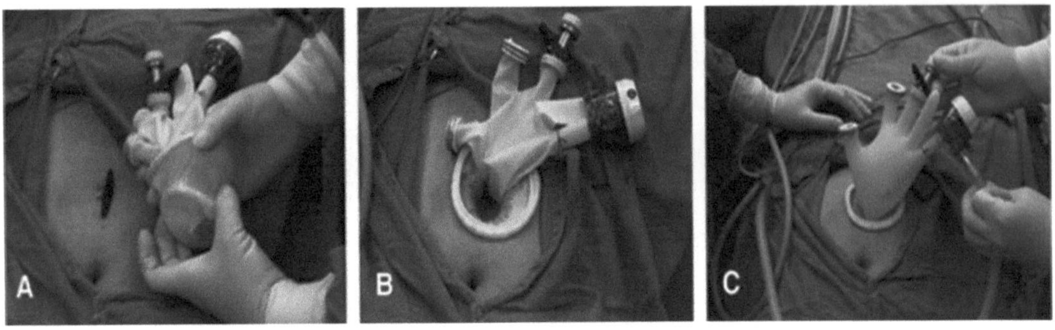

Fig. 20.4 (**a**) The incision and multichannel port. (**b**) The multichannel port was placed into the incision. (**c**) Insufflation with CO_2 created tension between the two rings and secured the device

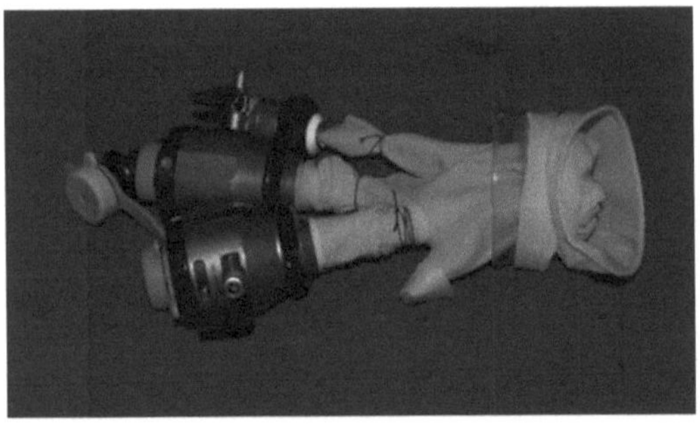

Fig. 20.5 Home-made single-port device. Ma LL et al. J Endourol. 2012 Apr;26(4):355–9

to standard laparoscopy or open surgery was required. There was no peri-operative mortality or port-related complications. Median operative time was 383 min (300–447) with median blood loss of 150 mL (120–400). Encouragingly, this group was able to retrieve a median of 25 lymph nodes (16–30), also with negative surgical margins. Continence rates were 80 % at 12-month follow-up. All patients were alive and tumour free at average follow-up of 16.1 months (range 9–20 months).

Ma et al. [8] also performed five LESS radical cystectomies using a homemade single-port device composed of an inverted cone device of polycarbonate and a powder-free surgical glove (see Fig. 20.5). The port was placed into a 5-cm peri-umbilical incision. The conventional laparoscope and laparoscopic instruments were inserted through the single port. No additional ports were needed for radical cystoprostatectomy and standard pelvic lymph node dissection. Cutaneous ureterostomy and ileal conduit urinary diversion were performed. The mean operative time was 208.2 (range 168–280 min) and estimated blood loss was 270 (100–500) mL. One patient needed a transfusion of 400 mL of red blood cells. The pathologic evaluation revealed negative margins and negative lymph node involvement. One patient had a bowel obstruction, while another patient died from cardiac disease.

Undoubtedly an extensive experience in laparoscopic surgery and stringent patient-selection criteria are fundamental for LESS radical cystectomy. Based on the available non-randomised evidence, these methods can be best regarded as experimental and hence strictly limited to centres with high volume laparoscopic, robotic and LESS practice.

All the studies discussed above are retrospective and are small case series (<20), with the majority having ≤T2 disease. Randomised prospective studies are needed to determine how this technique compares with the traditional open radical cystectomy (ORC) or multi-port robot-assisted radical cystectomy (RARC). Generally RC is often undertaken in an elderly population where cosmesis is not usually a priority, so there needs to be careful consideration as to whether this avenue should be pursued any further. It is possible that a further expansion of the indications and role of single-site surgery may occur with refinement of robotic technology, particularly, the development of more flexible instruments and this would influence our future surgical practice.

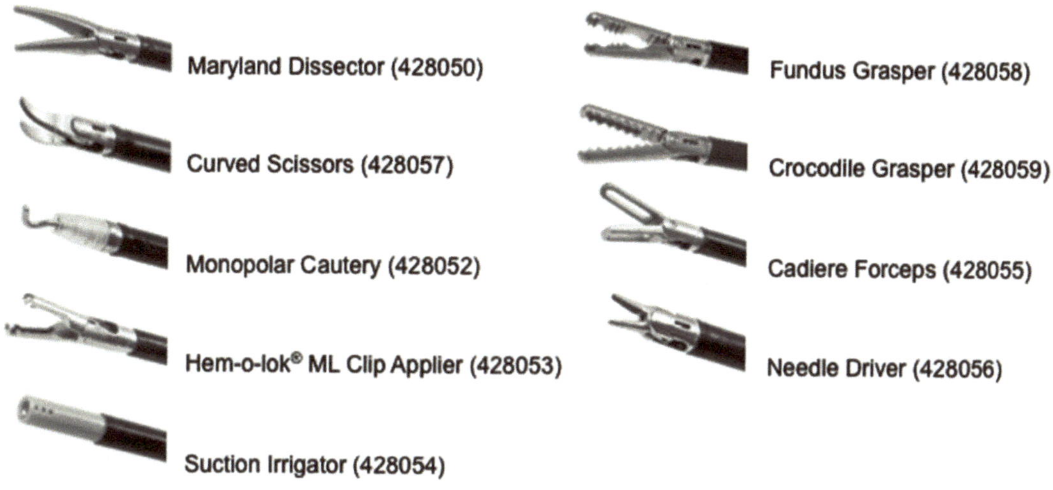

Fig. 20.6 Instruments for Single Port RS Da Vinci. Instruments are 5 mm in size, non wristed and semi-rigid. Intuitive surgical, Sunnyale, CA

Currently available robotic instruments for LESS robotic surgery (LESS-RS) are 5 mm in size, non-wristed and semi-rigid. These instruments (see Fig. 20.6) can be inserted into the abdominal cavity through a silicone port (see Fig. 20.7) which requires only a 2–2.5-cm skin incision. The trocars for the Da Vinci® single-port system are curved and marked with the same remote centre of motion (RCM) that can be found on each trocar used for a standard Da Vinci® procedure. In fact, each robotic instrument is able to rotate around a specific epicentre (RCM), marked as a black thick line on the port. The RCM provides a wide range of motion to operate the instruments and it is always located slightly lower to the level of the skin. In this way, the risk of collision between the instruments and the body of the patient is avoided. Thanks to the presence of the RCM and to the fact that the instruments are actually crossing within the silicone port, and not outside the body (as on the contrary happens during single port laparoscopic surgery), the risk for a collision of the instruments inside the abdomen is minimised.

However, knotting and suturing in LESS-RS is more difficult than in standard RS. The main limitation of the Da Vinci® Si system for LESS-RS is the lack of the endo-wrist technology. The presence of a wrist at the tip of the instrument allows

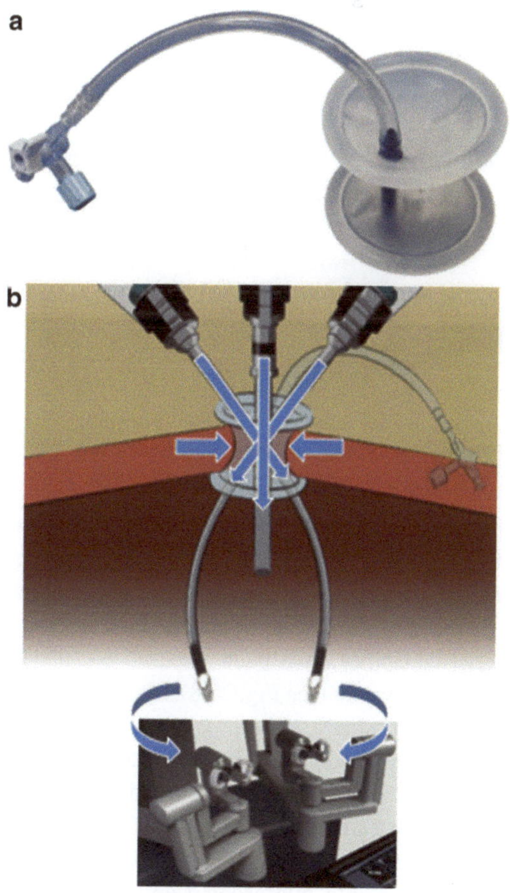

Fig. 20.7 (**a**) Silicon port for Single Port RS Da Vinci (**b**)

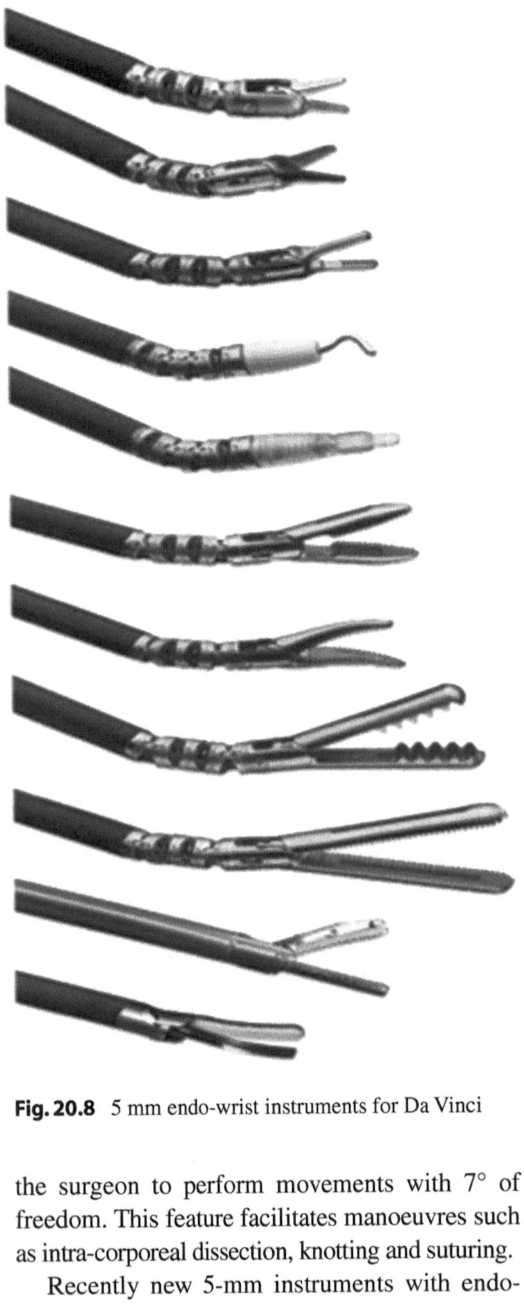

Fig. 20.8 5 mm endo-wrist instruments for Da Vinci

the surgeon to perform movements with 7° of freedom. This feature facilitates manoeuvres such as intra-corporeal dissection, knotting and suturing.

Recently new 5-mm instruments with endo-wrist capability have been released for the Da Vinci® Si system (see Fig. 20.8). These have been used for paediatric robotic surgery but are also suitable for standard RS. It is expected that in the future, LESS-RS will be performed with miniaturised instruments characterised by multiple joints, high flexibility and wristed tip.

Research into microscopic and miniaturised technology in clinical practice has been underway in the last decade. Miniature camera robots (microrobots) can provide a mobile viewing platform to enhance a surgeon's view, and nanorobots are also approaching clinical application. Interestingly, "in vivo robots"—which are miniature, dexterous, co-operative robotic devices can be deployed intra-corporeally to perform tasks such as imaging, retraction and tissue manipulation to enable precise movements [9]. These are the exciting developments and we eagerly await the outcome of research into their use in the oncological setting.

The future of RS will depend on the availability of new enhanced robotic systems. The current Da Vinci® Si system for RS is far from perfect and has several limitations:

- The robotic cart is still cumbersome. Although the arms are smaller in size compared to the original Da Vinci® (see Fig. 20.9), they are still quite heavy and are all attached to a cart. The cart itself is quite heavy and is not easily manoeuvred by the nurses. Development of lighter arms that could be attached independently to the operative table has been advocated as a possible solution to ease and reduce the time for docking.
- The robotic camera could be miniaturised. A miniaturised magnetic camera that could be inserted into the abdominal cavity through a 5-mm port would allow the surgeon to manoeuvre the camera from the outside by using a calamite. This would avoid the need of a port dedicated to hold the camera.
- The lack of tactile feedback is a significant deficiency of the system. Despite the presence of the endo-wrist technology, the robotic instruments are not able to transfer a tactile feedback to the hands of the surgeon who is operating at the console. This can be potentially dangerous. In fact, the accidental clashing of an instrument with an organ may result in a severe injury that could be avoided if the surgeon had the feeling of touching the tissues. However, it is possible to replace the lack of tactile feedback with an intensive training in the dry-lab.
- The number of instruments available is still low. Despite the recent introduction of new

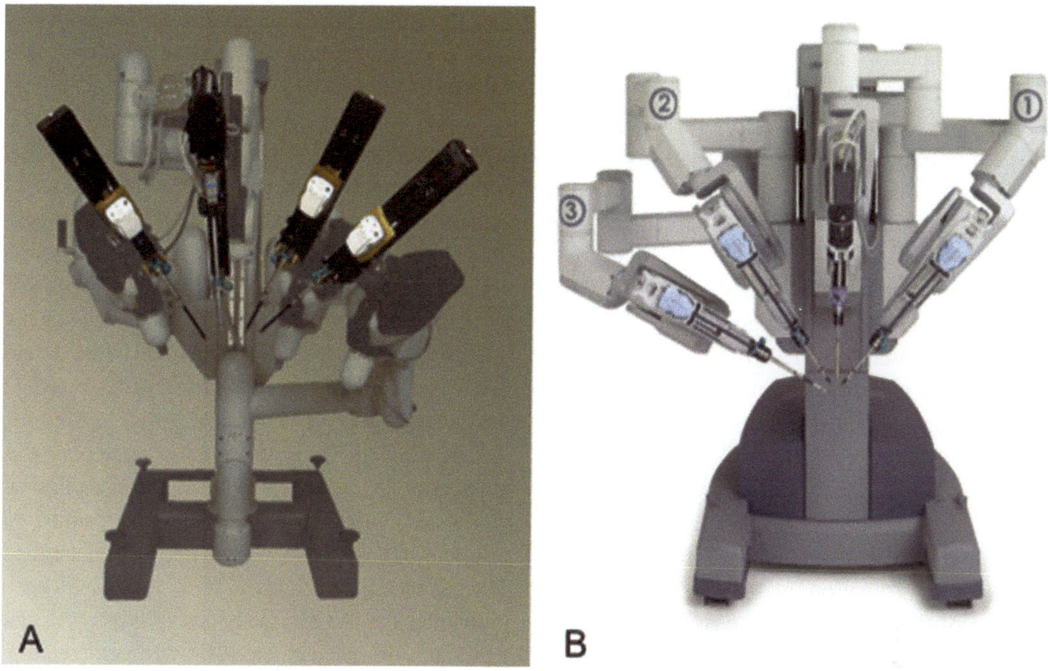

Fig. 20.9 (**a**) Da Vinci Standard patient Chart, 1999; (**b**) Da Vinci S and SI patient chart

instruments such as the Graptor, an 8-mm grasping retractor that allows atraumatic grasping of bowel and other delicate tissues, there are no instruments dedicated to specific procedures. As far as RARC is concerned, there is no miniaturised robotic stapler designed to perform an intra-corporeal diversion and there is no retractor specifically designed for RARC.

Intracorporeal Urinary Diversion

The majority of surgeons performing RARC recommend a combination of robot-assisted extirpative cystectomy and lymph-adenectomy, with subsequent extracorporeal urinary diversion, whether this be ileal conduit, orthotopic neobladder (ONB) or continent cutaneous diversion (CCD) formation [10–13]. As experience with RARC increases, intra-corporeal reconstruction of urinary diversion are emerging, in the expectation that this approach may confer benefits such as lesser incisional pain, with decreased bowel exposure and desiccation, thereby reducing the risk of ileus and resulting in faster recovery.

Approaches to reconstruction include extracorporeal ONB, re-docking of the robot with robot-assisted anastamosis of urethra to ONB and total intra-corporeal reconstruction. The intracorporeal approach is thought to be ergonomically beneficial in ONB formation, because the depth perception and optical magnification of the robot system facilitates formation of the anastamosis between urethra and reservoir. This minimises the risk of urinary leakage and may improve urinary continence [14].

Clearly, the learning curve in this approach is steep and current published studies on pure intracorporeal urinary diversion demonstrate longer operating times. However, these improve significantly over time [15]. This method of urinary diversion may be suitable for younger patients with fewer co-morbidities and a better performance status, as they would better tolerate the potential prolonged operating times. So far there appear to be lower inpatient narcotic requirements and comparable short-term clinical outcomes [16].

Existing published studies on intra-corporeal diversion feature small patient series (<50) and are non-randomised. Unpublished data from the

International Robotic Cystectomy Consortium (IRCC) have shown that, on retrospective analysis from 21 institutions (intra-corporeal $n=148$, extracorporeal $n=787$), patients undergoing intra-corporeal urinary diversion have lower readmission rates and experience fewer gastrointestinal complications and infections. Larger randomised studies are needed to determine superiority, or at least non-inferiority, before these techniques can be fully incorporated into RARC.

Total intra-corporeal urinary diversion is evolving, but majority of centres are still focusing on extracorporeal urinary diversion performed through the incision used to retrieve the specimen. A total intra-corporeal diversion would certainly be advantageous in females where the specimen can be retrieved trans-vaginally. Prior marking of the ileocecal junction and ileal conduit, and transfer of the left ureter to the right, all leads to a smaller incision and faster extracorporeal urinary diversion, therefore reducing operative time and the impact of Trendelenburg position and pneumo-peritoneum, especially in the elderly population.

The aim of robotic surgery is to reproduce the same steps of open surgery in a minimally invasive context. RARC is a totally intra-corporeal minimally invasive procedure that aims to remove the bladder with all the surrounding organs and lymph nodes. However, the procedure does not end with the removal of the specimen, but with the formation of a urinary diversion. Therefore, the formation of a diversion during RARC should by definition totally intra-corporeal. Bearing this logic in mind, we anticipate that in the next 5–10 years, all centres undertaking RARC will be performing total intra-corporeal urinary diversion. In order to make this feasible, it is crucial that there should be a significant further evolution of robotic instrumentations and training/simulation systems dedicated to RARC.

Sentinel Lymph Node Detection

Lymph node dissection (LND) during a radical cystectomy is a crucial step that can potentially lead to a wide spectrum of complications including vascular injuries, development of lymphoceles and deep vein trombosis leading to pulmonary embolism.

Extent of lymphadenectomy during radical cystectomy is still a subject of debate. In this context we are not focusing here on the controversies regarding the extent of LND, its therapeutic potential or the minimum number of lymph nodes to be removed, which it has been suggested to be at least >16 [17]. We will rather analyse the possible implications of the sentinel node detection during radical cystectomy and its possible future application in robotic surgery.

The concept of sentinel node detection was introduced by Gould in 1960 as the detection of lymph node that is suggested to be primed in receiving metastatic deposits at one time or another. The sentinel lymph node (SN) is specific in each individual and can be ideally described as "the first guardian" on the pathway of a cancer spreading throughout the lymphatic system of a specific organ. When a SN is identified during surgery, it is removed and sent for pathology. The absence of tumour cells in the SN would indicate the absence of further spread in the regional lymph node basin(s) and would therefore make LND not mandatory. The detection of the SN in oncologic surgery has been extensively investigated for many cancers, including breast [18], prostate [19], colorectal [20], esophageal [21], melanoma [22], thyroid [23] and penile cancer [24].

The current mainstay of the technique of SN detection is the combination of a gamma ray-emitting radiotracer (99-m technetium) with blue dyes. However, the use of gamma ray-emitting radiotracers requires involvement of a nuclear medicine physician, and the localisation of the SN can be technically very difficult using a hand-held gamma probe. On the contrary, the blue dyes can be injected in the peri-tumoral tissue and be identified without the need of specific probe. However, blue dye cannot be seen easily through the fatty tissue making it a sub-optimal technique particularly in obese patients.

Current evidence surrounding SN detection during radical cystectomy appears to be limited mainly to case series. Sherif et al. first reported the feasibility of the SN detection on a cohort of

13 patients [25]. The day before surgery, 2 ml of 99-m technetium were injected in the detrusor muscle peri-tumourally and a lymphoscintigraphy was performed. In addition patent blue dye marker was injected around the tumour with a cystoscope, prior cystectomy.

SNs were identified during surgery by combining the use of gamma-probe radiotracer with the visualisation of blue nodes. All SNs were removed, and a subsequent extended LND was then performed on both sides. SNs were sent separately for pathology and were compared histopathologically with all the other lymph nodes retrieved at LND. Detection rate for the SN was 85 %. A lymph node invasion was observed in four patients and in all cases the SN lymph was infiltrated by the cancer. Liedberg et al. also reported a detection rate of 87 % in a cohort of 75 patients [26]. The authors observed that the detection of a SN improved the staging accuracy in >25 % of cases.

More recently the green indocyanine (ICG) has been introduced as a new dye marker for the detection of SNs. ICG is a molecule with specific optical properties. The absorption and fluorescence spectrum of ICG is in the near infrared region, as it absorbs mainly between 600 and 900 nm and emits fluorescence between 750 and 950 nm.

Optical imaging using near-infrared (NIR) fluorescence is a novel technique that can be used to visualise structures in real time during surgery. Advantages of NIR fluorescent light (700–900 nm) include high tissue penetration (millimetres to centimetres deep) and low auto-fluorescence, thereby providing sufficient contrast [27].

Infrared ray observation based on the absorption characteristics of ICG has also been reported to make it easy to distinguish lymphatic vessels and lymph nodes containing ICG particle from surrounding tissue compared with naked eye observation [28].

Therefore, the use of NIR fluorescence imaging has the potential of great value in the intraoperative detection of critical anatomical structures and oncologic targets such as SNs [29]. ICG is currently used for the detection of SN during breast surgery for a localised cancer [30].

In a recent study, Wishart et al. combined ICG with blue dye and technetium to detect SN in a cohort of 104 women undergoing quadrantectomy for localised breast cancer [31]. SN detection rate was reported 100 % for ICG alone, 77.2 %, for ICG & radioisotope and 73.1 % for ICG & blue dye & radioisotope. Metastases were found in 25/201 SNs (12.4 %) and all positive nodes were fluorescent, blue and radioactive. The combination of the three markers had the highest nodal sensitivity at 95.0 %.

As far as urologic surgery is concerned, ICG has been recently introduced as a marker that can improve the accuracy of the resection of a tumour during a robotic partial nephrectomy [32–35]. ICG could find further future applications in urologic oncologic surgery. A valid example could be the use of ICG for the detection of SN during RARC.

At present there is not enough evidence to suggest that retrieval of a SN could have a role in the staging and/or in the treatment of a muscle-invasive bladder cancer. If the concept of the sentinal node proves to have high specificity, retrieval of SNs would reduce the theoretical risk of complications related to an extended LND.

The main risk of relying on the concept of sentinal nodal biopsy would be the possibility of missing skip lesions either because of the unpredictable biology of the cancer or the lack of accuracy of the technology available to date. To reduce the likelihood to missing skip lesions by improving the sensitivity of the techniques is vital.

The gamma probes currently available for open surgery are difficult to handle, are usually straight or angled and have a quite wide window for the detection of radiations. These features constitute their main limitation for the detection of a SN, especially within the narrow confines of the pelvis. Overall the accuracy of these probes is low as they can detect multiple inputs of radiation from different nodes which can be misleading and responsible for retrieval of nodes other than real SN.

Gamma probes that can be employed during laparoscopic surgery are also available. These are smaller in size but are not completely flexible and difficult to manipulate. So far, no gamma probes dedicated to a specific robotic system have been introduced in oncologic surgery. Hopefully development of a miniaturised light robotic flexible multi-jointed gamma probe with a smaller window for the detection of radiations will reduce the technical limitations of the probes available to date. It is expected that the surgeon will be able to move the probe easily in order to target a SN with greater precision. The ICG injected around a bladder tumour prior to RARC will further increase the accuracy of the detection of SN.

With new developments it will be possible to integrate the images of the preoperative lymphoscintigraphy with the intraoperative NIR fluorescence vision at the console during surgery. This combination will allow the surgeon to detect the SN with greater precision. The improvements in the technology will pave the way to set up RCTs that will hopefully answer the key question whether the SN detection has a role during RARC and whether it would influence the decision making to perform an extended LND during a RARC.

Simulation and Training

Robot-assisted radical cystectomy is a long and difficult procedure that requires a dedicated training targeted on acquiring high surgical skills and deep knowledge of the surgical anatomy of the abdomen and the pelvis [36]. An inexperienced surgeon may easily encounter severe bleeding due to an accidental injury to visceral organs or main pelvic blood vessels. The difficulty related to perform a radical cystectomy is also enhanced by the fact that the patients often present multiple co-morbidities or had previous abdominal/pelvic surgery, which could act as potential trigger that may further increase the risk of complications during surgery. Presence of anatomical and vascular variants and/or the local extent of the cancer within the pelvis or the lymph nodes are further variables that have to be considered when the surgery is planned, in order to reduce the risk of unexpected events.

During the last 10 years, we have witnessed an increasing interest for simulation projects in surgery. This new kind of research is becoming increasingly popular and is aimed to create simulators that are reproducing artificial surgical scenarios in a risk-free laboratory environment. Simulators enable trainees to practice at any convenient time and also outside clinical working hours. The simulation of a specific surgical setting favours the development of determined skills (e.g. endoscopic resection, intracorporeal knotting, etc.) and at the same time increases the safety of a specific procedure. In fact simulators have been found to decrease the learning curve especially for complex procedures [37, 38].

We can classify simulators in bench models, animal/cadaver models and virtual reality simulators.

Bench model simulators are made of materials with characteristics similar to human tissues. Although these simulators are relatively cheap and can also be easily reproduced in a home setting, they are considered to be of low fidelity when compared to human models or animal models. The latter are considered to be the gold standard because they represent the real-life scenario and allow the trainees to become familiar with real tissues.

Since animal and cadaver models are very expensive and not easily available for trainees in all the countries, virtual reality simulators have been recently introduced as sort of good compromise. In a virtual reality setting, the anatomic variants of a specific organ can be reproduced, and the level of complexity of each task can be easily modified in order to promote the progression of the learning curve. There are different simulators for TURP, TURB-t, Ureteroscopy or basic and advanced laparoscopic surgery.

In relation to robotic surgery a range of simulators are available: The Robotic Surgical Simulator (RoSS™) (Simulated Surgical Systems, Buffalo, USA) and the SEP Robot (SimSurgery®, Norway) the dV-Trainer® (Mimic Technologies Inc., Seattle, USA) and the Da Vinci® Skills Simulator (Intuitive Surgical, Sunnyvale, USA). These vary on the bases of different tasks and ergonomics but act as useful tools to learn basic or advanced skills in robotic surgery. None of these simulators include specific scenarios targeted on a determined surgical procedure like RARC.

If an experienced surgeon is asked about as to what is the ideal case scenario of a RARC, he would perhaps describe it as a relatively straightforward procedure, performed within a reasonable operative time and with a minimal blood loss. This could theoretically happen only if the surgeon who is sitting at a console knows in details the individual's pelvic anatomy, extent of the tumour and the lymph nodes. Although at a first impression this concept could sound utopic, it could become reality in the RS of the future.

The future of simulation will be based on the development of dedicated softwares that will integrate images obtained with a CT/MRI scan in a 3D virtual reality environment. It will therefore be possible to reproduce the entire anatomy of each patient and the trainees will be able to practice on the virtual case that will happen in reality a few days later. In this way, the likelihood of intra-operative complications would be significantly lowered and both operating time and blood loss would be optimised. In conclusion, the future of simulation and training on RARC will be lead and guided by the evolution of technology and engineering that will be targeting on dedicated softwares for specific virtual reality settings.

Conclusion

RARC is a procedure that duplicates the steps of the open technique. Currently there are no results from a RCT comparing RARC with the open and laparoscopic approaches. However, there are several randomised controlled trials in progress comparing RARC with open and laparoscopic radical cystectomy, including the randomised CORAL (Cystectomy Open Robotic and Laparoscopic) [39]. A Randomised Trial, University of Texas Health Science Centre, USA [40] and BOLERO, Cardiff University, UK [41]. The long-term outcomes of the first cohort of patients who underwent RARC will be available in the next 1–2 years.

The future of RARC will most likely be LESS-RS and the procedure will be likely performed with miniaturised instruments and new robotic systems. It will be possible to identify the extension of a bladder cancer through the SN by combining the data obtained with a very accurate robotic gamma probe and with intra-operative NIR fluorescence images.

Finally, the progression of technology will make training and simulation even more precise and it will be possible to simulate and perform a virtual RARC before it happens in reality. This will increase the safety of the procedure and will allow the trainees to improve the learning curve for a technically challenging procedure such as the radical cystectomy.

References

1. Smaldone MC, Kutikov A, Egleston B, Simhan J, Canter DJ, Teper E, et al. Assessing performance trends in laparoscopic nephrectomy and nephron-sparing surgery for localized renal tumors. Urology. 2012;80(2):286–91.
2. Pearl JP, Ponsky JL. Natural orifice translumenal endoscopic surgery: a criticial review. J Gastrointest Surg. 2008;12(7):1293–300.
3. Gill IS, Advincula AP, Aron M, Caddedu J, Canes D, Curcillo II PG, et al. Consensus statement of the consortium for laparoendoscopic single-site surgery. Surg Endosc. 2010;24(4):762–8.
4. Gettman MT, Box G, Averch T, Cadeddu JA, Cherullo E, Clayman RV, et al. Consensus statement on natural orifice transluminal endoscopic surgery and single-incision laparoscopic surgery: heralding a new era in urology? Eur Urol. 2008;53(6):1117–20.
5. Box G, Averch T, Cadeddu J, Cherullo E, Clayman R, Desai M, et al. Nomenclature of natural orifice translumenal endoscopic surgery (NOTES) and laparoendoscopic single-site surgery (LESS) procedures in urology. J Endourol. 2008;22(11):2575–81.
6. White MA, Autorino R, Spana G, Hillyer S, Stein RJ, Kaouk JH. Robotic laparoendoscopic single site urological surgery: analysis of 50 consecutive cases. J Urol. 2012;187(5):1696–701.
7. Lin T, Huang J, Han J, Xu K, Huang H, Jiang C, et al. Hybrid laparoscopic endoscopic single-site surgery for radical cystoprostatectomy and orthotopic ileal neobladder: an initial experience of 12 cases. J Endourol. 2011;25(1):57–63.
8. Ma LL, Bi H, Hou XF, Huang Y, Wang GL, Zhao L, et al. Laparoendoscopic single-site radical cystectomy and urinary diversion: initial experience in China using a homemade single-port device. J Endourol. 2012;26(4):355–9.
9. Lehman AC, Wood NA, Farritor S, Goede MR, Oleynikov D. Dexterous miniature robot for advanced minimally invasive surgery. Surg Endosc. 2011;25(1):119–23.

10. Wang GJ, Barocas DA, Raman JD, Scherr DS. Robotic vs open radical cystectomy: prospective comparison of perioperative outcomes and pathological measures of early oncological efficacy. BJU Int. 2008;101(1):89–93.
11. Murphy DG, Challacombe BJ, Elhage O, O'Brien TS, Rimington P, Khan MS, et al. Robotic-assisted laparoscopic radical cystectomy with extracorporeal urinary diversion: initial experience. Eur Urol. 2008;54(3): 570–80.
12. Pruthi RS, Wallen EM. Robotic assisted laparoscopic radical cystoprostatectomy: operative and pathological outcomes. J Urol. 2007;178(3):814–8.
13. Guru KA, Kim HL, Piacente PM, Mohler JL. Robot-assisted radical cystectomy and pelvic lymph node dissection: initial experience at Roswell Park Cancer Institute. Urology. 2007;69(3):469–74.
14. Jonsson MN, Adding LC, Hosseini A, Schumacher MC, Volz D, Nilsson A, et al. Robot-assisted radical cystectomy with intracorporeal urinary diversion in patients with transitional cell carcinoma of the bladder. Eur Urol. 2011;60(5):1066–73.
15. Guru K, Seixas-Mikelus SA, Hussain A, Blumenfeld AJ, Nyquist J, Chandrasekhar R, et al. Robot-assisted intracorporeal ileal conduit: Marionette technique and initial experience at Roswell Park Cancer Institute. Urology. 2010;76(4):866–71.
16. Pruthi RS, Nix J, McRackan D, Hickerson A, Nielsen ME, Raynor M, et al. Robotic-assisted Laparoscopic Intracorporeal Urinary Diversion. Eur Urol. 2010; 57(6):1013–21.
17. Leissner J, Hohenfellner R, Thuroff JW, Wolf HK. Lymphadenectomy in patients with transitional cell carcinoma of the urinary bladder; significance for staging and prognosis. BJU Int. 2000;85:817.
18. Gatek J, Vrana D, Hnatek L, Bakala J, Dudesek B, Duben J, et al. Sentinel node biopsy and neoadjuvant chemotherapy in the treatment of breast cancer. J BUON. 2012;17(2):265–70.
19. Meinhardt W, van der Poel HG, Valdés Olmos RA, Bex A, Brouwer OR, Horenblas S. Laparoscopic sentinel lymph node biopsy for prostate cancer: the relevance of locations outside the extended dissection area. Prostate Cancer. 2012;2012:751753.
20. de Haas RJ, Wicherts DA, Hobbelink MG, van Diest PJ, Vleggaar FP, Borel Rinkes IH, et al. Sentinel lymph node mapping in colon cancer using radiocolloid as a single tracer: a feasibility study. Nucl Med Commun. 2012;33(8):832–7.
21. Thompson SK, Bartholomeusz D, Jamieson GG. Sentinel lymph node biopsy in esophageal cancer: should it be standard of care? J Gastrointest Surg. 2011;15(10):1762–8.
22. Vidal M, Vidal-Sicart S, Torrents A, Perissinotti A, Navales I, Paredes P, et al. Accuracy and Reproducibility of Lymphoscintigraphy for Sentinel Node Detection in Patients with Cutaneous Melanoma. J Nucl Med. 2012;53(8):1193–9.
23. Kaczka K, Celnik A, Luks B, Jasion J, Pomorski L. Sentinel lymph node biopsy techniques in thyroid pathologies—a meta-analysis. Endokrynol Pol. 2012; 63(3):222–31.
24. Horenblas S. Sentinel lymph node biopsy in penile carcinoma. Semin Diagn Pathol. 2012;29(2):90–5.
25. Sherif A, De La Torre M, Malmstrom PU, Thorn M. Lymphatic mapping and detection of sentinel nodes in patients with bladder cancer. J Urol. 2001;166:812.
26. Liedberg F, Chebil G, Davidsson T, Gudjonsson S, Månsson W. Intraoperative sentinel node detection improves nodal staging in invasive bladder cancer. J Urol. 2006;175(1):84–8. discussion 88–9.
27. Frangioni JV. New technologies for human cancer imaging. J Clin Oncol. 2008;26:4012–21.
28. Miyashiro I, Miyoshi N, Hiratsuka M, Kishi K, Yamada T, Ohue M, et al. Detection of sentinel node in gastric cancer surgery by indocyanine green fluorescence imaging: comparison with infrared imaging. Ann Surg Oncol. 2008;15:1640–3.
29. Crane LM, Themelis G, Pleijhuis RG, Harlaar NJ, Sarantopoulos A, Arts HJ, et al. Intraoperative multispectral fluorescence imaging for the detection of the sentinel lymph node in cervical cancer: a novel concept. Mol Imaging Biol. 2011;13(5):1043–9. doi:10.1007/s11307-010-0425-7.
30. Hirche C, Murawa D, Mohr Z, Kneif S, Hünerbein M. ICG fluorescence-guided sentinel node biopsy for axillary nodal staging in breast cancer. Breast Cancer Res Treat. 2010;121:373–8.
31. Wishart GC, Loh SW, Jones L, Benson JR. A feasibility study (ICG-10) of indocyanine green (ICG) fluorescence mapping for sentinel lymph node detection in early breast cancer. Eur J Surg Oncol. 2012; 38(8):651–6.
32. Krane LS, Manny TB, Hemal AK. Is near infrared fluorescence imaging using indocyanine green dye useful in robotic partial nephrectomy: a prospective comparative study of 94 patients. Urology. 2012;80(1):110–8.
33. Patel HR, Linares A, Joseph JV. Robotic and laparoscopic surgery: cost and training. Surg Oncol. 2009; 18:242–6.
34. Patel TH, Sirintrapun SJ, Hemal AK. Surgeon-controlled robotic partial nephrectomy for a rare renal epithelioid angiomyolipoma using near-infrared fluorescence imaging using indocyanine green dye: a case report and literature review. Can Urol Assoc J. 2012;6(2):E91–4. doi:10.5489/cuaj.11250.
35. Tobis S, Knopf JK, Silvers CR, Marshall J, Cardin A, Wood RW, et al. Near infrared fluorescence imaging after intravenous indocyanine green: initial clinical experience with open partial nephrectomy for renal cortical tumors. Urology. 2012;79(4):958–64.
36. Dasgupta P. Robotic assisted radical cystectomy and urinary diversion. Int J Clin Pract. 2012;66(7):618–9. doi:10.1111/j.1742-1241.2012.02950.
37. Albani JM, Lee DI. Virtual reality-assisted robotic surgery simulation. J Endourol. 2007;21:285–7.

38. Stefanidis D, Korndorffer Jr JR, Sierra R, Touchard C, Dunne JB, Scott DJ. Skill retention following proficiency-based laparoscopic simulator training. Surgery. 2005;138:165–70.
39. Ismail AF, Elhage O, Rimington P, Kelly JD, Dasgupta P, Khan MS. Initial experience with a Randomised Controlled trial of Open, Robotic and Laparoscopic (CORAL) radical cystectomy. BJU Int. 2010;106 Suppl 1:7.
40. Open vs robotic-assisted radical cystectomy: a randomized trial. http://clinicaltrials.gov NCT01157676
41. Bladder cancer: open versus laparoscopic or robotic cystectomy. http://www.controlled-trials.com ISRCTN38528926

Index

E.P. Castle and R.S. Pruthi (eds.), *Robotic Surgery of the Bladder*, DOI 10.1007/978-1-4614-4906-5,

FSC
www.fsc.org
MIX
Papier | Fördert
gute Waldnutzung
FSC® C083411

Kolibri 360 GmbH
Ferdinand-Jühlke-Straße 7
99095 Erfurt, Deutschland
produktsicherheit@kolibri360.de